Conquering
Heart Disease

Also by Harvey B. Simon, M.D.

Staying Well
Your Complete Guide to Disease Prevention

The Athlete Within
A Personal Guide to Total Fitness
(with Steven R. Levisohn, M.D.)

Tennis Medic
(with Steven R. Levisohn, M.D.)

Conquering Heart Disease

New Ways to Live Well Without Drugs or Surgery

Harvey B. Simon, M.D.

LITTLE, BROWN AND COMPANY

BOSTON   NEW YORK   TORONTO   LONDON

Library of Congress Cataloging-in-Publication Data

Simon, Harvey B. (Harvey Bruce).
    Conquering heart disease: new ways to live well without drugs or
surgery / Harvey B. Simon. — 1st ed.
        p.   cm.
    Includes index.
    ISBN 0-316-79157-1
    1. Coronary heart disease—Popular works.   I. Title.
RC685.C6S547   1994
616.1′2—dc20   94-10367

10   9   8   7   6   5   4   3   2   1

MV-NY

Published simultaneously in Canada
by Little, Brown & Company (Canada) Limited

Printed in the United States of America

For Rita

Once again, and more than ever before

To ward off disease or recover health, men as a rule find it easier to depend on healers than to attempt the more difficult task of living wisely.

—René Dubos

You gotta have heart . . .

—*Damn Yankees*

Contents

Preface   *xi*

Acknowledgments   *xv*

Prologue   Heart Disease in America —
            A Needless Epidemic   3

Part I   Hearts in Health and Disease
          Chapter 1   The Causes of Heart Disease   9
          Chapter 2   Evaluating Your Risk for
                       Atherosclerosis   29

Part II   Fifteen Ways to Conquer Heart Disease
          Chapter 3   Smoking: Cardiac Enemy
                       Number One   71
          Chapter 4   Dietary Fat and Cholesterol:
                       You Are What You Eat   84
          Chapter 5   Exercise—The Best-Kept Secret
                       in Cardiology   136
          Chapter 6   Blood Pressure: Minerals Make
                       a Difference   171
          Chapter 7   Aspirin: An Old Medication with
                       New Uses   191

Chapter 8   Dietary Fiber: The Power of
Positive Eating   205

Chapter 9   Alcohol: Fighting Atherosclerosis
with a Smile   221

Chapter 10   Fish: Tipping the Scales to Health   236

Chapter 11   Antioxidants: New Help on
the Horizon   248

Chapter 12   Niacin: Natural Vitamin or
Powerful Drug?   271

Chapter 13   Chromium and Other Metals:
Can You Steel Yourself Against
Heart Disease?   281

Chapter 14   Stress Control: Winding Down for
a Happy Heart   290

Chapter 15   Weight Control: Slimming Down
for a Healthy Heart   316

Chapter 16   Estrogens: Keeping Women Young
at Heart   342

Chapter 17   Facts or Fads: Other Tips That
May Help   355

Part III   Conventional Cardiology Can Help

Chapter 18   Understanding Medical Tests
and Treatments   371

Epilogue   Healthy Hearts, Healthy Bodies   398

Appendix   Sources for Further Information   401

Index   403

Preface

Conquering Heart Disease is a book that should not have been necessary — but it is. Heart disease should be a rarity — but it's not. We understand what causes coronary heart disease, and we know how to prevent it. New research is adding important dimensions to this information, but the basics have been known for years. Yet many people do not incorporate these principles into their daily life, and many doctors do not incorporate them into their clinical practice, perhaps because they are so basic. *Conquering Heart Disease* will explain the basics, explore exciting new discoveries, and present a workable program that can help make coronary artery disease rare.

My own experiences, both personal and clinical, help explain why I feel so strongly about *Conquering Heart Disease.* I had the benefit of the best medical education available, but I had little idea of the hazards threatening my own health, much less how to confront them. I have the privilege of practicing internal medicine at one of the finest hospitals in the country, but I witness daily the way high-tech medicine can displace individual responsibility and self-care. I have the challenge of teaching at one of the greatest medical schools in the world, but I find that many students understand the intricacies of molecular biology without mastering the essentials of nutrition, exercise, and stress control.

I know that it can be hard to change. I didn't begin to make the changes that have saved my life until I was 34 years old, and I'm still changing 18 years later. I didn't begin to change the emphasis in my clinical practice until I'd been taking care of patients for 10 years, and I'm still learning how to improve clinically.

Conquering Heart Disease has grown from my life and my work. Having learned how to take care of myself in the mid-1970s, I joined with like-minded doctors and nurses to establish the Harvard Cardiovascular Health Center in 1979. Over the years we've used exercise, nutrition, and stress control to help treat thousands of patients. Each patient is also under the care of a cardiologist who, of course, continues to prescribe medications that are also important. But although our patients are getting the best care that cardiology can offer in the 1990s, and although they are highly motivated and intelligent, they often come to us without understanding how to take care of themselves. During the past few years, our patients have asked for more help in caring for their hearts. In response, I've been offering a series of talks and lectures, which have gradually grown into this book.

To my patients, I should explain that I am one of you — not because I have heart disease but because I was at high risk. My family history could hardly be worse. My mother and uncles died of heart attacks before age 45 and my father was disabled by cardiovascular disease in his 30s. At age 34, though I felt perfectly well and considered myself healthy, I was poised to join them: I was overweight (200 pounds), sedentary (unable to jog half a mile), hypertensive (156/91), hyperlipidemic (cholesterol 294), and highly stressed. And I had only recently quit smoking. All in all, I was a heart attack waiting to happen. But then I began to change.

The results have been wonderful. Even without prescription medications, all my numbers are better: weight 162, blood pressure 130/84, cholesterol 220 (with an HDL of 110!). My exercise capacity is enormous, as can be seen by the many marathons I've run. And, just as important, I feel better than ever.

To my medical colleagues, I should explain that I am one of you, too. On virtually every day of my professional life, I write prescriptions to treat hypertension or angina. Virtually every week, I order echocardiograms or stress tests. Nearly every month, I refer at least one patient for cardiac catheterization, angioplasty, or bypass surgery. I try to keep up with the latest developments in medicine and to provide my patients with the newest tests and treatments. But although I practice high-tech medicine, I recognize that each prescription and every treatment represents a failure, a necessary response to a disease that never should have occurred in the first place. If anything, my daily reliance on high-tech medicine has strengthened my belief in the importance of nonprescription approaches to cardiovascular disease. And unless I miss my guess, many of my colleagues would do well to incorporate these approaches into their personal life as well as their medical practice.

To my readers, I should express the hope that *Conquering Heart Disease* will help you bridge the gap between high-tech medicine and nonprescription programs. It's really not an either/or situation. Instead, you should have the best of both worlds, the most enjoyable and healthful lifestyle and the finest of medical care. Above all, if you follow this book's 15-point program to conquer heart disease, you'll find yourself needing very little medical care. Take care of your heart, so I won't have to.

Harvey B. Simon
Stockbridge, Massachusetts

Acknowledgments

HEART DISEASE is a formidable foe, and writing this book about its control was a formidable task. It was for me a labor of love, an opportunity to share with others the principles that guide my clinical practice and, indeed, my life. But my work is only a small part of a much larger effort; I have only myself to blame for the shortcomings of *Conquering Heart Disease*, but many, many to thank for its virtues.

I could not have written this book without the other members of the Harvard Cardiovascular Health Center. We began nearly 20 years ago; at that time, the idea of using diet, exercise, and stress reduction to treat heart disease seemed radical. By now, however, these ideas have been proved successful. Scientists from around the world have contributed to this exciting progress, and the doctors, nurses, nutritionists, and physical therapists of our Center have been among the leaders. It is a privilege to work with them and a pleasure to thank them for their intellectual stimulation, boundless enthusiasm, and personal support.

One of the wonderful things about a career in medicine is that it's a life of learning. I am deeply indebted to the many investigators and clinicians who continue to teach about hearts, both healthy and ill. Among my best teachers are my students; they earn an A plus for the questions and curiosity that keep us learning together.

My thanks, too, to my patients, both in the preventive cardiology program and in the internal medicine practice that has been the core of my professional life for more than 25 years. I'm grateful to them for allowing me to share in their health care, for helping me to understand the problems facing real people, and for working with me to find solutions to those problems. A special thanks to the wonderful people who work with me and who continued caring for our patients when I set aside my stethoscope to pick up a pencil: Grace Sjoberg, Sue Ward, R.N., Eileen Barrett, R.N., A.N.P., and John Goodson, M.D.; as he's done so often in the past, Dr. Richard Pingree has earned my special gratitude for the cheerfulness and skill with which he's treated our patients in my absence.

Kathleen Sweeney Laing made it possible for me to write this book without sacrificing my equanimity; I am grateful to her for the patience, speed, and skill with which she transformed my scrawl into a real manuscript. And I'm no less grateful to Jennifer Josephy and her colleagues at Little, Brown for their enthusiastic efforts that turned the manuscript into a book.

Ultimately, of course, I owe most of all to my lovely family. My daughter Stephanie is a skilled journalist and splendid writer who read the manuscript with care and insight, offering many wonderful suggestions. My daughter Ellie is a constant source of enthusiasm and joy who brought energy and happiness to my longest day. And my wife, Rita, is the guiding inspiration behind each page in the book, as she is to every one of my days.

Conquering
Heart Disease

Prologue

Heart Disease in America — A Needless Epidemic

AMERICAN HEARTS may be the warmest in the world, but they are not the healthiest. Despite our proud leadership in basic research, biomedical technology, and medical education, our rate of death from heart disease is more than twice as high as Japan's. Although we spend far more on health care than any other nation, only 13 countries have higher heart disease mortalities — and except for Ireland and New Zealand, all of them are former members of the Soviet bloc.

Cardiovascular disease is America's leading killer, taking nearly a million lives every year. Two out of every 5 Americans will die from cardiovascular disease, and 17 percent of them will be younger than 65. In all, one American dies from cardiovascular disease every 34 seconds.

It's tragic to die prematurely from heart disease — and it can also be difficult to live with cardiovascular disease. Nearly 1 of every 4 American adults has some form of cardiovascular disease. One and a half million heart attacks will occur in the United States this year alone, and more than 6 million people will be treated for angina or other forms of coronary artery disease. Add the 500,000 strokes that cripple Americans every year and the 60 million Americans with hypertension, and the total can only be described as an epidemic of atherosclerosis.

The atherosclerosis epidemic does not reflect a lack of medical effort. The United States boasts 16,478 cardiologists and more than 1,200 coronary care units. In 1990, we performed 285,000 angioplasties,

392,000 bypass operations, and even 1,935 heart transplants. Nor does the epidemic reflect a lack of financial effort. In fact, heart disease drains an estimated $128 billion from the American economy each year.

American medicine is wonderful, and its ability to diagnose and treat heart disease is the best in the world. Fine medical care is obviously essential to contain the atherosclerosis epidemic — but it is also part of the problem. Because our medical care is so good, many Americans put their faith in treatment and technology instead of putting their efforts into prudence and prevention.

Smoking, high blood pressure, high cholesterol levels, and lack of exercise are the four leading causes of atherosclerosis — yet more than 25 percent of Americans smoke, nearly 30 percent have high blood pressure, 50 percent have undesirable cholesterol levels, and more than 60 percent don't get enough exercise. For additional explanations of our atherosclerosis epidemic, just look to the high-fat American diet, the high-stress American lifestyle, and the high-profile American waistline.

Not all the news is bad. We are making important progress against heart disease; since its peak in 1966, in fact, the mortality rate has declined by more than 40 percent. Almost half the improvement can be traced to better medical therapy, the rest to better lifestyles. But if we are to improve further, we must attack the causes of heart disease instead of relying on technology to patch things up for another few years until the bypass graft closes or another heart attack occurs.

We can do better, much better. Perhaps the saddest aspect of the atherosclerosis epidemic is that it is so unnecessary. Heart disease is not an intrinsic component of human biology, nor is it an inevitable part of the aging process. Instead, atherosclerosis is man-made, a product of the bodily abuse and disuse that characterize modern life throughout the industrialized world.

Physicians can help control atherosclerosis, not by abandoning high-tech medical research and treatment, but by putting much more effort into patient education and counseling. But to succeed as teachers, doctors must first learn more about nonprescription, low-tech approaches to cardiovascular disease — and, not so incidentally, they should also learn to take better care of themselves!

Ultimately, however, atherosclerosis can be controlled only by personal commitment, responsibility, and effort. Don't rely on medicine or society — instead, rely on yourself. Understand the causes of heart disease and the lifestyle changes that can prevent it. Add the nonprescription supplements that can help, and the few medical tests and treatments that you really do need. Keep abreast of the newest developments in preventive cardiology. By incorporating these simple principles into daily life, Americans can defeat atherosclerosis, one heart at a time.

How to Use This Book

Atherosclerosis is a complex disease, and fighting it is a complex task. *Conquering Heart Disease* will show you how to do it in stages.

Part I explains the biology of atherosclerosis. In Chapter 1, you'll learn how the process affects the heart and blood vessels; you'll also learn about the mechanisms responsible for atherosclerosis itself. Chapter 2 explores the quantitative impact of atherosclerosis risk factors; using simple self-assessment tests, you'll be able to calculate your own risk.

Part II turns theory into practice. Each chapter presents one aspect of the 15 ways to conquer heart disease. Having determined your own needs, you'll be able to construct the program that suits you best. You'll also get the practical advice that will make your plan a success.

Part III will show you how your doctor can help; you'll learn about the major tests, treatments, and prescription drugs. But if you master the 15 steps in Part II, you won't have much need for Part III — or for a cardiologist!

Conquering Heart Disease will give you a comprehensive battle plan to fight atherosclerosis. In the final analysis, though, it will be up to you to wage the war. It's easier than you think, and your reward will be a life that is more vigorous and enjoyable as well as longer and healthier.

Let's get started.

PART I

Hearts in Health and Disease

Chapter 1

The Causes
of Heart Disease

To TAKE care of your heart, you must first understand it. You won't
need a medical degree, but you will need to spend a few minutes learning how a healthy heart works, what can go wrong, and how to spot the
early warning signs of heart disease.

The Healthy Heart

The human heart is a wonder. Weighing barely 10 ounces, it's no larger
than a clenched fist. Despite its diminutive size, the healthy heart is a
prodigious worker, pumping some 2,000 gallons of blood through
60,000 miles of blood vessels every day. On average, the human heart
beats 100,000 times daily; with proper care and feeding, it should be
good for 2.5 billion contractions over the course of a long and healthy
lifetime.

The body contains many strong muscles, but the heart muscle, or
myocardium, is unique. Its special structure of muscle fibers allows it to
beat automatically and continuously. But like the body's ordinary
muscles, it requires the proper mixture of exercise and nutrition to keep
it fit.

The heart's job, of course, is to pump blood. To do its job, the heart
is divided into four pumping chambers (Figure 1–1). Blood is collected
from the body's veins for delivery to the two chambers on the right side

of the heart; blood first enters the *right atrium,* which pumps it into the *right ventricle.* In turn, the right ventricle pumps blood into the lungs, where it is cleansed of carbon dioxide and enriched with life-giving oxygen. As oxygen is added to the blood in the lungs, its color changes from deep blue to bright red. The oxygen-rich blood is delivered to the left side of the heart, where it is pumped through two final chambers, the *left atrium* and the *left ventricle.*

As if things weren't complicated enough, two additional elements are essential for the heart to pump properly. First, the contractions of the four chambers must be perfectly coordinated. The rhythm and timing of the heart's pumping action depends on an electrical network composed of specialized cells that function as pacemakers and a conduction

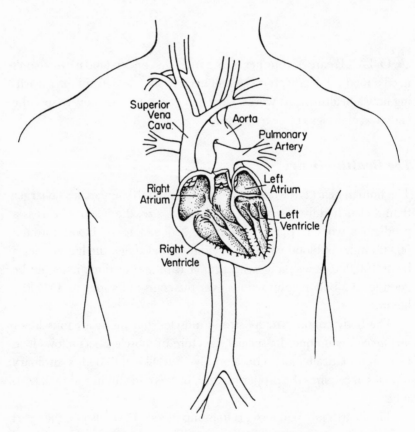

FIGURE 1-1: The Normal Heart and Circulation
The heart is pictured as if it were opened to look inside its pumping chambers.

system that carries the electrical impulses to muscle cells, triggering co-ordinated contractions. Second, to keep blood flowing in the proper direction, the heart's pumping chambers are separated by valves that open and close in sequence, allowing blood to flow only upstream.

After leaving the left ventricle, blood enters the body's largest artery, the *aorta*. Like the branches of a tree, the arteries divide into successively smaller vessels, finally bringing blood to the tissues. There, at last, the circulatory system does its real work, providing oxygen and nutrients to the tissues while gathering up carbon dioxide and waste products.

Blood from the left ventricle has a long way to go to carry vital oxygen to all the body's tissues. To go the distance, the left ventricle generates enormous force; the arteries that carry blood to the tissues must be strong and healthy to withstand this pumping pressure. But too much of a good thing can be harmful: while strong pumping pressure is needed to propel blood, excessive pressure can damage arteries. The left ventricle, too, can gradually weaken if it's forced to pump at excessive pressure levels.

Like all tissues, the heart muscle requires its own supply of oxygen-rich blood. The myocardium gets its blood from the *coronary arteries*. The coronary circulation begins with just two small vessels, the right and left coronary arteries, which originate in the root of the aorta, then quickly divide into a network of even smaller arteries (Figure 1–2).

The Types of Heart Disease

Sturdy and reliable in health, the heart can be jeopardized by disorders attacking any of its component parts.

Until 50 years ago, one of the most common heart disorders in this country affected the valves. *Rheumatic heart disease* produces inflammation, then scarring that prevents heart valves from opening or closing properly. In mild cases, the only consequence is a heart murmur, but in severe cases rheumatic heart disease can lead to congestive heart failure. In 1950, 22,000 Americans died from rheumatic heart disease, but in 1990, despite a much larger population, the number had fallen to 6,000. The reason: penicillin treatment stops strep throats from developing into rheumatic fever. Most of the 1.3 million Americans with rheumatic heart disease today are elderly, having contracted rheumatic fever decades ago in the preantibiotic era. But even today, rheumatic fever still

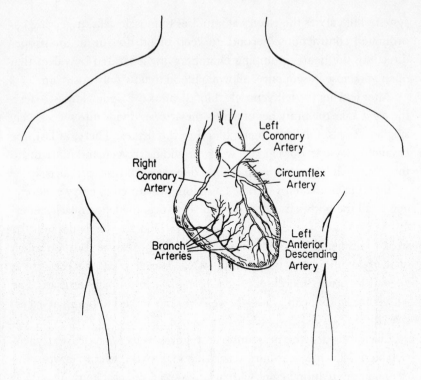

FIGURE 1–2: The Anatomy of the Coronary Arteries
The heart is pictured from the outside,
with the coronary arteries running through the heart muscle.

occurs from time to time, so it's important to treat strep throats with antibiotics, particularly in children.

Although rheumatic heart disease is on the wane, other heart valve disorders continue unabated. An example is *congenital heart disease* in which babies are born with abnormal valves. Another valve disease with potentially fatal consequences is *endocarditis;* in this infection, bacteria enter the blood and establish themselves on the heart valves, where they proliferate, causing progressive valve damage. Endocarditis can be cured by prolonged, intensive antibiotic treatment, but the best treatment of all is prevention; patients with abnormal heart valves should always take antibiotics before they undergo dental work, surgery, or certain medical procedures.

Another group of problems that can cause the heart to malfunction are *arrhythmias,* disturbances of the heart's orderly pumping sequence. Most arrhythmias are quite benign, causing only palpitations, a sensation of fast or irregular beats. But sometimes arrhythmias can cause fainting or even sudden death. Serious arrhythmias are usually caused by other underlying heart diseases, but they can also be caused by disorders of the body's metabolism (especially thyroid disease and abnormal potassium levels) or by human misbehavior (tobacco abuse, alcohol abuse, or even excessive caffeine consumption). Mild arrhythmias don't require treatment; fortunately, most serious arrhythmias can be treated successfully with medications or artificial pacemakers.

The heart muscle itself is also subject to a variety of disorders. In most, the myocardium gradually enlarges. Large muscles are usually strong muscles, but enlarged heart muscles eventually weaken, pumping blood less and less effectively. The ultimate result is congestive heart failure, signaled by fatigue, shortness of breath, and the accumulation of edema fluid in the feet and legs.

Congestive heart failure has many causes. Scarring of the heart valves, for example, causes the heart muscle to work extra hard, leading eventually to cardiac enlargement and failure. Less commonly, congenital diseases are linked to inborn disorders of the heart muscle. Metabolic abnormalities and toxins (including too much alcohol) can produce abnormalities of the heart muscle called *cardiomyopathies*. Another uncommon problem affecting the heart muscle is inflammation, or *myocarditis*. Myocarditis is often caused by viral infections; it's a good reason to avoid strenuous exercise during the flu or other viral infections.

Cardiomyopathies and myocarditis are nearly as exotic to doctors as to the public. But the most common causes of congestive heart failure are tragically familiar: *high blood pressure*, which causes the heart muscle to enlarge because it must pump abnormally hard, and *coronary artery disease*, which causes the heart attacks that kill heart muscle cells, replacing them with scar tissue. Intimately linked, high blood pressure and coronary artery disease form the core of the epidemic of cardiovascular disease ravaging the United States today.

Hypertension

In a sense, hypertension is simply too much of a good thing.

Blood pressure is the force that drives the circulation; without it, the tissues could not get the oxygen and nutrients that sustain life. Blood pressure is simply the product of two other forces, the pumping force of the heart's left ventricle and the resistance force of the arterial channels that carry the blood. If the heart does not pump forcefully enough or if the arterial channels are abnormally widened, the blood pressure will be too low. But if the heart's action is excessive, or if the arteries are abnormally constricted, the blood pressure will be too high. An excessive volume of blood can also raise the blood pressure. Whatever its cause, high blood pressure stresses blood vessels; over time, sustained hypertension can have terrible consequences, including stroke, eye damage, kidney failure, congestive heart failure, coronary artery disease, and diseases of the aorta and its branches.

Because of its central role in life, blood pressure is regulated by amazingly intricate interactions among the kidneys, the nervous system, the body's hormones, and the circulatory system. In healthy people, all these systems work together to keep the forces balanced and the blood pressure normal. But if the regulatory mechanisms malfunction, hypertension can result.

Affecting more than 63 million Americans, hypertension is as common as it is serious. Because of its great importance, high blood pressure has been the subject of intensive medical research for more than 50 years. Despite all these studies, the root causes of hypertension remain obscure; in a few patients, an underlying abnormality can be discovered, but in 95 percent of cases doctors disguise their ignorance by diagnosing "essential hypertension."

When it comes to figuring out what hormones and chemicals are responsible for hypertension, I'm no less ignorant than other doctors. But while I'm all for basic research, I think we'll all remain ignorant until we start asking the right questions. In most cases, hypertension is not caused by abnormal chemicals, but by aberrant behavior. It's a disease of the industrialized lifestyle, brought on by too much salt and too little potassium and calcium, too much dietary fat and too little fiber, too much body fat and too little bodily exercise, and by the mental stress of life in the fast lane.

Even if we don't understand the biochemical and physiological basis of hypertension, we do know how to diagnose and treat it. You'll learn much more about your blood pressure in this chapter and the next. Even more important, you'll learn how to control your own blood pressure (especially in Chapters 5, 6, 14, and 15) and how your doctor can help (Chapter 18).

Coronary Artery Disease

Saving the worst for last, we finally come to America's number one killer. More than 500,000 Americans die from coronary artery disease annually, and another 6.2 million are being treated for the condition. Countless others have coronary artery disease without knowing it — until they have a heart attack.

It's easy to see why coronary artery disease has such a dreadful impact. Like all tissue, the heart muscle requires a constant supply of blood and oxygen. It's one thing for the biceps to do without its blood supply, but quite another thing for the myocardium — there is just no such thing as a rest break for the heart, even the weary heart. All of the heart's blood supply passes through just two small coronary arteries, and because those arteries are so vital, blockages in either one can have disastrous consequences. The same is true even for the smaller coronary artery branches, each of which supplies blood to its own portion of the myocardium.

Vital as they are, the coronary arteries are vulnerable to disease. Nature has done its best to provide a margin of safety; although the main coronary arteries are small (about 4 millimeters in diameter, roughly the width of a pencil eraser), healthy arteries can widen to carry more blood when the myocardium needs it most. Diseased coronary arteries lose the ability to dilate, but even here there is a remarkable margin of safety: in general, blockages won't cause any trouble until they narrow the coronary channels by at least 70 percent.

But unless people fight back, atherosclerosis progresses relentlessly, eventually blocking the coronary arteries enough to produce clinical disease. After crossing the clinical threshold, coronary artery disease can declare itself in many ways:

Angina. When the heart muscle is happy, it does its work without complaint. But if it can't get enough oxygen, it may signal its distress with the pain of angina. Angina occurs when the myocardium's demand for oxygen exceeds its supply. The need for oxygen is increased by physical exertion, mental stress, exposure to cold temperatures, and even large meals — all classic triggers for angina. Sprinting to catch a bus, for example, may trigger angina, while walking to the bus stop may not. Even the most demanding circumstances won't precipitate angina in healthy hearts. But narrowed arteries can't meet these demands; most often the narrowing is caused by the fatty plaques of atherosclerosis, but spasm of the coronary arteries is the culprit in a few cases. Also uncommon is angina triggered by lung diseases that prevent the body from taking up enough oxygen, or by blood disorders that reduce the amount of oxygen that can be carried to the heart; exposure to very high altitudes can also threaten the heart's oxygen supply.

Angina can take many forms. Most often, it is experienced as a dull, heavy pressure deep in the center of the chest. The pain often radiates, typically to the neck, jaw, or left shoulder and arm. Shortness of breath and weakness may accompany the pain, as may palpitations, faintness, or lightheadedness. But in some cases, these ancillary symptoms are present without chest pain or pressure, in which case they are known as anginal equivalents. In most cases, angina is triggered by exercise or stress and relieved by rest or relaxation. In a variant called Prinzmetal's angina, however, the pain comes on at rest, usually because of coronary spasm rather than plaques. Both the classical and variant forms of angina respond favorably to medications such as nitroglycerin and to oxygen.

Silent ischemia. Angina can be mildly uncomfortable or very painful. Either way, it tells patients they need help. But some hearts experience oxygen deficiency, technically known as ischemia, without setting off any alarm. At first glance, silent ischemia might seem to be less of an evil than angina precisely because it's painless. But without pain as a warning signal, patients don't seek help, so silent ischemia actually presents a greater threat than angina. Silent ischemia may strike anyone with coronary artery disease, but diabetics are particularly vulnerable to this insidious manifestation of atherosclerosis. Patients don't recognize silent ischemia unless it progresses to the point of irreversible muscle damage, but doctors can recognize it earlier by its electrocardiographic abnormalities, which are identical to those produced by angina. (See Chapter 18.)

Heart attack. Ischemia is a critical threat to all tissues. Deficiencies of blood and oxygen, for example, can cause strokes if the brain is involved or gangrene if a leg is affected. The heart muscle responds to oxygen deprivation with angina or silent ischemia — or with a heart attack.

Heart attacks occur when the heart muscle's oxygen deprivation is severe enough to kill myocardial cells. The technical name for a heart attack accurately reflects the event: a heart attack is a *myocardial* (heart muscle) *infarction* (cell death due to ischemia).

Whereas most heart attacks are painful, resembling severe angina, they may also be painless, like silent ischemia. Often, heart attacks are accompanied by sweating, nausea, weakness, or intense apprehension and a feeling of impending doom.

Unlike angina, which usually occurs gradually when the heart is under stress, heart attacks often occur suddenly without apparent precipitants. The explanation for the difference lies in the coronary arteries themselves. Heart attacks usually result when a narrow artery becomes completely blocked either by the rupture of an atherosclerotic plaque or by a clot that forms on the plaque's surface (Figure 1 – 3).

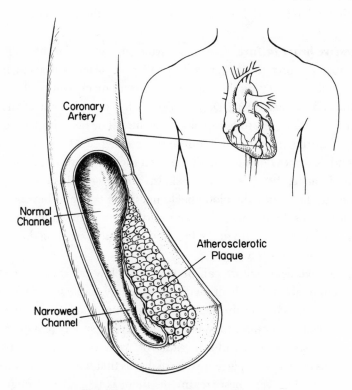

FIGURE 1–3: Coronary Artery Disease
The artery is partially blocked by an atherosclerotic plaque;
partial blockages produce angina and complete occlusions cause heart attacks.

Complete blockage of a coronary artery causes cell death. Doctors can recognize this by classic electrocardiographic changes or by blood tests that detect certain enzymes which are released by dying myocardial cells (Chapter 18).

How serious is a heart attack? Very serious. Each year heart attacks kill 300,000 Americans before they can even get to a hospital. Although modern treatment is excellent, 10 percent of all patients hospitalized with heart attacks will die within 3 days. The overall mortality is 30 percent, but 1 out of every 5 survivors will suffer a recurrence within 4 years. Heart attacks are also very expensive, averaging $50,000 each in medical costs and lost wages.

The consequences of a heart attack depend on how many cells die and where they are located. Even a small attack can be lethal if it damages the cells responsible for the heart's pumping rhythm. Large attacks cause disability and death more gradually by impairing the heart's pumping ability; multiple small attacks can cause the same effect.

Congestive heart failure. Coronary artery disease is the most important cause of congestive heart failure. Blocked arteries prevent heart muscle cells from getting the oxygen they need; myocardial cells die, to be replaced by scar tissue. Deprived of its full complement of muscle cells, the heart's ability to pump blood declines. The heart itself becomes enlarged as the chambers thin out and are distended by excess blood. The body's tissues don't get all the oxygen they need, resulting in exercise intolerance, then persistent weakness and fatigue. Instead of being pumped to the tissues, the blood backs up, filling the veins beyond their capacity. Excess fluid leaks from veins into tissues; in the lungs, this produces shortness of breath; in the legs and abdomen, swelling due to the accumulation of edema fluid.

Congestive heart failure can be treated. A low-salt diet will reduce fluid accumulation. Excellent medications are available to rid the body of excess fluid, to bolster the heart muscle's contractile force, to increase the heart's efficiency, and to maximize its oxygen supply (Chapter 18). In drastic cases, surgery can sometimes be used to remove scar tissue, but there is no way to replace myocardial cells that have been destroyed by ischemia. The very best treatment, then, is to prevent congestive heart failure by fighting atherosclerosis.

Arrhythmias. Coronary artery disease can cause arrhythmias by producing ischemia of the cells responsible for the heart's electrical apparatus, the pacemakers and conduction system. These disturbances can be transient if the ischemia is brief and reversible, or permanent if they follow heart attacks that produce cell death. Cardiac arrhythmias may be mild or serious; their consequences range from palpitations to dizziness to fainting — and, unfortunately, to sudden death.

Sudden death. Most people who have witnessed a loved one waste away slowly from congestive heart failure or die gasping for air because of fluid in the lungs express a preference for sudden death. Having cared for countless coronary care unit patients, I'd certainly prefer sudden death for myself — but not anytime soon, thank you.

About 250,000 sudden cardiac deaths occur in the United States each year, accounting for half of all cardiac deaths. By definition, these deaths are sudden and unexpected — but they are far from random events. Instead, the great majority occur in people who have diagnosed heart disease or who have experienced coronary symptoms but have neglected to get appropriate medical care.

Sudden death can occur anytime day or night, but its peak occurrence is in the early morning hours. The reason for this uneven distribution is not known. Most doctors postulate that it somehow depends on the cyclic variations in hormone levels, body temperature, and blood pressure that occur during everyone's day. Although these explanations may well be correct, I have another theory: new research has shown that a single large fatty meal can activate the body's clotting mechanism about 12 hours later. If these findings hold up, it may be that coronary arteries are clogged by clots in the morning because stomachs are clogged by fat the night before.

Sudden death can occur in bed or on the living room couch. We expect people to die in bed, but death during exercise makes headlines. Although many more people die from sudden cardiac death during rest than during exercise, physical exertion does increase the risk of sudden death. The increased risk is transient and is much greater in people who are out of shape than in regular exercisers. In fact, fit people are actually 60 percent *less* likely to suffer sudden cardiac death than couch potatoes. But the tragedy of exercise-induced death should remind everyone to get into shape gradually, follow appropriate precautions, and listen carefully for the body's warning signals (Chapter 5). With these provisos, exercise is safe, even in the early morning.

What causes sudden cardiac death? The usual explanation is a "massive heart attack," but that's not really the case. Instead the problem is most often a *small* amount of ischemia that happens to affect the heart's electrical impulses. The result is a critical arrhythmia, either ventricular tachycardia, in which the heart beats so quickly and inefficiently that it cannot propel blood, or ventricular fibrillation, in which the heart muscle quivers ineffectually, not really beating at all. Ventricular fibrillation is responsible for most cardiac arrests and sudden deaths.

In this truly remarkable era of modern medicine, it is possible to *survive* sudden death. Cardiac arrests can be treated, but only if cardiopulmonary resuscitation is initiated within four minutes. I heartily support the excellent Red Cross program to teach CPR to as many people as possible. But CPR is putting the cart before the horse — we could make CPR unnecessary if people would learn how to keep their coronary arteries healthy by conquering heart disease before it causes trouble.

What Causes Coronary Artery Disease?
Even in the midst of this book's very first chapter, it should be abundantly clear that the key to caring for your heart is caring for your coronary arteries. Cardiologists and cardiac surgeons are ready, able, and willing (perhaps sometimes a bit too willing) to help with medications to dilate coronary arteries, balloons to push plaques out of the way, and grafts to bypass blocked arteries. These are important techniques, and they require enormous training, technology, and skill. How can you possibly compete with the experts who take care of these small, delicate, and critically important arteries?

You can (and should) take care of your arteries even without a prescription pad, cardiac catheter, or bypass machine. In fact, you can do a better job than cardiac surgeons. The reason is simple — coronary artery disease is a symptom of a more fundamental disease that involves the whole body. Your job is not to fiddle with your coronaries, but to fight their real enemy: atherosclerosis.

Atherosclerosis

Medical terminology often seems willfully obscure, even to doctors. But atherosclerosis is a disease that's well named, indeed, thanks to the ancient Greeks. Two Greek words are combined in the name: *athere* (porridge) and *sclerosis* (hardening). And that's just what happens in coronary artery disease and other forms of atherosclerosis: the inner linings of arteries become filled with soft, mushy plaques that eventually make the artery narrow, stiff, and hard.

The plaques of atherosclerosis are, of course, composed not of porridge but of cholesterol. The story seems simple and familiar. High cholesterol levels start things off on the wrong foot. Excessive cholesterol is deposited on arteries, beginning first as fatty streaks, then gradually growing into plaques that can block the vital flow of blood. But while accurate, this scenario is far from complete. In fact, new research has revealed that atherosclerosis is far more complex. Complex or not, it's important to understand these new insights because they explain why fighting atherosclerosis requires much more than just lowering cholesterol levels.

How Atherosclerosis Develops

Atherosclerosis involves three basic elements: the blood cholesterol, the artery wall, and the body's clotting system. Each element is complex and delicate. A wide variety of problems can disturb the equilibrium of the blood cholesterol, the arterial walls, or the clotting system; abnormalities of any or all of these three systems can, in turn, dramatically increase the risk of atherosclerosis.

Cholesterol. Notorious as the cause of heart disease, cholesterol is much more complex than it's made out to be on TV and in the tabloids.

Although it's often included among the blood lipids, or fats, cholesterol is not technically a fat. Rather, it's a closely related, wax-like chemical belonging to a class of compounds called sterols.

Although it's often blamed for causing disease and death, cholesterol is actually essential for life and health. Entirely absent from the plant world, cholesterol is present in all animal tissues, where it is a vital part of cell membranes. In humans, cholesterol is also an essential building block of cortisone and the sex hormones.

Although it is often purged from health-conscious diets, most of the body's cholesterol does not come from food, but is made in the body itself. Because cholesterol is vital for cell membranes and hormones, the liver makes all the cholesterol the body needs, averaging about 1,000 milligrams per day; to keep our cells healthy we don't need to eat any cholesterol at all. In fact, consuming cholesterol-rich foods can cause the blood cholesterol to rise to abnormally high levels. But eating fat is even more dangerous, since dietary fat, particularly saturated fat, stimulates the liver to make much more cholesterol than the body needs.

Although excess cholesterol from the blood is deposited in the walls of arteries, not all blood cholesterol is bad cholesterol. In fact, there are many types of cholesterol in the blood, some bad but others good.

Cholesterol and fat do not dissolve in blood. To be carried in the blood, they are packed into spherical particles called *lipoproteins*. There are five major classes of lipoproteins: chylomicrons (the largest and lightest), very low density lipoproteins (VLDL), intermediate density lipoproteins (IDL), low density lipoproteins (LDL), and high density lipoproteins (HDL, the smallest and heaviest). To make things more involved and complex, each class of lipoproteins can be divided into subfractions that interact with each other in complex ways. That's the bad news. The good news is that to understand atherosclerosis, you need understand only two forms of cholesterol, LDL and HDL.

LDL cholesterol is the villain of the piece. About two-thirds of the blood cholesterol is in the form of LDL. The higher the LDL cholesterol, the greater the risk of atherosclerosis, coronary artery disease, and heart attack. That's because excess LDL cholesterol leaves the blood and enters artery walls. The newest research confirms that LDL cholesterol is harmful and that reducing LDL is an important way to fight atherosclerosis. But new research has also added an important twist to the story. It now appears that LDL itself is quite harmless; the damage comes not from natural LDL in the blood but from modified LDL, from LDL that is oxidized in the arterial wall.

Where a villain lurks, a hero can be found. When it comes to cholesterol, HDL is the good guy. Whereas low density lipoproteins deposit cholesterol in blood vessel walls, high density lipoproteins carry cholesterol *away* from the arteries. HDL transports cholesterol from arteries to the liver, where it's metabolized into bile salts that are eliminated harmlessly from the body through the intestinal tract.

The moral: down with LDL, up with HDL. But before learning how to put theory into practice, it's important to consider the artery wall, where LDL undergoes the oxidation that makes it so toxic.

The arterial wall. Every artery in the human body has three layers in its wall. The inner layer, or intima, is composed of a thin membrane of endothelial cells that are in direct contact with the blood stream and an underlying zone of protein, fluid, and cells. The middle layer, or media, is composed chiefly of smooth muscle cells and elastic fibers. The outermost layer, or adventitia, is composed of supporting tissues that are dense and strong in larger arteries, such as the aorta, but are nearly absent in the delicate blood vessels of the brain.

Not all arteries are equally vulnerable to atherosclerosis; unfortunately, the most vulnerable include the most vital: the coronaries, the aorta, the arteries that carry blood to the kidneys and to the legs, the carotid arteries that carry blood to the head, and the smaller arteries that supply blood to the eyes and brain.

Atherosclerosis begins in the intima, or innermost layer of the arterial wall. LDL cholesterol can pass directly from the blood into the intima, but injury to the endothelial layer (caused by high blood pressure or smoking, for example) accelerates the process. Once in the arterial wall some of the LDL is oxidized. Whereas normal LDL is harmless, modified LDL triggers a remarkable — and remarkably harmful — sequence of events (Figure 1–4).

Oxidized LDL produces inflammation and injury to the artery wall. In response, white blood cells arrive on the scene. These cells, called monocytes and macrophages, gobble up LDL cholesterol; in the process, they enlarge and are transformed into fat-laden foam cells. Unfortunately, the foam cells cannot dispose of all the toxic oxidized LDL. Instead, the cells themselves are injured by the LDL they have ingested; many die, releasing a soft and fatty gruel (not unlike the Greeks' porridge, I suppose) that provokes further inflammation. In an apparent attempt to seal off the inflammation, smooth muscle cells in the artery wall enlarge and proliferate. Growth factors released by injured endothelial cells and macrophages stimulate smooth muscle cell proliferation. The clotting mechanism comes into play as well, since blood platelets also release factors that stimulate smooth muscle cells. In turn, smooth muscle cells secrete collagen and other proteins into the enlarging plaque, or atheroma.

Although all this turmoil begins in the intima, it cannot remain contained in the delicate inner layer of the artery wall. Instead, the mix of

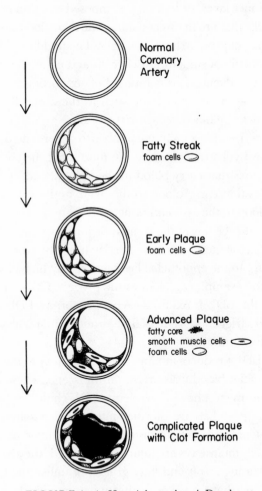

FIGURE 1–4: How Atherosclerosis Develops

The first stage is a small fatty streak composed of foam cells filled with oxidized LDL cholesterol. As the disease progresses, more cholesterol builds up, producing an early plaque. Eventually some foam cells die and rupture, releasing their fatty core and stimulating smooth muscle cells to enlarge; the result is an advanced plaque. Finally, the plaque itself ruptures, triggering the blood clot that blocks the artery.

foam cells, inflammatory cells, smooth muscle cells, collagen, and cholesterol enlarges and protrudes progressively into the arterial channel. Beginning as a small yellow dot, it gradually enlarges into a fatty streak, then into a full-fledged plaque, or atheroma. By then it's a disease — atherosclerosis.

The clotting system. Although atheromas enlarge relentlessly, their growth is slow and they rarely block arteries all by themselves. Instead, fissures form on the surface of the atheroma or the plaque itself ruptures. In either case, the smooth flow of the blood stream is disrupted, and this disruption activates the blood clotting system.

The first players in the clotting game are platelets, already familiar as a source of factors that stimulate smooth muscle cells in the arterial walls. Platelets are small cell fragments that are released from precursors (megakaryocytes) in the bone marrow, then travel in the blood stream to sites of vascular injury. Platelets are designed to control bleeding by triggering the clotting cascade. It's a vital job, but when the vascular injury is not a ruptured blood vessel, but a fissured atheroma, platelets can do more harm than good: they turn on the clotting system, quickly producing a mesh of fibrinous proteins and entrapped blood cells. And it is this mesh of clotting proteins that finishes the nasty job begun by the atheroma, blocking the artery and depriving the tissues of blood and oxygen vital to their survival.

The War Against Atherosclerosis

To conquer heart disease, you have to improve your blood cholesterol, keep your arterial walls healthy, and be sure your blood clotting system works for you, not against you. It sounds like an awesome task: lower LDL, raise HDL, protect arterial endothelium, suppress monocytes and foam cells, keep smooth muscle cells in check, and prevent excess platelet activation — while leading a happy and productive life.

Fortunately, you don't need a degree in cell biology to win the war against atherosclerosis. You don't even have to know an HDL from an atheroma. But you do have to understand that there's more to atherosclerosis than cholesterol; improving cholesterol *is* an important battle, but it's only part of the war. Part II of *Conquering Heart Disease* presents a comprehensive 15-point plan that will enable you to fight atheroscle-

Table 1-1
HOW THE 15-POINT PLAN FIGHTS ATHEROSCLEROSIS AND
CONTROLS HEART DISEASE RISK FACTORS

Atherosclerosis-Promoting Factor	Atherosclerosis-Fighting Strategies and Substances
High LDL cholesterol	Low-fat, low-cholesterol diet
	Exercise
	Dietary fiber
	Weight control
	Eating fish
	Niacin
	Various dietary supplements
Oxidation of LDL cholesterol	Antioxidant vitamins
	Vitamin E
	Beta-carotene
	Vitamin C
	Antioxidant minerals (?)
	Selenium
	Zinc
	Red wine (?)
Low HDL cholesterol	Avoidance of tobacco smoke
	Exercise
	Weight control
	Alcohol consumption
	Niacin
	Chromium
High blood pressure	Low dietary sodium
	Exercise
	Weight control
	Stress control
	Dietary potassium and calcium (?)
	Dietary fiber (?)
	Eating fish
Arterial wall damage	Avoidance of tobacco smoke
	Blood pressure control
	Exercise
	Aspirin (?)
Blood clotting system	Aspirin
	Exercise
	Eating fish
	Alcohol (?)

rosis without prescriptions, and Part 3 will explain how your doctor can help.

The first skirmish, though, is to assess your own risk so you can plan the program best suited to your personal needs. Chapter 2 will help you do just that. But before moving from the theory of atherosclerosis to the practice of prevention, it's worth spending a minute or two previewing the many ways that your 15-point plan will combat the fats, proteins, cells, and clots that are poised to produce atherosclerosis if you let them.

It's interesting to note that most of the 15 points appear on the list again and again, acting against atherosclerosis in areas as biologically diverse as cholesterol, arterial walls, and the clotting system. It's interesting, too, that strategies as disparate as eating fish and avoiding tobacco smoke act together to fight atherosclerosis.

The reason that such diverse strategies act together is that they are all part of the normal lifestyle that human evolution prepared us for. Atherosclerosis is *not* an inevitable aspect of human biology, nor is it an intrinsic element of the aging process. Far from it. Atherosclerosis is a rarity in many parts of the world today; coronary artery disease and heart attacks are almost unknown in societies that feature physical activity, vegetable-based diets, and smoke-free environments. Even in America, coronary artery disease was very uncommon until the industrial revolution; in fact, heart attacks were not described in the American medical literature until 1912.

What's changed? Not our genes, but our behavior. We've substituted mental stress for physical exertion and fat-rich animal foods for fiber-and-vitamin-rich vegetable foods — often adding salt, at that. We've filled our air and our lungs with tobacco smoke. We've gained weight. In sum, we've *created* the disease of atherosclerosis.

Atherosclerosis is produced by abnormalities of the blood cholesterol, the arterial wall, and the blood clotting systems. But don't blame your cells or your proteins. Instead, look in the mirror. In the words of Pogo, Walt Kelly's marvelous comic strip creation, "We have met the enemy, and he is us."

Atherosclerosis is a twentieth-century disease. How bad is it in twentieth-century America? Two 1993 studies provide a shocking answer. The first reviewed the autopsies of 1,532 teenagers and young adults who died from trauma in twelve American cities. All the subjects had fatty streaks in their aortas by age 15, and about half had fatty deposits in their coronary arteries by age 19. The second examined trauma victims who died at an average age of 26; nearly 80 percent had coronary blockages, and 20 percent had blockages that narrowed an artery by at least half. Far from being a degenerative disease of old age, atherosclerosis is a behavioral disease that begins at an early age in industrialized societies.

The enemy in atherosclerosis is human behavior. To win the war against it, recapture the basic human lifestyle that evolution intended for us. But you don't have to return to the farm, much less the trees, to do so. The much lower rate of coronary artery disease in Japan bears witness to the fact that it's possible to live in an industrialized society without producing an epidemic of atherosclerosis.

The fight against atherosclerosis employs natural techniques. Of our 15 points, only two, aspirin and alcohol, involve man-made chemicals — and alcohol has been part of human society for 10,000 years, while aspirin-like compounds present in tree bark have been used therapeutically for 2,500 years. Other strategies involve consuming vitamins, minerals, or food extracts in doses higher than even the best diet is likely to provide. But even these "artificial" weapons would be unnecessary if we avoided the bodily disuse and the nutritional, emotional, and environmental abuses that turn our bodies against us by creating atherosclerosis.

Chapter 2

Evaluating Your Risk
for Atherosclerosis

IT MAY TAKE only a few seconds to discover that you have coronary artery disease: angina may be subtle but heart attacks are swift, and sudden cardiac death is cataclysmic. But if coronary artery disease is swift and obvious, the underlying problem, atherosclerosis, is slow and insidious. Slow or not, atherosclerosis will progress relentlessly until it causes a heart attack, stroke, or sudden death — if you let it.

You can take action to prevent, halt, or even reverse atherosclerosis. Every person should adopt the basic principles that will conquer heart disease. But people with atherosclerosis should do more, ideally before they experience advanced clinical disease.

How can you tell if you have atherosclerosis before your doctor shows you your abnormal electrocardiogram or coronary arteriogram? You can't peer inside your coronary arteries to hunt out an early atheroma, much less a fatty yellow streak. But you can accurately calculate your risk of atherosclerosis by establishing a simple risk-factor profile.

Risk and Protection: A Primer

Before your risk factors are enumerated, you should know how to interpret them.

The Meaning of Risk

Simply having one or more atherosclerotic risk factors does not mean you're doomed to occupy a bed in a coronary care unit. But it does mean you are more likely to develop atherosclerosis than somebody without those risk factors. And the more risk factors you have, the greater your chances of developing heart disease.

There are 10 major coronary risk factors, but not all are equally dangerous. To compare the impact of various risk factors, you should employ the concept of relative risk — not, of course, the hazards posed by your in-laws, but a statistical measure of each factor's strength.

Here's how epidemiologists determine relative risk. They identify a group of people without evident disease. Next, they establish a health profile for each member of the group. The third step is to observe the group, called a cohort, over time. The final step is to compare members of the cohort who stay healthy with those who become ill, trying to identify factors that are associated with illness.

Cohort analysis has been used extensively to study heart disease. A cohort, for example, will contain both smokers and nonsmokers. Over time, the smokers will develop many more heart attacks than the nonsmokers. In fact, heart attacks are two and a half times more common in smokers than in nonsmokers. Smoking, the most potent risk factor, increases the risk of heart disease by 250 percent; in statistical terms, the relative risk of smoking versus not smoking is 2.5.

Cohort analysis is a powerful technique, but it's slow and expensive, typically involving thousands of subjects over many years. The famous Framingham Heart Study, for example, has been tracking more than 15,000 citizens of Framingham, Massachusetts, since 1948. The study has cost millions of dollars, but it has yielded reams of invaluable information. Still, in this era of fiscal constraints and diagnostic urgency, other investigative techniques are also being employed. One such tool is the case control study, in which doctors identify a much smaller number of subjects, who already have the disease in question, then compare them with an equal number of healthy people to see what risk factors may account for this difference.

Cohort analyses, case control studies, and other techniques have been used with great success to study atherosclerosis. Many factors that contribute to atherosclerosis have been identified, and a relative risk can be assigned to each; by comparing them, it becomes obvious that some are more hazardous than others. Although even a small risk can be important when your health is involved, relative risks below 1.2 should be interpreted with caution since they could represent statistical flukes.

Although the concept of relative risk is quite simple, subtle complexities abound. For example, how can risk factors be ferreted out when many are present simultaneously? If a smoker with hypertension has a heart attack, do we blame tobacco, high blood pressure, or both? It's tricky, but epidemiologists can sort it out with computers and a statistical technique called multivariate analysis. In this example, the answer is both.

Another potential pitfall in interpreting risk factors is more basic: it's the concept of causality. Although the human mind is quick to assign blame, the mere coexistence of two events does not necessarily mean that one is the cause of the other. Storks, for example, disappeared from Europe at the same time that the birth rate fell. Did the disappearance of storks cause the declining birth rate? No — the two events are associated without representing a cause and its effect. Heart attacks are 2.5 times more common in cigarette smokers than in nonsmokers. Does smoking cause heart attacks, or are the two merely associated?

Smoking *is* a *cause* of atherosclerosis. How can I be sure? By using standards that should be applied to all potential risk factors. First, be sure the observation that smokers get more heart attacks is based on sound data and that it is statistically valid. Next, be sure the observation is duplicated in additional population groups; if smoking causes atherosclerosis, it should be associated with heart attacks in Finland as well as Framingham. Finally, ask if a causal relationship is biologically plausible. Is it supported by test-tube data? By animal experiments? By what we know about the mechanisms of the disease? In the case of smoking and heart disease, the answers are yes, yes, and yes. In contrast, a 1993 study found that male pattern baldness is statistically associated with heart disease. Are they really cause and effect? In this case, the relative risk is low, the observation has not been duplicated, and biologic evidence fails to support the link. So for now I'm confident that baldness does not *cause* heart disease — a good thing, I might add, since I've been able to quit smoking but not to restore my hairline!

The remainder of this chapter will explain the 10 coronary risk factors that have been validated scientifically. The next 15 chapters will tell you what you can do about them. Remember, though, that decisions about treatment should be based on criteria just as strict as the standards used to assign blame.

Understanding Benefit

The very same techniques that can be used to establish risk can be used to determine benefit. Exercise, for example, has been the subject of more than 100 cohort analyses and case control studies in population groups from around the world. Exercise has been studied in mice, pigs, chimps, and dogs. Numerous laboratory tests have explained how exercise affects human tissues. The results all agree: exercise prevents atherosclerosis.

But scientists have an additional tool at their disposal when they are trying to establish benefit: to study a medication or treatment, for example, they can actually try it out. Needless to say, clinical trials must be careful and precise. The drug or treatment should be studied first in test tubes and then in animals (humanely, of course) prior to being tested in humans. Before large-scale human studies are done, pilot projects should monitor small groups. All subjects should understand the risks and benefits of the study, should consent freely to their participation, and should be free to withdraw at any time. And if at all possible, the clinical trial should be randomized and blinded; in such trials, volunteers are randomly assigned to receive the real study drug or to take an inert or dummy pill, called a placebo, that looks and tastes like the real thing. To eliminate bias, neither the subjects nor the scientists will know which pills are active and which are placebos until the trial is over.

A randomized, blinded clinical trial is the very best way to study a treatment, but it's not the only way. The U.S. Physicians' Health Study, for example, used this technique to see if low-dose aspirin could reduce the risk of heart attacks (it did, by 44 percent in men older than 50). But the Nurses' Health Study used a simpler cohort analysis to see if taking vitamin E was associated with a reduced risk of heart attacks (it was, by more than 40 percent). A randomized trial will be required to be sure that vitamin E is the *cause* of the protection observed. But clinical trials are painstaking, slow, and expensive; until one is completed, we can still derive lots of useful information from the strong *association* between vitamin E consumption and a reduced risk of heart disease, particularly since it's supported by other human studies and by animal trials (see Chapter 11).

Conquering Heart Disease is designed to provide the latest scientific data about strategies to fight atherosclerosis. Before planning your personal program, however, you should evaluate your personal risks.

Atherosclerosis Risk Factors

Medical students learn about coronary artery disease just as you have. In their first year of study, they master the normal heart and circulation; in the second, they tackle the cell biology of atherosclerosis. You've done both in Chapter 1, and now you'll join third-year medical students in moving from the lab to the bedside to grapple with the things that cause atherosclerosis in real, whole people.

Because atherosclerosis is so complex, there are many risk factors. It's no trick to master the list, and our students do it quickly. But they often lose sight of the relative importance of these risk factors and how they interact. It is a pitfall that can be avoided simply by stratifying the coronary risk factors into logical groups before considering them individually. (See Table 2–1.)

In addition to these 10 important risk factors, epidemiologists have linked many other abnormalities to an increased risk of coronary artery disease. Some, such as ear lobe creases, are curiosities of little biological significance. Others, such as infections with chlamydia, an unusual bacterium, are interesting and provocative but require further study. At

Table 2–1
CORONARY ARTERY DISEASE RISK FACTORS

Factors That Cannot Be Modified

Age
Male gender
Family history

Factors That Can Be Improved

The "big four"

Smoking
Abnormal blood cholesterol
Hypertension
Lack of exercise

The "little three"

Diabetes
Obesity
Mental factors

present, these extra factors seem linked to coronary artery disease by association rather than causality; we'll consider a few after dealing with the major risk factors.

Age

It's obvious that older patients get more heart attacks than younger people. Four out of every 5 heart attacks occur in people older than 65: age is a statistically important risk factor for coronary artery disease. It's a unique risk factor, though, since it's the only one that you want more of! Since age is a nonmodifiable factor, there is little point in worrying about it. But you should keep it in mind. If you are an American, your risk of coronary artery disease will begin to mount beyond age 45 if you're a man, and it will rise beyond age 55 if you're a woman. If you're in these risk groups, you'll want to take a little extra care in planning your diet and exercise programs, you may be a candidate for low-dose aspirin, and you'll need a few more medical checkups.

Careful readers may have caught me in an apparent contradiction. I stated earlier that to be valid, coronary risk factors should apply worldwide, yet I've now linked age to heart attacks specifically in America. In fact, age is a valid risk factor throughout the industrialized world, but it's much less potent elsewhere. It's not because people live longer in "advanced" societies — it's because preindustrial cultures do not incorporate the abusive lifestyles of modernity, so their old people are remarkably free of atherosclerosis.

Gender

Another nonmodifiable risk factor: throughout the industrialized world, men get more heart attacks than women, and they get them about 10 years earlier. But in twentieth-century America, women are, unfortunately, catching up. During each of the last 10 years, more American women than men have died of heart disease. Just as in men, heart attacks are the leading cause of death in American women, and female heart attack victims are actually more likely to have second attacks (20 percent versus 16 percent) and to die within 1 year (39 percent versus 31 percent).

The sad fact is that women are catching up to men because they are adopting some previously "male" living patterns such as tobacco abuse, sedentary living, nutritional neglect, and mental stress. Even so, women do have a biological advantage when it comes to atherosclerosis. The female sex hormone, estrogen, raises HDL cholesterol and lowers LDL cholesterol, thus reducing the risk of atherosclerosis.

Estrogen levels decline abruptly at the time of menopause; a few years later, the risk of heart attack begins to rise. Women can do better, staying happily behind men in the dubious category of cardiac risk. First, they should reduce other risk factors by eating properly, exercising regularly, relieving stress, and avoiding tobacco. Second, they should consider postmenopausal hormone replacement therapy. Estrogen replacement is very effective in fighting atherosclerosis; in fact, it reduces the risk of both heart attack and stroke by about 50 percent. Estrogen replacement does have drawbacks, and even risks, but these can be quantitated and minimized, allowing each woman to decide if postmenopausal hormones are right for her. From the cardiovascular point of view, estrogen replacement is a plus. (See Chapter 16.)

Family History

Coronary artery disease "runs in families"; since you can't trade in your ancestors any more than you can turn back the clock or alter your sex chromosomes, a family history of coronary artery disease is the third nonmodifiable risk factor.

Remember, though, that families share lifestyle traits every bit as much as they share genes. Families eat together; some exercise together; others sit in front of the TV together. Smokers often pick up the habit from a parent or sibling; even nonsmokers are at increased cardiac risk from passive smoke exposure if anyone in their household smokes. Stress, too, is a cardiac risk that tends to be shared among family members.

In addition to these acquired habits, some cardiac risk factors can be inherited. In particular, high cholesterol levels, hypertension, diabetes, and even obesity can have a genetic basis. Families with these traits do share an increased risk of coronary artery disease. Other families appear to inherit an extraordinary risk of premature atherosclerosis, with heart attacks striking 20- and 30-year-olds. Doctors studying such families have recently discovered the gene responsible for this terrible situation; it's been named ATH-S for atherosclerosis-susceptible. Fortunately, this type of family history is quite uncommon.

If your family tree includes branches felled by heart attacks, you should take extra care to prune your risks. Be sure everyone in your family adopts the elements of the 15-point program that are personally appropriate. Be sure, too, that your medical care includes tests for cholesterol, hypertension, and diabetes.

Are people with a family history of heart disease taking these important steps? A 1994 survey tells us the answer; unfortunately, it's no. Despite having a parent with heart disease before age fifty-five, 37 percent of the subjects smoked, 31 percent were overweight, less than half had had their cholesterol or blood pressure measured, and most were sedentary. Is it any wonder that heart disease runs in families?

How important is a family history of heart disease? By factoring out smoking and other shared lifestyle patterns, the Framingham Heart Study has determined that having a parent or sibling with coronary artery disease increases an individual's risk by about 25 percent. Genetics is important — but it has a much smaller impact than the "big four" modifiable risk factors.

Smoking
A positive family history of heart attacks may increase your risk by 25 percent, but smoking is 10 times worse, increasing your risk by *250 percent.*

Smoking is the most lethal cardiac risk factor, accounting for more than 20 percent of all heart attack deaths. That means that smoking causes fatal heart disease in 115,000 Americans each year; as many as 40,000 more suffer heart attacks because of passive smoking. Add the needless death and disability from lung cancer, emphysema, and many other problems, and you'll see why smoking is public health enemy number one.

That's the bad news. The good news is that quitting *will* help your heart. In fact, your risk of heart attack will decrease by 70 percent within just 5 years of quitting. Using a sophisticated computer model, Dr. Lee Goldman's group at Harvard Medical School found that, on average, a 35-year-old smoker who quits will gain 2.5 years of life expectancy.

We know how smoking affects the heart and circulation. We know the costs of tobacco abuse. We know that quitting is difficult — but we know what will help. If you need help, you'll find it in Chapter 3.

Cholesterol

Twenty-five percent of Americans need help with smoking, but at least 50 percent need help with cholesterol.

An elevated blood cholesterol level is a major cause of atherosclerosis, increasing the risk of coronary artery disease by a factor of 2.4. Nationally, 300,00 heart attack deaths can be attributed to high cholesterol levels. Even small improvements in cholesterol levels can produce big benefits; a 1 percent decrease in blood cholesterol will reduce the risk of heart attack by nearly 3 percent. The computer tells us that 35-year-olds who bring high cholesterol levels down to 200 will gain up to 6 years of life expectancy.

Interpreting cholesterol levels. The U.S. Public Health Service has set 200 milligrams per milliliter as the desirable blood cholesterol level for American adults. We are making progress toward that goal; the average American blood cholesterol level has come down by about 15 milligrams per milliliter, or 7 percent, over the past 40 years. But more than 50 percent of the adults in this country still have cholesterol levels above 200 milligrams per milliliter; 20 percent have levels above 240, and about 30 percent should be on therapeutic cholesterol-lowering diets.

While I'm grateful to the government for setting an easily understandable goal for blood cholesterol levels, I think we can be more precise. For one thing, the risk of atherosclerosis varies directly and continuously with blood cholesterol level; simply put, the lower the cholesterol level, the lower the risk. Bringing the average American cholesterol level down to 200 milligrams per milliliter will help — but there will still be far, far too many heart attacks. For example, a 1991 study of people with cholesterol levels below *190* found that reducing cholesterol levels by another 10 percent reduced cardiac risk by 20 percent. I'd vote for a target of 180 or even perhaps 160; it's a demanding standard, but it is doable—if not for the average American, then for the well-motivated person who follows this book's 15-point program.

The second problem with a simple goal of 200 is that it glosses over the complexities of the cholesterol problem. And complex or not, the details do matter. The first consideration is age. Both blood cholesterol and cardiac risk rise with age; a level of "just" 220 may not raise eyebrows in an 80-year-old, but it should set off alarms in a 20-year-old.

The second concern, of course, is the role of HDL cholesterol; since high HDL levels are protective, it's really impossible to interpret any person's cholesterol numbers without knowing at least the total cholesterol and the HDL cholesterol. A personal example: in the Preface I boasted of bringing my total cholesterol down from 294 to 220. By the government standard of 200, however, I'd hardly be a good advertisement for my own advice. Happily I am — because my HDL, or "good" cholesterol, is a very healthy 110.

Recognizing these complexities, the experts of the National Cholesterol Education Program offered more detailed guidelines in 1993. (See Table 2–2.) Once you've checked your total cholesterol, LDL cholesterol, and HDL cholesterol levels, you can see how you measure up.

These guidelines make the central message clear: to reduce cardiac risk, lower LDL and total cholesterol levels and raise HDL levels.

But what about people with high LDL (bad) *and* high HDL (good) cholesterols — should they buy life insurance or long-term bonds? Conversely, what is the risk when both LDL and HDL are low? You'll need to do a little math to sort out these factors and understand your cholesterol numbers. No need to panic — it's really quite simple: just divide your total cholesterol by your HDL:

$$\frac{\text{Total Cholesterol}}{\text{HDL Cholesterol}} = \text{Risk Ratio}$$

The cholesterol risk ratio provides a single number that measures the impact of both good and bad cholesterol (Table 2–3).

Using this technique, most authorities peg a ratio of 4.5 as desirable. Indeed, there's nothing wrong with being average — unless it means having the heart attack risk of the average American. You can, and

---

Table 2–2
NATIONAL CHOLESTEROL EDUCATION PANEL GUIDELINES
FOR BLOOD CHOLESTEROL LEVELS IN ADULTS

	Total Cholesterol	LDL Cholesterol	HDL Cholesterol
Optimal		Under 100	Above 60
Desirable	Under 200	Under 130	
Borderline	200–239	130–159	
Abnormal	Over 240	Over 160	Below 35

Source: Adapted from *Journal of the American Medical Association* 269:3015, 1993.

Table 2–3
YOUR CHOLESTEROL RISK RATIO

Ratio	Risk
6.0	High
5.0	Higher than average
4.5	Average
4.0	Lower than average
3.0	Low

should, do better. Reduce your ratio as much as possible by lowering your LDL and raising your HDL; Part II will show you how.

The other blood lipids. When you get your cholesterol results, you'll notice that the whole does not equal the sum of its parts; don't question your doctor, your lab, or your arithmetic — your LDL and HDL never add up to equal your total cholesterol. The reason is that your blood contains other lipids; they may or may not be measured and reported separately, but they always figure into the total cholesterol equation.

Chapter 1 described the five major lipoproteins; in addition to LDL and HDL, your blood contains fats and cholesterol carried in chylomicrons, VLDL, and IDL particles — to say nothing of lesser lipoproteins and their subfractions.

Few clinical labs are equipped to perform a complete lipoprotein analysis, but most do measure and report triglyceride levels. Triglycerides are transported in very low density lipoproteins (VLDL); they represent fatty acids that are being carried to the liver after they've been absorbed from food in the intestinal tract. Because blood triglyceride levels rise after meals, they should always be measured while you are fasting, ideally for 14 hours.

Normal triglyceride levels are below 150 milligrams per milliliter. Elevated triglyceride levels are common in patients with coronary artery disease; still, I don't recommend routine measurements of triglyceride levels. My reason relates to the discussion of risk and statistics that you skimmed over at the beginning of this chapter. Elevated triglyceride levels are more common in heart attack victims — but they are also associated with low HDL levels, obesity, sedentary living, and diabetes. When these proven, powerful risk factors are accounted for by the technique of multivariate analysis, triglyceride levels do *not* hold up as independent atherosclerosis risk factors, so they do not need to be measured to screen for risk.

Still, triglyceride measurements should not be completely abandoned; such measurements may be worthwhile for patients with familial heart disease, diabetes, chronic kidney disease, hypertension, peripheral vascular disease, and established coronary artery disease. And even if triglycerides don't cause atherosclerosis, very high levels can cause inflammation of the pancreas. Fortunately, the 15-point program to conquer heart disease will improve triglyceride as well as cholesterol levels.

Lipid research labs can measure many other blood components that have been linked to heart disease. It turns out that an increased risk of atherosclerosis is related to elevated levels of some of these components (apolipoprotein B, small dense LDL, LDL subclass B, Lp(a), IDL, oxidized LDL) and to low levels of others (apoA-I, apoA-II, HDL subfractions). I'm glad that research labs are sorting all this out. It sounds like an alphabet soup of lipids, but someday soon these studies may give even much more accurate predictors of risk. For now, though, all you really need to know is your total cholesterol and HDL levels — and you thought they were complicated!

Can your cholesterol be too low? It's a surprising but important question. Over the past 10 years, several trials of cholesterol-lowering drugs have disclosed that patients taking the medications had fewer deaths from heart disease but more deaths from trauma, including accidents, homicide, and even suicide. This unexpected finding remains unexplained, but few experts blame low cholesterol *per se*. For one thing, some of the drugs used in these trials have unpleasant side effects — the drugs, rather than the cholesterol levels, may be responsible. In addition, newer studies using detailed psychological testing have failed to link low cholesterol to depression or hostility. Keep cholesterol in perspective — a high level shouldn't drive you crazy, and a low level won't either.

Perhaps stimulated by these drug trials, Dr. Daniel Jacobs and his associates conducted an extensive review of 21 earlier studies of cholesterol and mortality. After analyzing more than 68,000 deaths from around the world, they released their findings in 1992. As expected, they confirmed the well-known rise in cardiovascular deaths with rising cholesterol levels. But they also found that low cholesterol levels — total cholesterol levels below 140 to 160 — were actually associated with increased mortality, not from heart disease, but from cancers, brain hemorrhages, digestive diseases, and trauma.

Predictably enough, this man-bites-dog story provided lots of fodder for the press — and, I suppose, some comfort for the steak-and-chop folks. But before you fry up some burgers, consider the details.

First, Dr. Jacobs's study used a sophisticated statistical technique called meta-analysis. It's a powerful technique, allowing small studies to be grouped together to increase their power. But statisticians have questioned the ground rules employed in this particular meta-analysis. My math is not good enough to say which group of statisticians is right, but I can see other limitations of the study. First, it measured mortality but not morbidity; in other words, it did not utilize the reams of data that link high cholesterol levels to the disability, expense, and suffering of nonfatal heart disease. Second, the low cholesterol levels linked to increased noncardiac deaths were really *very* low, below the levels that are generally attainable by even the most rigorous program of diet and exercise.

But the hoopla about the putative hazards of low cholesterol levels should recall an even more basic fact from the beginning of this chapter: even if two phenomena are associated, they don't necessarily represent cause and effect. In this case, it's very *un*likely that low cholesterol levels cause problems as diverse as cancer, digestive diseases, and brain hemorrhages. Quite the reverse: people wasting away from cancer or digestive disease eat poorly and their livers make less cholesterol. Although I can't prove it, it seems likely that low cholesterol levels are the result, rather than the cause, of the noncardiac diseases that crop up in mortality studies.

At the risk of belaboring the point, it may be worth considering a 1993 report by Dr. Carlos Iribarren of the University of Southern California. When men who abused tobacco or alcohol or had advanced diseases of the intestines or liver were accounted for by multivariate analysis, the 23-year study of 8,000 Japanese-Americans in Hawaii found no association between low cholesterol levels and deaths from trauma, violence or, indeed, any cause.

Two 1994 studies provide even more reassurance. In the first, Drs. Law, Wald, and Thompson performed a meta-analysis of the worldwide experience with cholesterol-lowering treatments in more than half a million subjects. They found that reducing blood cholesterol levels by just 10 percent could reduce the risk of coronary heart disease by 50 percent at age 40; the benefits are less dramatic in older people — but even 70-year-olds can achieve a 20 percent reduction in risk. More good news: the benefits of reducing cholesterol levels begin promptly, reaching full effect in just 5 years. And in the second study, this same team of scientists found *no* evidence that low cholesterol levels increase the death rate from cancer, trauma, digestive diseases, or any cause except brain hemorrhages. In all, the benefits of a low cholesterol level far outweigh the slight risk of brain hemorrhages, which are linked only to extremely low cholesterol levels in any case.

The moral: the lower your cholesterol, the better.

Measuring your cholesterol levels. America is preoccupied with cholesterol. It's a hot item for the media and a tasty tidbit for talk shows. It's on many food labels — sometimes even in the big print. It can be measured in doctors' offices or by portable equipment at health fairs; can corner drug store checks or home testing kits be far behind?

Cholesterol is on everyone's lips. Unfortunately though, it's often a case of lip service, as fatty foods pass on down to stomachs, hips — and arteries.

It may be silly to talk about your cholesterol over coffee and doughnuts, but it is important to know your cholesterol levels. How often should they be checked?

Atherosclerosis begins in childhood. The value of cholesterol screening for children is controversial in pediatric circles, but it seems reasonable to recommend a blood test for children as young as 2 if they have parents or siblings with early heart disease or abnormal cholesterol levels. In the absence of these warning signals, it's safe to delay an initial cholesterol test until age 20 — but even without blood tests, all children should be encouraged to enjoy healthful patterns of diet and exercise.

Adults should have their cholesterol levels measured on a regular basis. Healthy people with good results from their first test don't have to repeat the test every time they drive past a hospital — but cholesterol levels should be checked at least every 5 years, beginning at age 20. Although 5-year intervals are the recommendation of the expert National Cholesterol Education Panel, I recommend repeat tests every year if the initial results are unfavorable or if there are changes in diet, body weight, exercise patterns, or medications. Needless to say, patients with heart disease and those being treated for lipid disorders may require cholesterol tests even more often, sometimes even at intervals of just 8 to 10 weeks.

Cholesterol testing can be tricky. Because the results are so important, it's vital to have your test done by well-trained technicians using top-flight equipment. If possible, have your testing done by a medical center, hospital, or good commercial lab instead of by a community screening program, health fair, or even a doctor's office lab. Even in the best of labs, cholesterol levels can vary by up to 20 percent, so it's important to repeat the test if your results are out of line with previous findings or reasonable expectations. You don't have to fast for a screening test, but if your cholesterol levels are unfavorable, you should have a repeat test after a 14-hour fast. Last but not least, remember that a simple total cholesterol level will not give you the information you need; instead, be sure your HDL level is measured at every test.

Setting your cholesterol goals. Your cholesterol risk ratio should be as low as possible. This means that your LDL should be as low as possible and your HDL as high as possible.

But just how far should you go? In my view, everyone should avoid tobacco, exercise regularly, and follow a diet low in fat and cholesterol but high in fiber. Chapters 3, 4, and 5 will provide the details. In most cases this program will achieve a risk ratio below 3.5 or 4. If it doesn't, or if you have two or more cardiac risk factors in addition to cholesterol, you should work harder on your cholesterol. For starters, you should consider a stricter diet and the nutritional supplements discussed in Part II. They should do the trick; if not, Part III will discuss the pros and cons of prescription medications.

Above all, keep cholesterol in perspective. It's a major cardiac risk factor — but there are 9 others. Understand all the elements of risk so you can construct a comprehensive program to fight atherosclerosis on all fronts.

High Blood Pressure

Cholesterol gets all the attention, but high blood pressure is nearly as common and nearly as dangerous. The relative cardiac risk of hypertension is 2.1 — if you have high blood pressure, your risk of suffering a heart attack is increased 210 percent. Since 63 million Americans (including 3 million children!) have hypertension, it's surely a major cause of our atherosclerosis epidemic. In all, high blood pressure accounts for 195,000 heart attack deaths in the United States each year — to say nothing of all the death and disability from stroke and other hypertensive diseases.

Don't let all these gloomy statistics raise your blood pressure — hypertension can be prevented and treated. Reducing blood pressure by just 1 point will reduce the risk of a heart attack by about 3 percent. According to computerized estimates, 35-year-olds can gain more than 5 years of life expectancy just by reducing their blood pressures to normal levels, even just high normal.

If the blood pressure story reminds you of the cholesterol scenario, it's no accident: the two problems are really very similar in their frequency in America, in their impact on heart attack risk, and in the benefits that can be realized from their control. And there are other similarities as well. Like cholesterol abnormalities, high blood pressure does its damage slowly and silently over years. Like cholesterol, blood pressure can almost always be improved by simple lifestyle changes; as with cholesterol, medications are available if backup treatment is needed. As with cholesterol, there is no single level of normal; instead, all the data suggests that the lower the blood pressure, the better. And like cholesterol abnormalities, the first challenge is to measure your blood pressure and understand its meaning so you can use your 15-point program to optimize your readings.

Understanding blood pressure. In Chapter 1 you learned (I hope) that blood pressure is the force that propels blood through the circulation and that it is simply the product of two forces: the contractile force of the heart's left ventricle and the resistance force of the body's arteries. But even if you stayed awake through all this theory, it would not be enough to enable you to understand the numbers that are recorded when your blood pressure is measured.

Two numbers are monitored with each blood pressure check. The higher number is the *systolic blood pressure;* it's the pressure in your arteries during the time your heart is pumping blood into your arteries. After each contraction, your heart muscle relaxes so it can refill with blood.

The pressure in your arteries during this relaxation phase is your *diastolic blood pressure,* the lower number of the blood pressure pair. By convention, the systolic pressure is given first. For example, a systolic blood pressure of 110 and a diastolic of 70 would be announced as "110 over 70" and written as "110/70."

Doctors have been measuring blood pressure for more than a century, and the hazards of hypertension have been clear for many decades. But despite all these years of study, two very important facts about blood pressure were not recognized until the past few years.

First, it's clear that both the systolic and the diastolic blood pressures contribute to the risk of heart attack and stroke. Formerly, doctors overlooked systolic readings, concentrating therapy on the diastolic pressure alone. It didn't make much sense, and it wasn't the right thing to do. Both numbers count.

Second, we've learned that there is no "safe" or "normal" blood pressure. Instead, the risk of disease is continuously related to blood pressure over its entire range. Put simply, the lower your blood pressure, the lower your risk; the higher your pressure, the higher your risk.

Interpreting your blood pressure. Armed with this new data, the National High Blood Pressure Education Program issued a brand new blood pressure classification system in 1992 (Table 2–4). It's more complex than the old system ("normal, borderline, and high") but it's much better because it demonstrates that systolic and diastolic pressures both impose a continuum of risk.

Measuring your blood pressure. Hypertension has been called the silent killer. It's a dramatic name but a good one. Most people with hypertension do *not* have headaches, ruddy complexions, nosebleeds, or high-powered personalities. In fact, most people with hypertension feel perfectly well — until they have a heart attack or stroke. Forty-six percent of all Americans with hypertension don't even know it.

The only way to know your blood pressure is to have it measured.

Having your blood pressure taken may seen formidable, but it's really very simple. First, an inflatable cuff is wrapped around your arm. Next, the cuff is filled with air until it's snug enough to block the flow of blood in the artery beneath it — but the blockage is temporary, harmless, and painless. The final step is to gradually release air from the cuff

Table 2-4

BLOOD PRESSURE CLASSIFICATION

Diastolic Blood Pressure	Systolic Blood Pressure						
	Lower than 120	120–129	130–139	140–159	160–179	180–209	210 or higher
Lower than 80	Optimal						
80–84		Normal					
85–89			High normal				
90–99				Stage 1 hypertension			
100–109					Stage 2 hypertension		
110–119						Stage 3 hypertension	
120 or higher							Stage 4 hypertension

while sounds are monitored over your artery. Your blood flow will resume when the cuff pressure drops below your systolic blood pressure; the blood flow is silent to your ears but it creates a sound that can be detected easily with a stethoscope. When the cuff pressure drops below your diastolic pressure all sounds will disappear. Because the earliest blood pressure machines used columns filled with mercury to calibrate the cuff pressure, blood pressure units are reported in millimeters of mercury, or mmHg.

It's simple enough — the appearance and disappearance of blood pressure sounds reflect respectively your systolic and diastolic blood pressures. The practice is as simple as the theory — but there are potential pitfalls. First, the cuff size must match your arm size; bigger arms demand bigger cuffs. Second, you should be relaxed; anxiety can raise your blood pressure, producing misleading results. Even if you feel calm, the simple act of having your blood pressure checked may be enough to raise it; this phenomenon is so common, in fact, that it has a name: white coat hypertension. Don't let a single high reading label you as having hypertension — instead try to relax by reading, sitting back with your eyes closed, or meditating, then have your pressure checked again.

Because exercise, caffeine, and nicotine can produce temporary changes in blood pressure, you should avoid all three before having your pressure taken. If your pressure still seems high, have it checked again on another day. Blood pressure is notorious for its peaks and valleys, but these swings ("labile hypertension") are not harmful, so you should be sure that high readings reflect sustained hypertension, particularly before you consider medication.

You don't have to see a doctor to have your blood pressure checked. Because of the anxiety factor, in fact, the readings obtained by nurses or technicians are often more reliable, particularly if you are checked in familiar surroundings at home or work. You can even learn to check your blood pressure yourself. Home monitoring devices that meet the standards of the Association for the Advancement of Medical Instrumentation are best. Serviceable cuffs and stethoscopes are available for about $30, and easier-to-use electronic monitors can be purchased for $60 to $150. It's a small price to pay if you have hypertension and need to monitor your treatment — but frequent monitoring is not at all necessary for people who are able to maintain good blood pressure.

Because hypertension usually begins gradually and insidiously between ages 20 and 50, all adults should have their blood pressure checked regularly. One check every 3 years may suffice for people with normal and optimal pressures (see Table 2–4). But higher results call for more frequent measurements, at least once a year for people with high normal blood pressures. All hypertension — even Stage 1 high blood pressure — mandates treatment, and everyone being treated for hypertension — even if the treatment is diet, exercise, and stress reduction — should be monitored closely to be sure they are getting good results. People who are at increased risk for developing hypertension (including African-Americans, relatives of hypertensives, and patients with kidney disease) should have their blood pressure checked at least once a year, even if their own numbers are "normal."

Check your blood pressure early and often. It's as easy as it is important. Take advantage of routine doctor's appointments, community screening, health fairs, and other opportunities to have this quick and easy risk factor measurement.

Can your blood pressure be too low? It's similar to the question we asked about cholesterol, and since the answer is the same, I won't keep you in suspense: no.

That's the short answer, but as usual there's a long answer as well. There are two circumstances in which blood pressure can be too low. The first occurs in the setting of acute medical illnesses, which may be mild (diarrhea, dehydration) or very serious (infection, bleeding, heart attacks). An abrupt or drastic decline in blood pressure can produce lightheadedness, fainting, coma, and critical organ dysfunction. When dehydration is the cause, fluid replacement is a simple and effective treatment, but more serious causes of low blood pressure require urgent medical therapy.

The other situation in which blood pressure may be too low is in patients who are on *drug* therapy. If overtreated, they can feel dizzy or faint. In addition, while appropriate treatment is of great benefit, reducing the risk of heart attack and stroke, mortality actually begins to rise a bit in patients who are treated so intensively that their diastolic blood pressures fall below 70 or so. It's another reason to control your blood pressure with lifestyle changes rather than medication, if at all possible.

Setting your blood pressure goals. Like cholesterol, the lower your blood pressure the better. As with cholesterol, the mainstay of blood pressure reduction should be lifestyle change rather than medication. Use the 15-point program to bring your blood pressure down as much as possible; the higher it starts, the harder you should push diet, exercise, weight control, and stress reduction. If you have other cardiac risk factors, your blood pressure goals should be even more stringent than if blood pressure is your only concern. In any case, if you can't get below Stage 1, turn to Chapter 18 to see how your doctor can help.

Lack of Exercise

Sedentary living may be fourth on the risk factor hit list, but it's a close fourth. Despite its importance, it is the most often neglected cardiac risk factor.

The relative cardiac risk of a sedentary lifestyle is 1.9 — people who don't get enough exercise increase their risk of heart attack by 190 percent. Since at least 60 percent of American adults do not exercise at recommended levels, it can be argued that sloth causes more heart attacks than any other risk factor, accounting for more than 205,000 heart attack deaths in the United States each year. But sedentary living is a modifiable risk factor; even people who don't get started until middle age can benefit, gaining more than 13 months of life expectancy and feeling much better in the process.

Many people with risk factors turn immediately to their doctor for help, seeking nicotine patches for smoking or pills for cholesterol and blood pressure. I'm pretty quick to prescribe nicotine patches (in conjunction with other smoking cessation techniques) but I ask patients to establish their own 15-point lifestyle program before seeking a quick fix for cholesterol or blood pressure with medication. When it comes to exercise, though, there's no room for debate: your doctor can't do it for you.

Exercise is up to you — and it's up to you to do it right, so it will be safe, effective, and enjoyable. Chapter 5 will explain it all; for the moment let's determine if sedentary living is a risk factor for you.

What exercise is best? When considering the impact of smoking, cholesterol, and blood pressure on cardiac risk, the bottom line was simple: the less the better. When it comes to exercise the reverse is true — up to a point.

Exercise has many benefits: it strengthens the heart muscle, improves cholesterol levels, lowers blood pressure, fights obesity and diabetes, controls excessive blood clotting, and reduces stress. Since regular exercise improves so many cardiac risk factors, it's no surprise that it reduces the risk of heart attacks and extends life.

Many studies have confirmed these benefits, and many have discovered *what type* of exercise is best for health. It's aerobic exercise, in which the heart is working at 70 to 85 percent of maximum. Brisk walking, jogging, biking, swimming, cross-country skiing, and aerobic dance are examples of aerobic exercises that will help prevent atherosclerosis if they are performed on a regular basis.

Many studies explain how exercise works and what type of exercise is best, but few have explored the optimal *amount* of exercise. It is clear that every little bit helps, which is probably why the goal of 20 minutes 3 times a week has gained widespread currency. An hour of exercise each week will help — but it's not enough.

How much exercise is enough? The best answer comes from the observations of Dr. Ralph Paffenbarger and his colleagues at Stanford University and the Harvard School of Public Health. The good doctors evaluated 16,936 graduates of Harvard College, comparing their exercise levels with their risk of heart attacks and death. Physical activity was measured in numbers of calories burned up by exercise each week. As little as 500 exercise calories per week was helpful, but optimal benefits occurred in men who exercised enough to consume 2,000–3,000 calories per week. And the benefits were substantial, amounting to a 26 percent reduction in heart attack risk. Beyond the 3,000 calorie level, however, additional exercise did not produce additional gains in life expectancy. And to be effective, exercise had to be performed on a regular basis; winning a varsity letter in college was not helpful unless it was followed up by a lifetime of exercise.

Even without a Harvard degree, you can use Dr. Paffenbarger's data to establish your exercise goals: you will consume 2,000 calories with about 20 miles of walking or jogging, 80 miles of biking, or 4 miles of swimming. It sounds like a lot, but it's not so daunting if you spread it out over the course of a week. In fact, a good rule of thumb is to aim for an average of 30 minutes of moderately brisk aerobic exercise per day.

Table 2–5
TIME REQUIRED TO BURN 2,000 CALORIES

Strolling	10 hours
Bowling	8¹/₂ hours
Golf	8 hours
Raking leaves	7 hours
Doubles tennis	6 hours
Brisk walking	5¹/₂ hours
Biking (leisurely)	5¹/₂ hours
Ballet dancing	4¹/₂ hours
Singles tennis	4¹/₂ hours
Racquetball or squash	4 hours
Biking (hard)	4 hours
Jogging	4 hours
Downhill skiing	4 hours
Aerobic dance	¹/₂ hour
Brisk calisthenics	3¹/₂ hours
Cross-country skiing	3 hours
Running	3 hours

Evaluating your exercise level. Is sedentary living a risk factor for you? You won't need a doctor or lab to answer this question. Instead, you can use two simple methods to evaluate your own exercise level.

The first method is easier: just tally up the time you spend exercising each week, then check Table 2–5. Remember that your goal is to burn 2,000 calories per week; you can do it with 3 to 4 hours of moderately intense exercise. For greater precision, use Table 5–1 to compare your exercise with the aerobic intensity of representative activities.

The second way to evaluate your exercise pattern is to take a fitness test. If you are getting enough exercise, the results will show up in increased physical capacity as well as in reduced cardiac risk. To see if you are fit, just head for a neighborhood high school track. Be sure that you haven't eaten for 2 hours prior to the test and that you are feeling well. Warm up for 10 minutes and then simply see how much distance you can cover in 12 minutes of walking or jogging. Don't push yourself too hard, and back off if you don't feel well. Cool down after you complete your test, then use Table 2–6 to evaluate your results.

Setting your exercise goals. Unless your goal is athletic competition, you don't have to aim for superior physical fitness. Instead, your goal

Table 2-6
AEROBIC FITNESS TEST

Distance Covered	Fitness Level
More than $1^3/_4$ miles	Superior
$1^1/_2$–$1^3/_4$ miles	Excellent
$1^1/_4$–$1^1/_2$ miles	Very good
1–$1^1/_4$ miles	Good
$^3/_4$–1 mile	Fair
Less than $^3/_4$ mile	Poor

for optimal cardiac risk reduction and maximal longevity should be to exercise aerobically for 3 to 4 hours each week, burning 2,000–3,000 calories in the process. If you have low HDL cholesterol levels or excess body fat, you may want to push to higher levels. If you have other medical problems, you may have to settle for lower levels. If you have cardiovascular disease or even just major risk factors, you'll need medical clearance and supervision. Even without such problems, you'll have to go slowly, using the guidelines in Chapter 5 to construct a personal exercise program that is safe, effective, and enjoyable.

Diabetes
Diabetes is a major atherosclerosis risk factor. It's every bit as serious as the "big four" modifiable risk factors but is included with the "little three" just because it's numerically less prevalent in America than smoking, high cholesterol levels, hypertension, and sedentary living.

Numbers aside, you may be surprised to find diabetes listed as a modifiable risk factor. Indeed, it's true that diabetes can be inherited — but it's also true that in many cases diabetes can be prevented or controlled by exercise, diet, and weight reduction.

Fourteen million Americans have diabetes, but not all are equally vulnerable to complications. One million have the more serious Type I diabetes, which is characterized by its onset early in life, its requirement for daily insulin injections, and its very high risk for atherosclerosis, visual loss, and kidney disease. Type II diabetes is much more common and much less serious; occurring later in life, it is often linked to obesity, and it can often be treated with diet, weight loss, exercise, and — if needed — oral medications. Because Type II diabetes is so strongly linked to obesity, hypertension, high cholesterol levels, and sedentary living, its independent impact on cardiac risk is unclear. But the overall cardiac impact of diabetes is clear, and it's substantial: diabetics are 2 to 3 times more likely to die of heart attacks than nondiabetics. In all, diabetes accounts for 30,000 cardiac deaths in the United States each year.

Evaluating your blood sugar. Are you at increased risk of diabetes? Like gender or smoking, this risk factor would seem to have an all-or-nothing, yes-or-no answer. But a true picture of atherosclerosis risk cannot be painted in black and white; when it comes to diabetes, too, there are shades of gray.

Virtually all patients with Type I diabetes know they have it. They became ill rather abruptly, typically suffering weakness, weight loss, blurred vision, remarkable thirst and hunger, excessive urination, and dehydration. Without prompt diagnosis and insulin treatment there is a substantial risk of coma and death.

Type II diabetes is different. In a typical case, it develops very slowly, producing no symptoms at first, then gradually causing fatigue, blurred vision, increased thirst and hunger, increased urination, and dehydration.

It's no trick to diagnose Type II diabetes once symptoms have developed. But since diet and exercise can prevent these symptoms from developing, it would be nice to discover diabetes in an earlier, clinically silent stage.

The traditional screening test for diabetes is to check for sugar in the urine. Ancient Greek physicians did this simply by tasting urine; being less courageous and smarter, we now use a simple chemical test. Smarter or not, our urine tests are not accurate enough to diagnose diabetes — many patients with the disease test negative, and some people without diabetes have traces of sugar in their urine samples.

Blood tests are the best way to test for diabetes. A new test (the glycosylated hemoglobin) is being used to monitor blood sugar levels in diabetics, but it has not yet been standardized for diagnostic purposes. It's easy enough, however, to measure the blood sugar itself — the difficulty comes in interpreting the results.

To interpret your blood sugar levels, you'll need two additional facts. First, it is normal for blood sugar levels to rise after meals; the more carbohydrates in the meal, the higher the blood sugar level. In healthy

Table 2-7
INTERPRETING YOUR BLOOD SUGAR

Diagnosis	Fasting Blood Sugar	Blood Sugar within 30-90 Minutes after a Sugar-Rich Meal	Blood Sugar 2 Hours after Eating or Drinking Sugar
Healthy	Less than 115	Less than 200	Less than 140
Impaired glucose tolerance	115-140	Over 200	140-200
Diabetes	Over 140 (on more than one test)	Over 200	Over 200
Diabetes of pregnancy	Over 105	Over 190 (at 90 minutes)	Over 165 at 2 hours or over 145 at 3 hours

people, however, the blood sugar doesn't go as high, nor does it stay high for as long, as in diabetics. But even abnormally high blood sugars don't automatically imply diabetes; some people can have mild elevations ("impaired glucose tolerance") without having diabetes. Finally, pregnancy is a special case, with its own diagnostic standards.

With all this in mind, you can now use Table 2-7 to interpret your blood sugar levels.

How often should you have your blood sugar tested? Symptoms of diabetes, of course, call for prompt testing. All pregnant women should be tested between weeks 24 and 28. Other people do not need to schedule special tests; instead, the blood sugar can be monitored along with cholesterol levels at the time of ordinary checkups.

Obesity
A weighty subject in America, obesity has earned its place among cardiac risk factors only after years of study and debate. The delay will surprise anyone who has visited a coronary care unit: heart patients surely are more likely to be portly than svelte. But obesity is strongly linked to other cardiac risk factors, including high LDL and low HDL cholesterols, hypertension, diabetes, and sedentary living. At last, however, the sophisticated statistical technique of multivariate analysis has confirmed everyday common sense: obesity *is* an independent risk factor for coronary artery disease.

Obesity is so common that it may be hard to think of it as a medical disorder; more than one-third of all Americans have excess body fat, and 1 in 5 are more than 20 percent overweight, thus meeting the medical definition of obesity. Obesity has many effects on the mind and body; few are good. In terms of cardiac risk, a 10 percent gain in body fat increases the likelihood of heart attack by about 25 percent.

Obesity is very hard to control, but reducing body fat has important cardiac benefits; 35-year-olds who correct their obesity will gain about a year of life expectancy. But the benefits of weight reduction, like the benefits of all lifestyle changes, depend on keeping up (or in the case of weight, down) the good work. The Framingham Heart Study, which has taught us so much about heart disease, discovered that cyclical weight changes actually increase cardiac risk. Don't be a yo-yo; instead, try to keep your weight down.

Good fat, bad fat, worse fat. Whether your concerns are medical or aesthetic, the real problem in obesity is not high body weight, but excess body fat.

Like cholesterol, some body fat is essential for health. Fat is an important energy depot, storing calories and vitamins in time of plenty for use in time of need. Fat insulates the body, conserving heat. Body fat cushions and protects the internal organs, and fat cells are essential for the metabolism of sex hormones.

Like cholesterol, fat comes in two varieties. But while blood cholesterol can be good (HDL) or bad (LDL), excess body fat is either bad or worse.

Although all fat cells look the same under the microscope, they can behave quite differently. Fat cells around the abdomen and upper body have high levels of an enzyme called lipoprotein lipase; in everyday terms, this means they are geared up to store energy when the body has an excess of calories — when people gain weight, fat tends to accumulate first around the waist. In contrast, fat cells in the lower body enlarge more slowly—but when weight comes off, they are also a lot slower to shrink.

There are also other differences between upper and lower body fat cells. The former are more responsive to adrenaline, the stress hormone; the latter are more responsive to estrogen, the female hormone. Men tend to have more upper body fat (hence the "beer belly"), women more lower body fat (the "pear shape").

Abdominal fat is easier to gain but easier to lose, an aesthetic advantage, perhaps, for men (who find it easier to slim their waists) compared to women (who have more difficulty slimming down their buttocks and thighs). But in medical terms, the advantage goes to women, since abdominal obesity is a much stronger predictor of cardiac risk than is lower body fat.

Evaluating your body fat. Does your body weight increase your cardiac risk? The answer is not quite as obvious as you might think, since an accurate response depends on evaluating fat rather than weight and on determining the location of the excess fat cells in your body.

The simplest way to answer this question is to take the "mirror test" — just have a look. Easy or not, it's not an accurate method; body image is just too subjective to serve as your standard.

The traditional way to answer the question is to check yourself against the norms established by the Metropolitan Life Insurance Company. Height-weight tables are handy, and I've included one in Chapter 15 — but this method is not accurate enough for a question as important as cardiac risk.

The fanciest way to answer the question is to have your body fat measured. Health clubs often use calipers to measure skin fold thickness, a fairly accurate indication of fat. For greater precision visit your hospital — but bring your wallet as well as your waist; tests such as bioelectric impedance and magnetic resonance imaging are accurate but expensive.

The best way to answer the question is to take two simple self-assessment tests in the convenience (and privacy) of your home. You'll need a scale, a tape measure, and (if your math is anything like mine) a calculator.

Your *body mass index* provides an accurate reflection of your body fat. To calculate your index, just follow four steps: (1) Measure your height (without shoes) in inches and your weight (without clothing) in pounds. (2) Multiply your weight by 700. (3) Divide that number by your height. (4) Finally, divide again by your height. Or if you don't like arithmetic, you can approximate your BMI by looking it up in Table 15−2.

To interpret your body mass index, compare your result with standards developed by the Second National Health and Nutrition Examination Survey. (See Table 2−8.)

Table 2–8
INTERPRETING YOUR BODY MASS INDEX

	Body Mass Index	
	Women	Men
Average	23.1	24.3
Obese	Above 27.3	Above 27.8
Severely obese	Above 32.2	Above 31.1

Your body mass index will tell you if you have too much fat. To find out if it's in the wrong place, medically speaking, just determine your waist-to-hip ratio:

1. With your abdomen relaxed, measure your waist at its narrowest (usually at the navel).
2. Measure your hips at their widest (usually at the bony prominence).
3. Divide

$$\frac{\text{waist size (in inches)}}{\text{hip size (in inches)}}$$

How does your ratio translate into cardiac risk? The risk of heart attack and stroke is increased in women with ratios above 0.8 and in men with ratios above 1.0. And the risk is substantial. For example, men with ratios above 1.0 have twice the death rate of men with ratios below 0.85; women who add 6 inches to 40-inch hips increase their death rate by 60 percent.

Can you be too thin? Not for your heart. In fact, the risk of dying from heart disease is lowest with BMIs as low as 18 to 19. But like the low cholesterol and low blood pressure stories, there's more to the reply than a simple no.

Experienced orthopedists insist that you can't be too thin for your back. The Duchess of Windsor proclaimed that you can't be too thin or too rich. The diet industry seems to agree, often achieving the latter at the expense of the former. But the mortality data tell a different story: as expected, the death rate increases with increasing body weight, but mortality also rises at the other end of the spectrum, as body weight declines below average.

You don't have to be a cardiologist, much less a statistician, to sort this one out. In all probability, being thin does not *cause* death rates to increase. Instead, people with cancer, liver disease, digestive diseases, and other chronic conditions tend to lose weight — they become thin because they are sick, not the other way around. The same is true for tobacco abuse, since smokers tend to be thin and they certainly have increased death rates. Simply excluding smokers from the analysis makes the relationship between body fat and mortality crystal clear: thinner people live longer (see Figure 15–1).

Even if being thin doesn't harm the heart, extreme weight loss can have adverse consequences. Very thin people tend to feel cold, and they may have fewer reserves to call on when energy is needed for prolonged effort. More important, women with very little body fat have low estrogen levels; as a result, they lose their menstrual periods and are prone to osteoporosis (thin bones) and fractures. Most important, drastic weight loss using extreme caloric restriction and liquid-protein diets *can* harm the heart, causing arrhythmias that may be fatal. BMIs below 18.5 reflect protein-energy malnutrition.

Setting your goals for body weight. From a medical point of view it's a simple task: reduce your body mass index and waist-to-hip ratio to healthful, low-risk levels. But from your individual point of view, nothing is more personal than your body image, and few things are more difficult than achieving sustained weight loss.

Difficult or not, you can lose weight. If your medical needs include weight loss or if your personal goals include slimming down, use Chapter 15 to construct a sensible, balanced program for gradual, sustained weight loss. But keep things in perspective. If you have other cardiac risk factors, particularly diabetes, hypertension, or unfavorable cholesterol levels, your weight is especially important to your health. But even with these problems, weight is only one element in the cardiac risk equation. Weight loss should be one goal among many, a sensible part of a comprehensive, multifaceted plan to take care of your heart and your health.

Psychological Factors
As a firm believer in the unity of mind and body, I'm quick to point out that your mental state can affect your cardiac risk. Unfortunately, the results are not always heartwarming.

Mental factors are the last of the 10 major cardiac risk factors. Psychological factors probably deserve tenth place on the list, but it's hard to be sure, since they are difficult to measure and quantify with statistical precision. Perhaps because of these methodological difficulties, the importance of stress is hotly debated by cardiologists and psychologists. Although the details do require further study, the main point is clear: psychosocial factors can increase cardiac risk.

Heartfelt emotions. Even authorities who agree that psychological factors contribute to cardiac risk don't always agree about which factors matter most.

It's easy to see that psychological factors produce important short-term effects on cardiovascular function. Stress, anger, and hostility are the most potent. They provoke a surge of adrenaline and other stress hormones; the result is a dramatic rise in blood pressure and pulse. Patterns of blood flow and certain blood clotting factors also change for the worse, as do blood sugar levels. Contrary to popular belief, however, stress does not appear to have an adverse impact on blood cholesterol levels.

There is debate about the psychological profile that adds most to cardiac risk. The pioneering 1959 studies of Drs. Meyer Friedman and Ray Rosenman implicated the Type A personality, characterized by ambition, drive, impatience, perfectionism, and a short temper. More recent studies have emphasized the importance of free-floating, or undirected, hostility. And the newest research asserts that the lonely heart is the most vulnerable, that depression, isolation, and the lack of a social support network increase the risk of recurrent heart attacks.

More research will be needed to sort this out. For now, however, two things seem clear: first, there is no single "coronary prone personality"; second, psychological factors are important to your heart, to say nothing of your overall health and happiness.

Evaluating your emotions as risk factors. It's not as precise as having your cholesterol measured or as easy as having your blood pressure checked. It may take longer than a 12-minute fitness test and be even more painful than calculating your waist-to-hip ratio. Inexact and difficult to be sure — but it's still worth a try. Use Table 2−9 to ask yourself a few questions that may help evaluate your emotional state. Even bet-

Table 2-9
EMOTIONAL SELF-ASSESSMENT TEST

	Column A: Rarely or Never	Column B: Sometimes	Column C: Often or Always
1. I drive in the left lane.			
2. I prefer to be alone.			
3. I feel pessimistic or sad.			
4. I get angry or tense when even little things go wrong.			
5. I keep my watch set ahead.			
6. I like to plan out all my time as far ahead as possible.			
7. I feel my heart pounding or my breathing speeding up without exercise.			
8. I sleep poorly and feel tired in the morning.			
9. I blame myself when things go wrong.			
10. I prefer to keep worries to myself.			
11. I honk my horn in traffic jams.			
12. I dread weekends and vacations.			
13. I feel guilty.			
14. I wake up before I have to, even on weekends.			
15. I dwell on details.			
16. I eat more quickly than other people.			
17. I worry about my heart.			
18. I do two things at one time.			
19. I frown, grimace, or clench my teeth.			
20. My speech is louder or faster than other people's.			
21. I arrive at meetings early or "on the dot."			
22. I keep an eye on people to make sure they're doing the right thing.			
23. People tell me to slow down or take it easy.			
24. I sigh more often than other people.			
25. I shout or use expletives when I'm frustrated.			

ter, review your answers with your spouse, a close relative, or a dear friend to make sure they're objective. Think about each question carefully, then put a check mark in the column that fits you best; it's important to answer each question, even if you are not sure of the answer.

Add up the check marks in each column. Give yourself one point for each mark in column A, two for each in column B, and three for column C. Add up your total score. A grand total below 35 suggests low cardiac risk from personality factors, a score between 36 and 50 suggests a moderate role for emotions, and a score above 50 suggests the possibility that psychological factors might increase your cardiac risk.

Setting your goals for hearty emotions. It can be every bit as hard to set goals for your emotions as it is to evaluate your personality. But stress control should be part of your 15-point program to fight atherosclerosis; Chapter 14 offers some help. Above all, get control of *all* your risk factors; as your body improves, your self-confidence will rise and your spirits will soar. Because your mind and body are inseparable, your physical and mental goals are congruent: health and happiness.

Risk or Rumor: Other Factors Possibly Associated with Coronary Artery Disease

Ten risk factors may be enough for your mind — and they are surely more than enough for your heart. But tens of other factors have been investigated over the years. Most have been rejected as erroneous or unimportant, but a few persist as possible predictors of cardiac risk.

Some of these putative risk factors are little more than statistical curiosities. Studies tell us, for example, that people with deep horizontal earlobe creases, frequent dental infections, or male pattern baldness are more likely to have heart attacks. But the increased risk is small, and the biological significance of such factors borders on the trivial.

Some risk factors have short-lived notoriety. Elevated iron levels caused great alarm in 1992, only to be downgraded by studies in 1993 and 1994. Still worrisome but poorly understood is a 1993 report that links infections by a respiratory bacterium, *Chlamydia pneumoniae,* to an increased rate of heart attacks years later.

Metabolism may be even more important. Gout, for example, may be a marker for increased cardiac risk. People who eat more animal protein have a greater risk of heart disease than people who eat vegetable protein, even taking their differences in dietary fat into account. People with tissue resistance to insulin are unusually prone to heart attacks, even if they don't have clinical diabetes; still a bit mysterious, this disorder has earned the appropriate name "Syndrome X." Similarly, people with high levels of the blood clotting protein fibrinogen have a higher-than-usual rate of heart attacks, even if they have normal platelet counts and clotting functions; if additional research confirms this observation, fibrinogen may join the list of modifiable risk factors, since exercise (Chapter 5) and weight loss (Chapter 15) reduce blood fibrinogen levels. Finally, people with high blood levels of the amino acid homocysteine have an increased risk of atherosclerosis; the mechanism behind the link is not understood, but new studies suggest that it can be corrected by vitamin supplements. (See Chapter 17.)

These metabolic abnormalities may provide additional clues to the causes of atherosclerosis. All deserve further study, but none is well enough documented to earn a place on your already formidable worry list. Stay tuned — as long as we allow heart disease to ravage American society, we'll need scientists to figure out just how we're doing ourselves in.

Your Diet and Your Heart

Diet has a major role in atherosclerosis. Poor nutrition, however, is not an independent cardiac risk factor. That's because bad eating habits contribute to obesity, high blood pressure, diabetes, and high cholesterol levels, and these major risk factors are traditionally monitored in place of diet itself.

Still, poor dietary habits add to risk factors and promote cardiovascular disease. Good nutrition, on the other hand, is central to the fight against atherosclerosis. Nutrition is so important, in fact, that it contributes to 10 of 15 ways to fight atherosclerosis that you'll find in Part II. Before constructing your program, spend a few minutes answering the questions in Table 2–10 to evaluate your current diet.

Circle the answer that applies to you best, and add up your points. Interpreting your diet score is easy: the higher your score, the more you need to change, particularly if you have other cardiac risk factors. But don't try to go from a score of 132 to 33 all at once — instead, make changes slowly and thoughtfully, so they'll stick. Part II will help you

Table 2–10
DIETARY SELF-ASSESSMENT

	Rarely or Never	Sometimes	Often	Very Often
1. I use 1% or skim milk.	4	3	2	1
2. I eat more than 8 oz. of red meat in an average week.	1	2	3	4
3. I eat whole grain rather than white bread.	4	3	2	1
4. I eat hot dogs, bacon, or luncheon meats more than once a month.	1	2	3	4
5. I eat fish at least twice a week.	4	3	2	1
6. I eat fried foods.	1	2	3	4
7. I eat beans or other legumes at least three times a week.	4	3	2	1
8. Given a choice, I select muffins over doughnuts.	4	3	2	1
9. I remove the skin from poultry.	4	3	2	1
10. I eat bran cereals for breakfast.	4	3	2	1
11. I snack on chips, crackers, or pretzels.	1	2	3	4
12. I use margarine or butter on bread.	1	2	3	4
13. I eat at least 2 portions of fruit in an average day.	4	3	2	1
14. I cook with olive oil or canola oil.	4	3	2	1
15. I use nonfat salad dressings or mayonnaise.	4	3	2	1
16. I eat 3 portions of vegetables in an average day.	4	3	2	1
17. I snack on fruit or vegetables.	4	3	2	1
18. I eat canned soups.	1	2	3	4
19. I add salt to my food.	1	2	3	4
20. I eat dinners without meat or poultry three or more times in an average week.	4	3	2	1

continued

Table 2–10 *continued*

	Rarely or Never	Sometimes	Often	Very Often
21. Given a choice, I choose bagels or toast over muffins.	4	3	2	1
22. I eat ice cream.	1	2	3	4
23. I choose fruit rather than pastry or cake for dessert.	4	3	2	1
24. I add nuts or seeds to my salads, baked goods, or other foods.	4	3	2	1
25. I eat cheese or pizza.	1	2	3	4
26. I generally order fish in restaurants.	4	3	2	1
27. I generally order salads in restaurants.	4	3	2	1
28. I eat at a fast-food restaurant at least once in an average week.	1	2	3	4
29. When I snack on popcorn, I eat it without salt, butter, or margarine.	4	3	2	1
30. I eat four or more egg yolks in an average week.	1	2	3	4
31. I eat deep green or yellow-orange vegetables at least once in an average day.	4	3	2	1
32. I eat chocolate.	1	2	3	4
33. I eat citrus fruits or drink juice at least once in an average day.	4	3	2	1

construct a good nutrition program to protect your heart and enhance your health. Try it — you really will like it.

Your Heart Attack Risk Profile

It may have surprised you to learn that so many things can jeopardize your coronary arteries. The reason, of course, is that atherosclerosis is a multisystem metabolic disease involving blood cholesterol, arterial walls, and the clotting system, each of which is complex, delicate, and easily deranged — so easily deranged, in fact, that a 1994 study revealed that 4 of every 5 Americans have at least one major modifiable risk factor.

Not all risk factors are equally dangerous, and not all are present at once. How can you evaluate your overall risk in the face of competing influences? Is a 37-year-old woman with a blood pressure of 104/68 but a cholesterol ratio of 5.8 at high risk? Is a 59-year-old man protected by a cholesterol ratio of 4 despite smoking 10 cigarettes per day? There are no sure answers — but you can get a picture of your overall risk from the test in Table 2–11.

To interpret your result, total up your point score from Table 2–11. A score below 25 suggests a very low overall risk for heart attack; 26–50 suggests low risk; 51–75 suggests moderate risk; 76–100 suggests high risk; above 100 suggests very high risk.

Interpreting your risk profile. Your risk profile gives you an index of your vulnerability to atherosclerosis, but you should interpret it with care. A high score doesn't mean that you are doomed to suffer a heart attack or stroke, nor does a low score mean that you are immune to atherosclerosis. You should also know that this risk profile test does not have the statistical predicting power of its more precise components. Finally, remember that individual risk scores should not be compared arithmetically; a score of 100 certainly places you at higher risk than someone with a score of 50, but your risk is not necessarily twice as high. Above all, understand the central message of a high score: it's an invitation to do more to conquer heart disease.

Setting your lifestyle goals. So many risks, so many worries. It's true that there is a lot to think about. But each risk factor in your profile represents an opportunity for improvement. Think of each as a challenge. You can lower your risk — in the process you'll protect yourself against atherosclerosis, you'll enhance your overall health, *and* you'll enjoy life more.

Although change appears daunting, it's really much easier than it seems — if you go about it in the right way. And the right way includes consideration of your personal preferences and pleasures as well as your

Table 2–11
YOUR CARDIAC RISK PROFILE

Category	Score	
	Add	Subtract
Age		
Men 45–54	1	0
55–65	2	0
over 65	3	0
Women 55–65	1	0
over 65	2	0
Gender		
Male	3	0
Female	0	0
premenopausal or using estrogen replacement	0	2
Family history		
Parents or siblings with heart attacks		
1 or 2	2	0
more than 2	4	0
attacks before age 50	4	0
Smoking		
Smoking by a household member	3	0
Personal cigarette use		
none for 10 or more years	0	0
quit within 10 years	3	0
5–10 cigarettes/day	6	0
10–20 cigarettes/day	12	0
21–40 cigarettes/day	15	0
more than 40 cigarettes/day	20	0
Cholesterol ratio (see Table 2–3)		
Lower than 2.0	0	6
2.0 to 2.9	0	3
3.0 to 3.9	0	0
4.0 to 4.9	3	0
5.0 to 5.9	10	0
6.0 to 6.9	12	0
7.0 or higher	20	0
Blood pressure (see Table 2–4)		
Optimal	0	6
Normal	0	0
High normal	3	0
Stage 1	6	0
Stage 2	12	0
Stage 3	18	0
Stage 4	20	0

continued

Table 2–11 *continued*

Category	Score	
	Add	Subtract
Aerobic exercise level (see Table 2–5 & 2–6)		
4 or more hours per week	0	5
3 to 4 hours per week	0	0
2 to 3 hours per week	3	0
1 to 2 hours per week	8	0
30 minutes to 1 hour per week	12	0
Less than 30 minutes per week	18	0
Diabetes (see Table 2–6)		
Type I diabetes	20	0
Type II diabetes	10	0
Body weight		
Body Mass Index (see Table 2–7)		
Below 23	0	3
23.1–24.9	3	0
25.0–28.9	6	0
Above 29	10	0
Waist-to-hip ratio (see page 57)		
Men above 1.0	5	0
Women above 0.8	5	0
Up-and-down weight fluctuation of 10 pounds in 1 year	3	0
Psychosocial profile (see Table 2–9)		
Low stress	0	0
Moderate stress	3	0
High stress	6	0

cardiac risk factors and medical needs. Lifestyle change will help you live longer, not just feel like you're living longer. On the contrary, you'll *enjoy* your extra months and years.

Although certain basic principles should be incorporated into everyone's fight against atherosclerosis, each person should construct a personal program tailored to individual needs and priorities. Part II will help you do just that. Now that you understand where you're starting from, you can learn what each of the 15 points can do for you. You'll also learn the possible drawbacks of each, enabling you to construct your own risk-benefit appraisal. The decisions will be up to you. I may not eat eggs, but if you are one of the few who really cannot enjoy your

Table 2–12
15 WAYS TO REDUCE 7 RISK FACTORS

Smoking	Smoking cessation
High LDL/low HDL cholesterol	Low dietary fat and cholesterol
	Exercise
	High dietary fiber
	Niacin
	Alcohol
	Postmenopausal estrogen replacement
	Chromium
	Weight control
	Other nutritional supplements
Hypertension	Smoking cessation
	Exercise
	Low dietary sodium
	High dietary potassium and calcium
	Stress control
	Weight control
	Eating fish?
	Antioxidant vitamins?
Lack of exercise	Exercise
Diabetes	Diet
	Exercise
	High dietary fiber
	Weight control
Obesity	Low dietary fat
	Exercise
	High dietary fiber
Psychological factors	Behavior modification
	Behavior modification and stress control
	Exercise

day without them, then they're a risk you should take. The choice is yours — but it will be an informed choice.

It's time to get started. To preview how each of the 15 points can improve the 7 modifiable risk factors, have a look at Table 2–12; then start putting theory into practice with Chapter 3.

PART II

Fifteen Ways to Conquer Heart Disease

Chapter 3

Smoking: Cardiac Enemy Number One

As A WRITER, I crave readers. But as a doctor, I hope this chapter is largely unread: if you don't smoke — and if you understand why tobacco smoke is our nation's leading heart hazard — you can skip to Chapter 4. But if you are at all tempted by smoking, if you live with a smoker, or if you want to help free our society from its leading cause of preventable death, read on.

How Smoking Affects the Heart

Heartburn, indeed.

Smoke a cigarette, just one. Better yet, don't smoke it, but take my word for what would happen if you did. Your heart rate would increase and your blood pressure would rise. As a result, your heart would be working harder, but just when it needs more oxygen, that single cigarette could narrow your coronary arteries by up to 35 percent, and the narrowing might last for as long as 30 minutes. Smoke a few more cigarettes and your blood carbon monoxide level would rise, reducing your blood's oxygen-carrying capacity. If you were a heart patient, just a few cigarettes could trigger serious arrhythmias, angina, or even a heart attack. And if you really were a smoker, the effects of each cigarette would be far from hypothetical; the Centers for Disease Control calculates that each cigarette shortens the life of a smoker by 7 minutes.

Healthy people can, of course, survive a cigarette or two. But repeated tobacco abuse causes cumulative damage. Smoking lowers the HDL cholesterol. It damages the walls of arteries. And smoking increases the stickiness of platelets, activating the blood clotting mechanism. Damage to blood cholesterol components, blood vessel walls, and the clotting system is a powerful formula for atherosclerosis — and that's exactly why smoking is the most potent coronary artery disease risk factor, increasing the chance of suffering a heart attack by 250 percent. Toxic to the heart on its own, tobacco smoke also acts synergistically with other cardiac risk factors, so it's extra dangerous for people with diabetes, high blood pressure, and high cholesterol levels.

Smoking and Cardiovascular Disease

Tobacco abuse causes one of every 3 nonfatal heart attacks in the United States. Cigarette smoking also accounts for 20 percent of all cardiac deaths; that means 115,000 Americans die every year from heart disease caused by smoking. These deaths are all the more tragic because they are completely unnecessary.

Atherosclerosis is not confined to the coronary arteries, and the vascular damage caused by smoking is not confined to the heart. Smoking damages the body's largest artery, the aorta, weakening its walls. The result can be a bulge, or aneurysm, which can rupture without warning, almost always with lethal consequences. Smoking damages the arteries that carry blood to the legs, often leading to cramps that make walking difficult or impossible; in advanced cases, atherosclerosis of these arteries leads to gangrene. Smoking also damages the carotid arteries, which carry blood to the head, and the arteries of the brain itself; the results are predictable and predictably terrible: strokes and brain hemorrhages.

Every year smoking causes more than 200,000 American deaths from cardiovascular disease alone.

Smoking and Health

Smoking would be a tragedy even if its impact were confined to the cardiovascular system. Since it's not, smoking is a disaster.

Smoking accounts for *1 of every 6 deaths in the United States*; that's

435,000 a year, or more than 1,100 per day. Nor are we alone. In fact, 20 percent of *all* deaths in developed countries are caused by tobacco abuse; in the industrialized world, *a quarter of a billion people* who are alive today will eventually die because they smoke. Smoking is considerably less prevalent in developing countries, but as "advanced" societies continue to export their tobacco products, the third world will catch up, eventually sharing the full impact of the global smoking epidemic.

Why does smoking cause so many diverse diseases? Tobacco smoke contains more than 4,700 chemicals, at least 43 of which are proven causes of cancer. These chemicals are rapidly absorbed by the lungs and are then carried in the blood throughout the entire body. The tissue damage caused by this internal pollution is slow but sure; Table 3–1 lists the many organ systems damaged by tobacco smoke.

It takes many chemicals to produce so many diseases, but among the thousands of toxins in tobacco smoke, one stands out: nicotine. What is nicotine doing in tobacco leaves in the first place? It's an insecticide, protecting tobacco plants from insects. Poisoning insects is one thing, poisoning people quite another — why can't modern manufacturing techniques remove the nicotine from tobacco? They can — in fact, they do. The process that transforms tobacco plants into cigarettes actually removes most of the nicotine — but the cigarette makers spray nicotine back into their product. FDA commissioner David Kessler believes that this is done to enhance the addictive properties of cigarettes, and I agree. Let's hope that Dr. Kessler succeeds in his 1994 initiative to classify the nicotine in cigarettes as an additive that can be regulated as a dangerous drug.

Passive Smoking

Smoking is responsible for nearly one death a second in the United States alone. Although it's small consolation at best, people who kill themselves by smoking have only themselves to blame. But for every *8 smokers* who are killed by their habit, *one nonsmoker* will die from effects of environmental tobacco smoke. If smoking is suicide, it's also murder.

After reviewing many careful scientific studies, the Environmental Protection Agency has determined that environmental tobacco smoke, or passive smoking, is a carcinogen, accounting for more than 3,000

Table 3–1
HEALTH CONSEQUENCES OF SMOKING

Heart	Coronary artery disease
	Angina
	Heart attacks
	Sudden cardiac deaths
	Arrhythmias (irregular heart beats)
Circulation	Hypertension
	Blockages of arteries
	Aneurysms of the aorta
	Thrombophlebitis (blood clots in veins) in women taking oral contraceptives
Central Nervous System	Strokes
	Brain hemorrhages
Lungs	Lung cancer
	Mesotheliomas (cancers of the lung lining) in conjunction with asbestos exposure
	Bronchitis
	Emphysema
	Pneumonia
	Asthma
Head and Neck	Cancers of the mouth, tongue, and larynx (voice box)
	Allergies
	Sinusitis
	Periodontal disease
	Tooth loss
Digestive Tract	Cancers of the esophagus, stomach, colon, and pancreas
	Gastritis
	Ulcers
Urinary Tract	Cancers of the kidneys and bladder
Male Reproductive System	Impotence
	Cancer of the prostate gland
Female Reproductive System	Cancer of the cervix
	Tubal pregnancies
	Miscarriages
	Premature deliveries
	Low-birthweight babies
	Fetal abnormalities
	Sudden infant death syndrome
Skeletal System	Osteoporosis
	Fractures
Skin	Premature wrinkling

continued

Table 3–1 *continued*	
Psychiatric	Addiction
	Depression
Trauma	Burns and smoke inhalation
Blood	Decreased oxygen-carrying capacity
	Increased white and red blood cell counts
	Leukemia
	Multiple myeloma
Metabolism	Decreased HDL cholesterol
	Increased waist-to-hip ratio (truncal obesity)
	Altered metabolism of various medications

deaths from lung cancer in the United States each year. The 1993 EPA decision produced a flurry of well-deserved concern, along with predictable lawsuits by the tobacco industry. Surprisingly enough, there has been much less publicity about the impact of passive smoking on heart disease; in fact, passive smoking kills 10 times more people from heart attacks than lung cancer. Every year nearly 40,000 Americans die of heart disease because they are the passive victims of someone else's smoking.

Environmental tobacco smoke is actually even dirtier than smoke inhaled. That's because only 15 percent of environmental smoke comes from exhaled mainstream smoke; the other 85 percent is sidestream smoke that is emitted directly from the burning end of the cigarette without passing through the cigarette or the filter. Sidestream smoke contains three times more benzopyrene, five times more carbon monoxide, and fifty times more ammonia than does mainstream smoke. That's dirty indeed.

Tobacco smoke is the most dangerous form of indoor air pollution. And if heart attacks and lung cancer are not bad enough, passive smoking also increases the incidence of childhood brain cancer, bronchitis, nasal irritation, and other ailments. According to the 1994 report of the American Heart Association, smoking by mothers is responsible for 26,000 new cases of asthma in American children each year. Nonsmoking women who are exposed to environmental tobacco smoke have an increased risk of fetal loss. The children of smokers have reduced scores on intelligence tests; even worse, they have more leukemias and lympho-mas than the children of nonsmokers.

Many of the 4,700 chemicals in tobacco smoke are capable of dam-aging blood vessels and accelerating cardiac risk factors. All of the car-diotoxic chemicals found in the blood of smokers can also be found in the blood of passive smokers. Passive smoke exposure raises the heart rate and blood pressure. Passive smokers have higher carbon monoxide levels and lower oxygen levels. Exposure to environmental tobacco smoke reduces HDL (good) cholesterol; just 20 minutes in a smoke-filled room is enough to increase platelet stickiness. With all those insults, it's no surprise that passive smoking produces injury: exposure to environ-mental tobacco smoke will lower the lung capacity and decrease the exercise tolerance of healthy people, and it can trigger arrhythmias, an-gina, and silent ischemia in heart patients.

People who live with smokers suffer the most damage from passive smoking; simply sharing living quarters with a smoker increases the risk of heart attack by 30 percent. People who work in smoke-filled rooms are also vulnerable; that's why nonsmoking waiters are one and a half times more likely to develop lung cancer than other nonsmokers. But environmental tobacco smoke is shockingly ubiquitous, and no Ameri-can is immune to its effects. In 1993, the EPA used a sensitive blood test to survey 800 Americans older than 4; traces of cotinine, a sure sign of nicotine exposure, were found in *100 percent* of the subjects.

Smoking is the leading cause of preventable death in the United States. *Passive* smoking is our third leading preventable killer, ranking just behind alcohol abuse.

There ought to be a law. Fortunately in many communities, there is.

The Costs of Smoking

Smoking costs lives. On average, smokers die 6 years younger than nonsmokers.

Smoking costs health. Smokers experience much more illness, dis-ability, and suffering than nonsmokers. The leading cause of social se-curity compensated disability is coronary artery disease, 30 percent of which is smoking-related. Emphysema is the second leading cause of disability. Ten million Americans have this slowly progressive chronic lung disease, and 1 million new cases are diagnosed each year; more than 90 percent of emphysema patients owe their daily respiratory distress to smoking.

Smoking also costs money. The amount is staggering. Each smoker can expect to run up a lifetime total of more than $20,000 in medical bills and lost wages. Every year smoking drains more than $200 billion from the American economy; it's a hidden tax that forces each nonsmoker to pay $220 a year to support tobacco abuse in America.

Because the numbers are so very large, the costs of smoking often seem abstract, unreal, or even surreal. A group of five epidemiologists and statisticians headed by Willard Manning have helped clarify the impact of smoking by calculating its costs on a daily basis. Their fascinating book, *The Costs of Poor Health Habits,* shows that each pack of cigarettes will cost the average smoker *137 minutes of life expectancy* and $1.10 in medical expense and lost productivity. Since the economic impact of smoking is distributed throughout society, each pack of cigarettes will cost nonsmokers $.18. Eighteen cents may not seem like much, but smokers don't stop with one pack; over the years each person who smokes will cost the nonsmoking public $1,185.00. Keep that in mind when you vote on tobacco taxes!

Is Safer Smoking Possible?

No.

You can't have your health and smoke too. The low-tar, low-nicotine cigarette is a boon to the tobacco industry but not to health. Quite the reverse; it's a medical bane because it lulls smokers into a false sense of security. People who smoke "low-yield" cigarettes light up more, puff more, and inhale more to satisfy the nicotine craving. After reviewing all the evidence, the British Health Education Council put it best: switching to so-called low-yield cigarettes is "like jumping from the 36th floor instead of the 39th." Suicide is suicide.

Is cutting down on the number of cigarettes helpful? Perhaps. It is true that the hazards of smoking are dose-dependent; the more you smoke, the more you'll damage your heart and blood vessels, to say nothing of your lungs and the rest of your body. Theoretically, the converse should also be true — smoking less should be less dangerous. The theory is sound, but the practice is dubious because nicotine is highly addictive; as a result, smokers who cut down on cigarettes usually creep up again, gradually returning to their habitual nicotine dose. Remember, too, that even low doses of this powerful toxin are harmful; women who smoke as few as 4 cigarettes a day will double their lifetime heart attack risk.

The only safe cigarette is the one that's unsmoked.

The Other Forms of Tobacco Abuse

The cigarette is a relative newcomer. Tobacco was cultivated first in the New World about 5,000 years ago. In the age of exploration it became one of the first American exports; tragically enough, it has remained one of our most successful exports. But for centuries tobacco was used mostly in snuff and pipes; hand-rolled cigars and cigarettes followed, but the "brown plague" of the tobacco epidemic didn't really get rolling until the early twentieth century, when mass-production techniques were developed. It's no coincidence that heart attacks and lung cancers, both of which were very rare in nineteenth-century America, began to increase dramatically soon thereafter.

In many respects, fighting atherosclerosis amounts to turning back the clock by adopting elements of an older lifestyle and adapting them to the contemporary world. Is it wise to return to the older forms of tobacco usage?

Every rule has its exceptions; when it comes to health, the original forms of tobacco are an exception to the rule that basic is better. Pipes and cigars are less likely to cause lung cancer and heart disease than cigarettes, but they are clearly a major cause of oral cancers. Particularly worrisome is the trend of young people using old-fashioned snuff and chewing tobacco. Smokeless tobacco was nearly snuffed out by the anti-spitting campaigns of the early twentieth century, but it's making a comeback. Twelve million American men now use snuff or chewing tobacco; alarmingly, 25 percent are teenagers. Boys are probably enticed to use smokeless tobacco by the example of professional baseball players, but they won't reap a reward of fame and fortune. Instead, they'll suffer a 50-fold increase in oral cancer, gingivitis, periodontal disease, and tooth loss. Most users also become addicted, since smokeless tobacco users have blood nicotine levels that are every bit as high as cigarette smokers'. And a 1994 study found that using smokeless tobacco increases the risk of heart attacks nearly as much as cigarette smoking.

The only safe tobacco leaf is the one that's unharvested.

The Benefits of Smoking Cessation

Some good news, at last: quitting helps. The earlier you quit, the better — but it's never too late to benefit from smoking cessation. And the benefits are substantial.

Your body will begin to improve as soon as you stop smoking. Your blood nicotine levels will begin to fall right after your last puff. Within minutes, your heart rate and blood pressure will return to normal. Within hours your blood carbon monoxide levels will fall and your blood oxygen levels will rise. Within days, your lung capacity will begin to improve; as time goes on, your lung function numbers will actually look younger and younger.

The cardiac risks that smokers accumulate over the years are slower to improve, but improve they will. In just 1 year, people who quit smoking will cut their excess heart attack risk in half; in 15 years, their risk will be no higher than it is for people who have never smoked.

The other vascular toxicities of tobacco abuse are also quick to diminish. For example, current smokers are twice as likely to die from strokes than nonsmokers; within 5 years of quitting, the risk for former smokers is no higher than for people who have never smoked.

Cancer risk, too, improves with quitting. Men who smoke are 22 times more likely to die from lung cancer than nonsmokers; within 10 years of quitting, however, their risk falls by nearly 70 percent. In just 5 years, quitting will cut the risk of oral cancer in half; the incidence of cancers of the throat and esophagus declines at a similar rate. Cancers of the bladder and cervix also begin to diminish within just a few years of quitting.

Pregnant women who quit smoking will have healthier babies even if — heaven forbid — they delay quitting until the second trimester. People who quit smoking raise less phlegm and get less pneumonia and influenza. Their stomach ulcers heal faster. They have more energy and "wind." They discover the real taste of food. They even smell better to the nonsmokers of the world.

Smoking cessation is lifesaving. On average, tobacco abuse robs each smoker of 6 years of life. People who quit by age 45 recover 5 of those 6 years; even at age 65, quitting will extend life expectancy by more than 3 years.

The best time to quit smoking is now; the only better time was yesterday.

Smoking Cessation and the Treatment of Atherosclerosis

The ultimate test of any technique used to conquer heart disease is its ability to treat patients who already have the disease. It's a test that we'll apply to other aspects of the 15-point program in the chapters ahead. How does smoking cessation meet this test?

Very well. Even patients who have *already had heart attacks* benefit greatly from smoking cessation, reducing their risk of suffering another attack by more than 50 percent compared with heart attack survivors who continue to smoke.

It is, of course, best to stop smoking before you have a heart attack. Even after an attack, however, smoking cessation is a vital part of a comprehensive program to fight atherosclerosis.

Techniques of Smoking Cessation

Smokers should quit early; unfortunately they may have to quit often to get the job done once and for all.

Smoking cessation is difficult because nicotine is highly addicting. Animal studies, in fact, show that it's more addicting than cocaine and even heroin. The average smoker gets more than 50,000 nicotine "hits" in just a year.

Nicotine, which is found only in tobacco, is a potent stimulant. It's rapidly absorbed from smoke, reaching the brain in less than 6 seconds, twice as rapidly as mainlined heroin. Faster than heroin, nicotine is also as toxic as cyanide; as little as 60 milligrams will produce lethal respiratory paralysis if given in a single dose.

Because nicotine is addicting, it's hard to quit smoking. Because nicotine is poisonous, it's essential to quit. Because help is available, it's possible to quit.

More than 44 million Americans, in fact, have quit smoking. At the time of the first Surgeon General's report on smoking and health in 1964, more than 42 percent of American adults were smokers; now, only 25 percent smoke. That's impressive progress, but it's not enough. For the first time in a decade the percentage of smokers did not fall in 1991. Forty-six million Americans still smoke, and they are being joined by new teenage smokers at the rate of 1 million per year; each day, 5,000 American children light up for the first time.

As with so many battles in the war against atherosclerosis, the best way to quit smoking is without prescriptions. Try quitting on your own. If it's difficult, turn to support groups or hypnosis. If these fail, turn to your doctor for prescriptions that can help.

About 90 percent of successful quitters have used self-help strategies, most by adopting the "cold turkey" approach of quitting abruptly. Here are a few tips:

- Make a list of the health hazards and personal disadvantages that frighten you most.
- Make a list of the benefits of quitting.
- Make a list of people you know who have kicked the habit. You'll see that they are not any smarter or stronger than you are. If you don't know any successful quitters, feel free to list my name.
- Keep your lists handy and refer to them often to bolster your resolve.
- Pick a quitting date and stick to it. Birthdays and other special occasions are good choices. Another good day: The American Cancer Society's Great American Smoke Out in November. Holidays, though, can be tricky if they're accompanied by smoke-filled parties.
- Try to get other smokers in your household to join you in quitting. If smoking is still allowed in your workplace, try to recruit colleagues who smoke as well. Sign a mutual quitting contract; incidentally, a written pledge makes a great gift for loved ones who don't smoke.
- Commit yourself to your quit date: throw out your ashtrays, clean your house and car, clean your clothes, and clean your teeth.
- Plan ahead. To minimize weight gain (which only averages 5 pounds, in any case) start an exercise and nutrition program before you quit. Stock up on healthful, low-calorie snack foods; sugarless gum and candy can also help keep your nonsmoking mouth occupied.
- Keep your nonsmoking hands busy as well. Consider knitting or carving, doodling, or using worry beads.
- Reward yourself. Put all the money you *don't* spend on cigarettes into a special account, and use it for a special treat.

- Avoid high-risk situations like cocktail parties or stressful encounters until you are secure in your success.
- Find other ways to relieve tension; aerobic exercise, meditation, and deep-breathing exercises can all help.
- Think positively — you *can* quit. If you start to falter, read over your lists of smoking's hazards, quitting's benefits, and successful quitters.
- Above all, take one day at a time. Every cigarette that you don't smoke is another step forward. Don't delude yourself into thinking that you can smoke "just one." Because nicotine is so addictive, just one puff can sabotage your success, even after months or years.
- If you don't succeed in your first try, quit, quit again. You'll be in good company — most people who kick the smoking habit have logged several failures before their final success.

If you can't quit on your own, try again — and again. But if you really can't quit on your own, get help. First, try a smoking cessation group or clinic offered by your local hospital, school, civic group, or organization; the American Heart Assocation or the American Cancer Society will be glad to provide referrals. Commercial smoking cessation plans can also be very helpful; they tend to be more expensive but they're a good investment, both medically and financially. Hypnosis, too, has helped many people. Consider acupuncture. Try anything — but beware of expensive plans with exaggerated claims. If it seems too good to be true, it's probably not true.

If you are still hooked on cigarettes despite all this, you should turn to your doctor for help. In fact, your physician should have already tried to help by explaining the hazards of smoking and by offering advice and encouragement for quitting. Like many patients, however, many physicians are tempted by the quick fix of the prescription pad.

In this case it's a prescription for nicotine. You're right: nicotine is addicting, and it is toxic. But if you're hooked, it's better to get nicotine in a controlled, regulated dose while avoiding all the other toxins in smoke. Several forms are available; nicotine gum has largely been abandoned in favor of the nicotine patch, and a nicotine inhaler is on the way. All are expensive, and all require careful use to avoid nicotine toxicity. Finally, prescription nicotine should always be used in conjunction with behavior-modification techniques; it's a temporary tool that should be tapered and withdrawn so you'll be nicotine-free as well as smoke-free.

Smoking and Society

Smoking is everyone's problem.

It's obvious that we need collective action to protect involuntary smokers from environmental tobacco smoke. Not so obvious, perhaps, is the need to protect voluntary smokers from themselves.

Tobacco abuse is not as voluntary as it seems. The tobacco manufacturers know this well — which is why they spend $1.37 to advertise each carton of cigarettes they sell. In all, the industry spent $3.6 billion to promote cigarettes in the U.S. in 1991 alone. That's a lot of money; but it's rewarded by more than $7 billion in annual profits.

Even as many Americans struggle to control tobacco abuse, the industry giants are seeking new markets. As taxes rise, they cut prices. As adults quit, they target youth. As smoking declines in men, they promote the habit to women. As the affluent and well educated quit smoking, they sell more cigarettes to the poor and less educated. As overall smoking declines, it is promoted in minority communities. And as Americans quit smoking, American companies ship their deadly products abroad, especially to new markets in developing countries. It's no accident that worldwide smoking has *increased* by 75 percent since the U.S. Surgeon General's report in 1964. In all, more than 1 billion people smoke, consuming more than 5 trillion cigarettes annually. Among the costs: 2.5 million excess or premature deaths each year. Smoking, a creation of the human mind, causes 5 percent of all human deaths.

To win the war against atherosclerosis, we'll have to win the fight against smoking. And to reach the goal of a smokeless society, we'll have to work together through education and publicity campaigns, economic policies and tobacco taxes, antismoking laws and regulations, and new research into quitting techniques. Using the defense industry as a model, we should also help tobacco farmers convert to "peaceful" pursuits. But in the final analysis, smoking cessation is an individual's responsibility. Start helping others by setting an example: help yourself by quitting.

Chapter 4

Dietary Fat
and Cholesterol:
You Are What You Eat

BACON AND EGGS. Burgers and fries. Pie à la mode. What could be more American?

Heart attacks. Strokes. Colon cancer. Obesity. What could be more American?

We are what we eat.

Dietary Fat in the United States

Americans are hooked on fat. Each year, the typical American eats 261 eggs, 70 pounds of beef, and 11 gallons of ice cream. Each day, the average person consumes one-third of a cup of pure fat, the equivalent of 22 pats of butter. Each time we stop in for a quick cheeseburger with fries and a shake, we'll consume 75 grams of fat.

By any measure, the average American eats too much fat. To make matters worse, it's the wrong kind of fat; since so much of our food comes from animal products, much of the fat we eat is saturated fat.

It wasn't always that way. In 1900 only 30 percent of the calories in the typical American diet came from fat. By the 1960s, however, our fat intake was up to 44 percent. Since then, of course, we've become a cholesterol-conscious society, and we have started to improve. At present, Americans get 37 percent of their daily calories from fat. It's progress, to be sure, but it's not good enough, particularly since half our daily fat is the saturated variety.

How much fat should we be eating? It's a complex question that each person will have to answer individually; in these pages I'll do my best to help you set your own goals. But we can get some important clues by looking back into human history and by looking around the world today.

Dietary Fat in Human History

As a species, human beings first appeared on earth 40,000 years ago. It seems like a long time ago, but it's just a quick tick on the evolutionary clock — so quick, in fact, that human genetics has remained nearly unchanged throughout the history of our species. Since primitive humans ate a diet that was truly natural, anthropologists may be able to determine what nature intended for us to eat today.

Early humans lived in small bands, depending for survival on their ability to hunt, fish, and gather. As hunters, they did eat animal foods, but the wild game they consumed was very different from the domesticated cattle of the twentieth century. Instead of being penned up, stuffed with grain, and treated with hormones, wild game grazed on grasses and ranged over large areas; as a result, the meat consumed by primitive humans was much lower in fat than today's steaks and chops. Not only was wild game lean, but it was also hard to hunt down; as a result, the early human diet depended largely on gathering wild fruits, nuts, seeds, and tubers. Life must have been hard for our earliest ancestors, but their diet was healthful, deriving only 21 percent of its calories from fat and providing lots of fiber, about 45 grams a day.

With the advent of farming about 10,000 years ago, things began to change. Domesticated cattle replaced wild game and dairy products arrived on the scene. Vegetable foods also changed, as cultivated grains began to replace wild fruits and vegetables. The diet of the agricultural era had more fat, less fiber, and less diversity than the diet of the hunter-gatherer — but it was still much more healthful than the daily fare in our contemporary industrialized world.

The industrial revolution that began a mere 150 years ago swept away many aspects of the traditional human lifestyle. We enjoy the enormous advantages of our brilliant, rapidly changing technological advances — but we also suffer the consequences of the environmental pollution, mental stress, and physical inactivity that have accompanied each breakthrough. We suffer, too, from a diet that has shifted from natural foods to processed foods, from vegetable-based foods to animal-based foods, from low-salt foods to high-salt foods, from complex carbohydrates to refined sugars, from high dietary fiber to low fiber, and from low fat consumption to today's nutritional infatuation.

The American Heart Association tells us that 30 percent of the average American's caloric intake should come from fat. In a sense, they would turn back the nutritional clock by 100 years. As a national average, it's an excellent goal, at least for starters. But my patients, friends, and readers are not necessarily average folk, and I'd like to see well-informed, well-motivated people do better. I don't want to turn the clock back 40,000 years, but I would like to see certain aspects of the basic human diet incorporated into our daily fare, including an average fat intake of 20 percent, with most of it coming from vegetable or marine sources. And people with heart disease, atherosclerosis risk factors, or obesity might aim for significantly less dietary fat. In fact, low-fat, high-fiber, vegetable-based diets are the norm in much of the world today; it's a wide, wide world but not a universally fat, fat world.

Dietary Fat Around the World

Even as we enter the twenty-first century, there are peoples who eat and live much as our hunter-gatherer ancestors — and, like all humans before the industrial revolution, these people are virtually free of atherosclerosis. In industrialized Western societies, too, there are wide variations in the amounts and types of fats in typical national diets. These variations parallel differences in the risk of atherosclerosis. For example, the landmark Seven Countries Study tracked more than 12,000 men for over 10 years; it found that the men who ate the most fat had the highest blood cholesterol levels and the most coronary artery disease. Finland led the way in both dietary fat and heart attacks, with the United States close behind. In Greece, though, things were much better; the average Greek diet contained less than 30 percent of its calories in fat, and the average Greek was only one-third as likely to suffer a heart attack as the average American.

There is, of course, much more to atherosclerosis than dietary fat intake; genetics, smoking, lack of exercise, obesity, diabetes, and stress all contribute to cardiac risk, while dietary fiber, vitamins, fish, and alcohol are protective. Still, we can and should take a lesson from the Greeks, not only because their fat intake is lower than ours, but because it consists largely of unsaturated vegetable fat from olive oil.

We can also look beyond the West to learn about diet and atherosclerosis. For example, the typical diet in China derives just 7 percent of its protein from animal sources, compared to 70 percent in the typical American diet. The diet in China is much lower in fat and much higher in fiber. Although the Chinese consume 20 percent more calories than Americans, Americans have 25 percent more body fat and average cholesterol levels that are 100 points higher. Is it any wonder that heart attacks kill only 4 of every 1,000 Chinese men but 67 of every 1,000 American men?

The Mediterranean diet features olive oil and pasta, the Oriental diet, rice and fish. We can learn from both, while constructing a uniquely American diet to keep us healthy and free of atherosclerosis. But first we must learn more about dietary fat and cholesterol.

What Are Fats?

Not all fats are created equal; some fats are more harmful than others, and a few special types of fat may even be on your side in the fight against atherosclerosis. To understand these distinctions, it's important to recognize the differences between saturated and unsaturated fats.

Cooks tell us it's simple: saturated fats are solid at room temperature, whereas unsaturated fats are liquid. Fats of animal origin are generally saturated, whereas fats from vegetable sources are generally unsaturated. That's why beef tallow and lard come in jars while safflower and olive oils come in bottles.

The cooks are right, but chemists can teach us a thing or two as well. In fact, we need a bit of chemistry to understand the important exceptions to the wisdom of the kitchen. Carbon atoms are more complicated than cookies, but when it comes to fats, every bit of information is important indeed.

In terms of their chemical structure, fats are actually rather simple molecules. All fats are composed of carbon and hydrogen atoms joined together in structures known technically as fatty acids. The carbon atoms are linked into a chain at the core of every fatty acid. Each carbon atom is surrounded by hydrogens. In saturated fats, each carbon is surrounded by the maximum number of hydrogens; all of the slots available for hydrogen are occupied. But in unsaturated fats, some of the hydrogen slots are vacant. In monounsaturated fats, the missing hydrogens are replaced by one double bond between neighboring carbons, whereas in polyunsaturates two or more double bonds are present (Figure 4–1).

Having completed your chemistry lesson, you can understand two important exceptions to the cook's rule. First, some vegetable oils are saturated — all their carbon atoms are surrounded by a full complement of hydrogens. Coconut oil, palm oil, palm kernel oil, and cocoa butter belong in this category. Because they are plentiful, inexpensive, and stable, tropical oils have found their way into many "cholesterol-free" foods and baked goods. Because it's tasty, cocoa butter has become a mainstay of the chocolate-lover's dessert menu. But because they are saturated, these fats behave more like animal fats rather than vegetable oils; of the four saturated vegetable fats, cocoa butter appears to be the least harmful. In contrast, an important group of fats from animal sources are unsaturated. These fatty acids don't come from land animals, but from marine animals; because they are unsaturated, fish oils behave more like vegetable oils than animal fats.

Cooks have figured out what to do with fats, and chemists have explained the structural differences between the many fatty acids in foods. Medical researchers have determined that saturated and unsaturated fats have very different effects on human health. New studies, in fact, are showing that important distinctions exist even among the unsaturated fats; although we still have much to learn about the relative merits and drawbacks of the unsaturates, we've already learned enough to warrant some changes in the traditional guidelines for low-fat diets. Before confronting these important issues, though, use Table 4–1 to see which foods contain saturated and unsaturated fats.

What Is Cholesterol?

Americans are preoccupied with cholesterol. More than 15 million blood cholesterol tests are performed in the United States every year. Food labels trumpet "No Cholesterol" in large print. Restaurant menus are emblazoned with little hearts to symbolize "low-cholesterol" meals.

All this concern is justified — yet I've not mentioned cholesterol in

FIGURE 4–1: The Structure of Fat and Cholesterol: A Primer.

Fats are simple molecules composed of many carbon (C) and hydrogen (H) atoms which are joined to a few oxygens (O) to form *fatty acids*. The carbons are linked to each other in a chain; each carbon atom is also bonded to hydrogen or oxygen atoms.

Saturated fatty acids have all the slots that are available for hydrogen filled by hydrogen atoms:

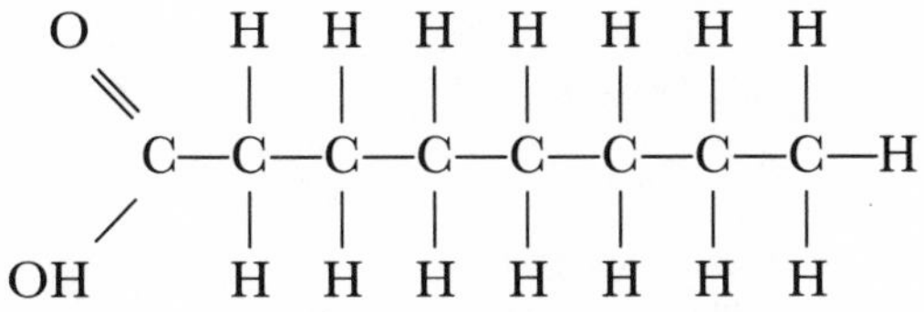

$$
\begin{array}{c}
\text{O} \qquad \text{H} \quad \text{H} \quad \text{H} \quad \text{H} \quad \text{H} \quad \text{H} \quad \text{H} \\
\diagdown \qquad | \quad\; | \quad\; | \quad\; | \quad\; | \quad\; | \quad\; | \\
\text{C}-\text{C}-\text{C}-\text{C}-\text{C}-\text{C}-\text{C}-\text{C}-\text{H} \\
\diagup \qquad | \quad\; | \quad\; | \quad\; | \quad\; | \quad\; | \quad\; | \\
\text{OH} \qquad \text{H} \quad \text{H} \quad \text{H} \quad \text{H} \quad \text{H} \quad \text{H} \quad \text{H}
\end{array}
$$

Unsaturated fatty acids are missing some of their hydrogen atoms. Because each carbon atom must have 4 bonds, a double bond between neighboring carbon atoms replaces the missing hydrogens.

Monounsaturated fatty acids have one double bond between carbons:

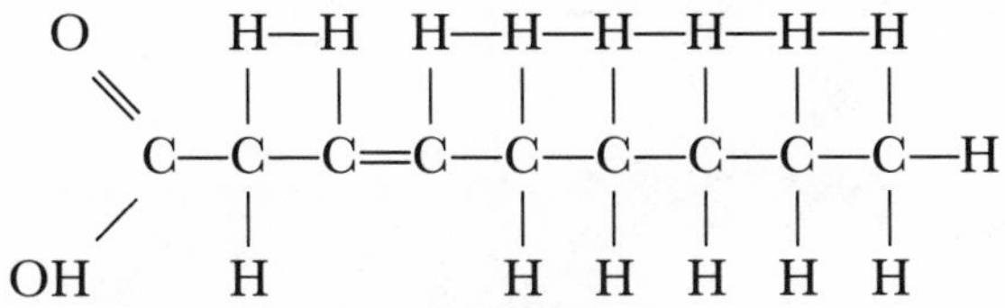

$$
\begin{array}{c}
\text{O} \qquad \text{H}-\text{H} \quad \text{H}-\text{H}-\text{H}-\text{H}-\text{H}-\text{H} \\
\diagdown \qquad | \quad\; | \quad\;\; | \quad\; | \quad\; | \quad\; | \quad\; | \\
\text{C}-\text{C}-\text{C}=\text{C}-\text{C}-\text{C}-\text{C}-\text{C}-\text{C}-\text{H} \\
\diagup \qquad | \qquad\qquad | \quad\; | \quad\; | \quad\; | \\
\text{OH} \qquad \text{H} \qquad\;\; \text{H} \quad \text{H} \quad \text{H} \quad \text{H}
\end{array}
$$

Polyunsaturated fatty acids have two or more double bonds:

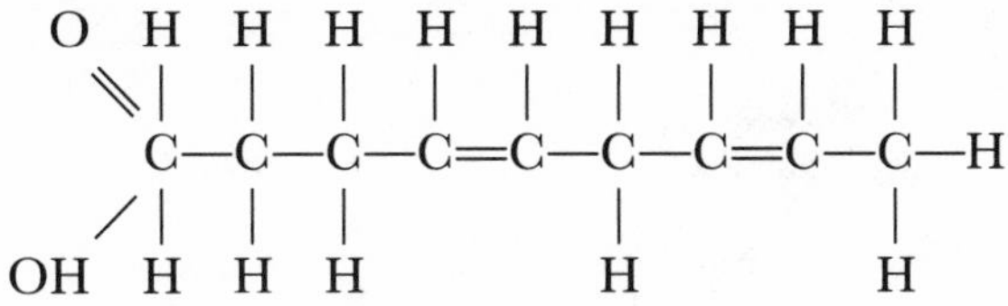

$$
\begin{array}{c}
\text{O} \quad \text{H} \quad \text{H} \quad \text{H} \quad \text{H} \quad \text{H} \quad \text{H} \quad \text{H} \quad \text{H} \quad \text{H} \\
\diagdown | \quad\; | \quad\; | \quad\; | \quad\; | \quad\; | \quad\; | \quad\; | \quad\; | \\
\text{C}-\text{C}-\text{C}-\text{C}=\text{C}-\text{C}-\text{C}=\text{C}-\text{C}-\text{H} \\
\diagup | \quad\; | \quad\; | \qquad\quad | \qquad\qquad | \\
\text{OH} \;\text{H} \quad \text{H} \quad \text{H} \qquad\;\; \text{H} \qquad\quad\;\; \text{H}
\end{array}
$$

Omega-3 unsaturated fatty acids have one of their double bonds located on the third carbon from the end of the chain. Marine oils are rich in omega-3s; in contrast, most vegetable oils contain unsaturated fatty acids that have their last double bond on the sixth carbon from the end of the chain.

Partially hydrogenated fatty acids have some of their missing hydrogens added back during processing. This changes the three-dimensional structure from the natural curved "cis" configurations to a straighter "trans" configuration. *Trans-fatty acids* are shaped like saturated fats; as a result, they can be packed together tightly into solids or semisolids that resemble saturated fats. But they also mimic the way saturated fats affect the body, contributing to atherosclerosis.

Cholesterol is not a fat, but a waxy substance with a complex ring-like structure:

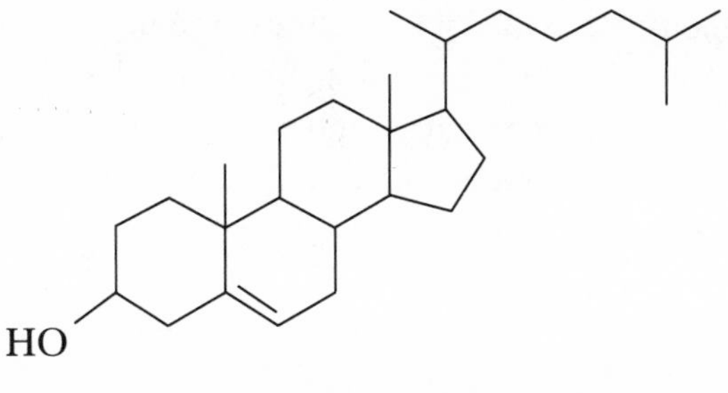

Table 4–1
FATTY ACIDS IN FATS AND OILS

High in Saturated Fat		Saturated Fat (as % of fat content)
Vegetable	Coconut oil	92
	Palm kernel oil	81
	Cocoa butter	63
	Palm oil	51
Animal	Milk, butter, cream	66
	Beef tallow	52
	Lard (pork fat)	42
	Chicken fat	30

High in Monounsaturated Fats		Monounsaturated Fat (as % of fat content)
Vegetable	Olive oil	77
	Canola oil	58
	Peanut oil	48
Animal	Fish oil	30

High in Polyunsaturated Fats		Polyunsaturated Fat (as % of fat content)
Vegetable	Safflower oil	78
	Walnut oil	70
	Sunflower oil	69
	Corn oil	62
	Soybean oil	61
	Cottonseed oil	54
Animal	Fish oil	40

Principal source: "Nutritive Value of Foods." U.S. Department of Agriculture.

our discussion of dietary fat. A glaring omission? Not at all. The explanation for considering cholesterol separately is perhaps the best-kept secret in nutrition.

Cholesterol is not a fat. Instead, it's a complex molecule with waxlike properties (Figure 4–1). The distinction may seem academic, but the food industry has used it to confuse consumers, since many products are *cholesterol-free* yet *high in fat*. To fight atherosclerosis, it's important to eat foods *low* in both cholesterol and fat, particularly saturated fat. Saturated fat, in fact, is even more harmful than cholesterol.

It may come as a surprise that cholesterol ranks below saturated fat as a cause of heart disease. But your surprise will vanish when you consider the distinction between the cholesterol in your food and the cholesterol in your blood.

Reducing blood cholesterol levels is a crucial aspect of the fight against atherosclerosis. More precisely, the villain is LDL cholesterol. Chapter 1 explains that LDL cholesterol moves from the blood into the walls of arteries; in the arterial wall, LDL cholesterol is oxidized, thus initiating the formation of atherosclerotic plaques that may eventually block coronary arteries. The more LDL cholesterol in the blood, the higher the risk of atherosclerosis.

Eating cholesterol-rich foods will raise blood LDL cholesterol levels. But a low-cholesterol diet, while important, is not enough to reduce blood LDL cholesterol levels. That's because only about a third of the cholesterol in blood comes from the cholesterol in food — the rest is made right in the human body. And the most potent stimulus to cholesterol production by the liver is saturated fat in the diet.

To lower blood cholesterol levels, reduce the saturated fat in your diet. But don't go overboard by neglecting cholesterol; instead, take care to reduce your intake of both saturated fat and cholesterol.

Where is the cholesterol in food? Remember that cholesterol is a vital constituent of all animal cells. Vegetable cells, on the other hand, get along perfectly well without any cholesterol. Cholesterol is found only in foods from animal sources; all vegetable foods are cholesterol-free. If you reduce your intake of animal fat, you'll automatically reduce your intake of cholesterol. But to lower your blood LDL cholesterol, you'll also have to avoid eating saturated fats from vegetable sources (Table 4–1).

The cholesterol in blood comes in two varieties, good (HDL cholesterol) and bad (LDL cholesterol). But the cholesterol in food comes in one form only — and it's all bad. Use Table 4–2 to identify foods that are bad for your health because they are high in cholesterol.

Dietary Fat, Cholesterol, and Atherosclerosis

So far it's fairly simple.

Dietary cholesterol raises blood LDL cholesterol, contributing to atherosclerosis. The average American diet contains nearly 500 milligrams of cholesterol per day; the major sources are eggs, beef and pork

Table 4–2
CHOLESTEROL IN FOODS

Very High in Cholesterol	Egg yolks (274 mg each) Liver (389 mg/3½ oz.) Lamb chops (215 mg/3½ oz.) Shrimp (195 mg/3½ oz.)
High in Cholesterol	Veal (128 mg/3½ oz.) Chuck roast (99 mg/3½ oz.) Ham (92 mg/3½ oz.) Bacon (85 mg/3½ oz.) Steak (80 mg/3½ oz.) Bologna, beef (58 mg/3 slices) Salmon (87 mg/3½ oz.) Lobster (72 mg/3½ oz.) Turkey (117 mg/3½ oz.) Chicken (91 mg/3½ oz.) Ricotta cheese, whole milk (58 mg/oz.) Waffles (102 mg/each) Pound cake (64 mg/slice) Ice cream, premium (88 mg/cup) Ice cream, regular (59 mg/cup) Pizza (56 mg/slice)
Moderate in Cholesterol	Tuna (49 mg/3½ oz.) Ricotta cheese, part-skim milk (25 mg/oz.) Whole milk (33 mg/8 oz.) Cheddar cheese (30 mg/oz.) Yogurt (plain) (21 mg/8 oz.) Chocolate cake (37 mg/slice) Bran muffin (24 mg/each)
Low in Cholesterol	1% milk (10 mg/8 oz.) Yogurt, low-fat (3 mg/6 oz.) Cottage cheese, low-fat (5 mg/4 oz.) Pancakes (16 mg each)
Very Little or No Cholesterol	Egg whites Skim milk Yogurt, nonfat Cottage cheese, nonfat Margarine All vegetable oils Fruit and vegetables Grains and pastas Bread and English muffins

products, liver, hot dogs and sandwich meats, cheese and whole dairy products, baked goods such as doughnuts, cookies and cakes, and poultry.

Saturated fat is even worse, raising blood LDL cholesterol levels by stimulating the human liver to produce cholesterol and pour it into the bloodstream. Not all saturated fats, however, are equally harmful; for you chemists, the most harmful are palmitic (16 carbons), myristic (14 carbons), and lauric (12 carbons) acids; for you cooks, they are found principally in red meat, lard, and dairy fat. Although it's saturated, stearic acid (18 carbons) does not appear to raise blood cholesterol levels; it's the main fat in dark chocolate — but before you rush out to the candy store, consider a 1994 report that found that stearic acid activates the blood clotting system, thus increasing heart attack risk. Unfortunately, the average American diet derives 18 percent of its calories from saturated fat; the major sources are beef and pork products, cheese and whole dairy products, hot dogs and sandwich meats, and commercially prepared baked goods such as doughnuts, cookies, and crackers.

Unsaturated fats do not increase blood cholesterol levels. Over the years, various medical studies have even suggested that unsaturated fatty acids may actually *lower* blood LDL cholesterol levels. As a result, traditional "heart-healthy" diets have lumped unsaturated fats together as "acceptable if eaten in moderation." In the past few years, however, the data have become more interesting (and more complex). For one thing, polyunsaturates seem to lower HDL cholesterol levels, hardly a desirable result. And, in animals at least, diets high in polyunsaturates may increase the risk of cancer. Finally, various unsaturated fats have very different effects on blood cholesterol levels, atherosclerosis, and human health. It now appears that we must take note of three special classes of unsaturated fats. One, partially hydrogenated vegetable oil, is bad for health (even in moderation); the other two, olive oil and fish oil, may actually help fight atherosclerosis and improve health (if used in moderation).

Partially Hydrogenated Vegetable Oils

Even in a book about the human heart, a few words of tribute to the human brain seem appropriate. It is, after all, the power of the mind that separates humans from all other animals. Humanity's inventions provide us with innumerable boons for our spirits and our bodies. The hydrogenation of vegetable fats surely seems insignificant among human discoveries — but it now appears to be a significant contributor to atherosclerosis.

Chemistry, cooking, and commerce all contribute to the hydrogenation story. Unsaturated fats are liquid at room temperature. Their chemical properties also limit their culinary uses; in particular, their low melting points make them undesirable for baking. No problem, the chemists tell the cooks — if we just add a little hydrogen, you'll be able to do all sorts of new things with unsaturated vegetable oils. Sensing a huge market for products that are inexpensive, plentiful, and stable, the giants of commerce get into the act. In the end, the collaboration is a success: margarine and other partially hydrogenated vegetable oils are born.

Margarine has long been a mainstay of standard "heart-healthy" diets. Indeed, it's nice to recommend food substitutes that look and taste like the real thing. To make margarine look like butter, hydrogen is added to polyunsaturates such as corn or safflower oil. In the process, the oils undergo two important changes: they become more nearly saturated with hydrogen and their configuration is altered, changing from their normal curved shape to a straightened structure. Chemists call it a shift from the "cis" to the "trans" configuration. Food manufacturers call it progress since the straighter trans-fatty acids can be packed more densely, giving margarine a semisolid texture that feels like butter. Cooks, too, are delighted since trans-fatty acids make margarine smooth and raise its melting point. Heart patients are reassured since they can use a "no-cholesterol" spread without guilt. But now doctors and nutritionists are putting all this happiness into doubt. New data reveal that trans-fatty acids raise LDL cholesterol levels and increase heart attack risk. The chemists have achieved more than they expected: margarine *is* like butter.

A group of Dutch scientists first raised the alarm about trans-fatty acids. Their study, published in 1990 in the *New England Journal of Medicine*, compared the effects of trans-fatty acids with those of saturated fats. It reported that trans-fatty acids raised LDL cholesterol levels nearly as much as saturated fat. Even worse, trans-fatty acids lowered HDL cholesterol levels, while saturated fat did not. The result: cholesterol ratios were even worse on trans-fatty acids than on saturated-fat diets.

Although the Dutch report was worrisome, American physicians reacted conservatively. Holland is a long way off; even more importantly, the short-term effects of experimental diets on blood cholesterol levels do not necessarily translate into long-term effects on the heart. But our complacency has been brought to an end by five new American studies.

In a 1993 study of 14 men being fed carefully monitored diets, researchers from Tufts University compared the effects of liquid corn oil and corn oil margarine on blood cholesterol levels. The changeover from liquid oil to margarine increased LDL cholesterol by 7 percent, even though all other aspects of the diet, including total fat intake, remained the same.

A study from Texas, also published in 1993, took the Massachusetts observations one step farther: healthy middle-aged men who were placed on diets containing stick margarine suffered a fall in their HDL cholesterols and a rise in their LDL levels.

A much larger study evaluated the effect of dietary trans-fatty acids in 748 men. Even after carefully accounting for other cardiac risk factors, including age, body-mass index, waist-to-hip ratio, smoking, exercise, and dietary saturated fat and cholesterol intake, the study found that trans-fatty acids raised LDL and lowered HDL cholesterol levels. In all, men eating small amounts of partially hydrogenated vegetable oils had average overall cholesterol ratios of 4.4, while men eating lots of trans-fatty acids had average ratios of 4.9. That may not sound like a big difference, but the authors of this 1992 report predicted that it would raise heart attack risk by 27 percent.

It didn't take long to confirm this prediction. In 1993, a team of investigators from Harvard reported the results of a detailed analysis of diet and heart disease in 85,095 American nurses. Even after accounting for other risk factors, trans-fatty acids were significantly linked to heart attacks. In fact, women who consumed the largest amounts of partially hydrogenated vegetable oils had *70 percent* more heart attacks than women who consumed little of them. The increased risk occurred across the board, occurring whether the trans-fatty acids came from margarine or from the vegetable shortening used in cookies, cake, or white bread.

Most recently, a 1994 study from Boston evaluated the impact of dietary trans-fatty acids on heart attacks in men. The results were striking: the men eating the most trans-fatty acids had 2.4 times more heart attacks than the men eating the least. The message: partially hydrogenated vegetable oils are even worse for men than for women.

It's time, I think, to take note of partially hydrogenated vegetable oils, moving them into the same category as saturated fat. That doesn't mean that you have to give them up altogether — but it does mean that you should use them very sparingly; the higher your cardiac risk profile (Table 2–11), the less you should use.

Should you use margarine or butter? The short answer, I'm afraid, is neither — but there is a lesser evil. The total fat and caloric content of butter and its closest imitator, stick margarine, is identical, but butter has 31 milligrams of cholesterol and 7 grams of saturated fat per tablespoon, while margarine has no cholesterol and only 1 gram of saturated fat. But stick margarines contain 25 percent trans-fatty acids; tub margarine has only 17 percent, and liquid margarine even less. So if you use margarine, use the least solid form that meets your needs, and use it sparingly. Even better, use the new *non*fat margarine or olive oil on bread — or learn to enjoy your bread dry or with jam or honey.

Margarine is only the tip of the trans-fatty acid iceberg. Partially hydrogenated vegetable oils are used in many prepared foods, including imitation cheese, nondairy creamers, frosting, candy, cereals, and hydrogenated peanut butter. In fact, as consumers have learned to avoid tropical oils in processed foods, manufacturers are replacing them with partially hydrogenated vegetable oils. They are now used as the major shortening in many commercially prepared baked goods, such as cakes, cookies, crackers, and white bread; a doughnut, for example, has about 6 grams of trans-fatty acids, while even a "heart-healthy" bran muffin has 4 grams. Fast foods are worrisome for their trans-fatty acids as well as their saturated fat, salt, and calories; a typical order of French fries contains 8 grams of trans-fatty acids, and an order of fried chicken or fish has 10 grams.

It's discouraging news; margarine and other partially hydrogenated vegetable oils and shortenings are sacred cows of nutrition that have been overturned by new research — just as cows themselves were downgraded by earlier studies. But don't let this new data turn you off. Don't give up on nutritional research; even though the rules seem to be changing every time you look up, the margarine story represents a change in the details but not in the basic principle: eat less fat, particularly saturated fat. In a sense, margarine actually fits both rules, since it is partially saturated. Perhaps it even fits another rule — since it's man-made, it seems fitting that it's now being grouped with undesirable animal fats instead of with desirable natural vegetable oils.

Above all, don't let concern about trans-fatty acids turn you away from the goal of using your diet to conquer heart disease. You'll find many tips for healthful and delicious eating later in this chapter. And you'll also be glad to know that there is some good news about the unsaturated fats in olives and fish.

Olive Oil and Other Monosaturates

Is any form of fat safe for the heart? Saturated fats are not, nor are the trans-fatty acids in partially hydrogenated vegetable oils. But how about natural vegetable oils?

Like the butter versus margarine controversy, there has been lots of debate over the relative merits of various vegetable oils (see Table 4–1). The early favorites were the polyunsaturates, such as safflower, sunflower, and corn oils. Some studies suggest that they may actually lower LDL cholesterol levels, but there is a catch: they also tend to reduce HDL cholesterol levels. The current consensus is that polyunsaturates neither raise nor lower the risk of atherosclerosis and heart attack.

Attention is now turning to the monounsaturates, particularly olive oil. In the 1950s, before the Greek diet became Americanized, middle-aged American men had 8 times more heart attacks than Greek men; Greeks had much less colon and breast cancer, and their average life expectancy was 4 years longer than in America and Western Europe. Perhaps, the argument goes, it's because most of the fat in the Greek diet is in the form of olive oil. Nor is the lower rate of heart attack and cancer confined to Greece; in fact, it extends throughout the "olive belt," including southern Italy, the south of France, Spain, Portugal, and parts of Northern Africa and the Middle East.

It's hard to be sure that olive oil is the protective element in the traditional Mediterranean diet, which is also high in vegetables, nuts, and grains and low in meat. Another protective candidate is wine (see Chapter 9). And protection may depend on genetics, exercise habits, or other factors as much as on diet itself. Granting these uncertainties, though, olive oil does have some intriguing properties.

Like polyunsaturated fatty acids, the monounsaturates seem to reduce LDL levels; unlike the polys, however, olive oil and other monos may not reduce HDL levels. As a result, people consuming olive oil appear to have better overall blood cholesterol ratios.

Olive oil may also be helpful in other ways. It's too early to be sure, but a 1993 study from Israel provides a hint: olive oil appears to have antioxidant properties. Remember from Chapter 1 that atherosclerosis depends on events in the arterial wall as well as on the cholesterol in blood. Olive oil seems to counteract two events that promote atherosclerosis in the arterial wall, decreasing the susceptibility of LDL to oxidation and reducing the uptake of LDL cholesterol by macrophages. More research will be needed to confirm these findings. And if olive oil is protective, we'll want to find out how it works; for example, the protection could depend on the high vitamin E content of olive oil rather than on the oil itself. It will also be important to learn if other monounsaturates share these properties.

Until the answers are available, what should you do about olive oil? I'm not ready to recommend a *high* intake of any kind of fat, even monounsaturated vegetable oils. Among other things, at 9 calories per gram, olive oil has the same high caloric content as all other fats. Still, in constructing a low-fat diet, I recommend favoring monounsaturates over polyunsaturates. Olive oil (77 percent monounsaturated) heads the list, but canola oil (58 percent monounsaturated) is another interesting possibility. We know less about canola oil; it isn't part of any regional diet, but it's already very popular in Canada, and as its use increases, we'll see how it measures up.

A 1994 study suggests it will measure up very well indeed; patients who consumed extra canola oil had many fewer heart attacks than patients eating traditional Mediterranean diets. The additional benefit of canola oil may depend on its high content of linolenic acid, an omega-3 fatty acid with properties similar to those of fish oil.

Fish Oils: The Omega-3 Polyunsaturates

The Greeks have moderately high dietary fat but moderately low cardiac risk; olives may be the explanation. Eskimos have high-fat diets but low rates of heart attacks; fish may be the reason.

Marine animals have fats that are very different from those present in land animals. Land animals have saturated fatty acids; the palmitic, myristic, and lauric acids found in red meat, lard, and dairy fat are particularly harmful. Fish and marine mammals, in contrast, have monounsaturated (30 percent) and polyunsaturated (40 percent) fatty acids. Called omega-3s, these fish oils are structurally distinct from other fats and oils from animal and vegetable sources. The omega-3s of greatest importance are eicosapentaenoic and docosahexaenoic acid; you can call them EPA and DHA so you'll have room for a mouthful of fish instead of a mouthful of chemical names.

The omega-3s may improve blood cholesterol levels, but they don't seem to be consistently helpful. They do not act as antioxidants. Instead, they appear to fight atherosclerosis by reducing inflammatory damage to arterial walls and by inhibiting the third step in the process that causes heart attacks, blood clotting.

Eating fish is an important tactic in the fight against atherosclerosis, so important, in fact, that it's the subject of Chapter 10. You can turn ahead for the details or settle for the bottom line now: eat fish. Think of fish as the olives of the sea — make them part of your low-fat diet, but don't consume fish oil as a dietary supplement.

Low-Fat Diets in the Treatment of Atherosclerosis

The ultimate test of any technique used to fight atherosclerosis is its ability to treat patients who already have the disease. How does dietary fat restriction meet this test?

Very well.

Doctors who treat patients with coronary artery disease have many goals. We want to reduce the pain of angina and improve the functional capacity of patients with heart disease. We want to halt the progression of the disease, preventing recurrent heart attacks and prolonging life. We can do all this with various medications, ideally combined with the 15-point attack on heart disease found in this book. But an even more ambitious goal has proved elusive: can treatment actually shrink existing plaques? Can treatment cause atherosclerosis to regress?

Animal experiments by Dr. David Blankenhorn and others have demonstrated that it is possible to halt progression and even to induce regression of coronary atherosclerosis by administering cholesterol-lowering drugs. Several trials have demonstrated similar benefits from prescription drugs in humans. And now new studies allow us to evaluate the effects of diet on coronary artery disease in humans.

These new studies rely on precise measurements of the diameter of coronary arteries and the size of atherosclerotic plaques blocking the channels. Even in the era of marvelous technology we can't actually see into the heart. But doctors can introduce tiny plastic catheters into coro-

nary arteries; they inject dye through the catheter, then take x-ray pictures of the arteries and the plaques. (See Chapter 18, Understanding
Medical Tests and Treatments.) Computer programs allow accurate
and objective measurements of plaque size. The technique is called
quantitative coronary angiography. It's an invasive test that should not
be overused, but in expert hands it's remarkably safe.

The studies that have evaluated diet and plaque size in humans depend first on identifying patients with coronary artery disease who volunteer to undergo angiography. The subjects must also agree to accept
random assignment to the diet treatment group or to a control group
that receives the best of medical care without the special diet. After a
specified period of time, the diet-treated and control patients undergo
repeat angiography and the results are compared. To ensure objectivity,
the doctors evaluating the x-rays and computer data don't know
whether the subjects were in the diet-treated or control group. This
study design is known as a randomized clinical trial; because they are
difficult and expensive, only a few have been performed with diet and
angiograms — but their results are encouraging.

The standard American Heart Association "Step Two" therapeutic
diet for patients with high cholesterol and heart disease calls for reducing dietary fat below 30 percent, saturated fat below 7 percent, and
cholesterol below 200 milligrams per day. These are modest goals at
best; for example, even though I'm perfectly healthy, I consume only
half as much fat and cholesterol, and the 15-point program in this book
recommends a target of 20 percent fat for healthy people. And while
the Step Two diet limits saturated fat, it does not regulate unsaturated
fat either by reducing harmful trans-fatty acids or by encouraging a shift
to moderate amounts of monounsaturates or omega-3s. Still, even the
mild Step Two diet has been successful in lowering blood cholesterol
levels; the benefits are modest to moderate but they're greatest in people
with high cholesterol levels who need them most.

Even modest Step Two diets can halt the progression of atherosclerosis. The subjects in Dr. Blankenhorn's Cholesterol Lowering Atherosclerosis Study (CLAS) who adhered to the diet developed fewer new
plaques than did the patients who ate more fat. The 3-year St. Thomas
Atherosclerosis Study (START) of 90 patients showed that a similar diet
was effective in halting the progression of atherosclerosis; even more
impressively, plaques actually *improved* in 38 percent of the diet-treated

subjects compared to 4 percent of the control subjects on "normal" diets. A 1992 German study of 113 patients used a Step Two diet plus exercise; over a 1-year period, the diet and exercise program produced regression in 32 percent of the patients, while only 17 percent of the control subjects improved.

If even modest dietary fat restriction can produce disease regression, can more demanding diets do even better? They can. The Leiden Intervention Trial used a vegetarian diet containing less than 100 milligrams of cholesterol per day; the patients who lowered their cholesterol most had no progression of disease over a 2-year span.

The most impressive evidence of all comes from Dr. Dean Ornish's Lifestyle Heart Trial. It used a nearly vegetarian diet providing only 8 percent of calories from fat and virtually no cholesterol (5 milligrams per day); modest exercise and stress reduction programs were also prescribed. The diet-treated patients dropped their blood cholesterol levels dramatically, with average values falling from 213 to 157. More important, coronary angiograms showed that atherosclerotic plaques regressed in 18 of the 22 patients who completed the program.

By now many studies have demonstrated that various combinations of diet, exercise, stress reduction, and cholesterol-lowering medications can actually produce regression of human atherosclerosis. But even the most encouraging studies found that although plaques may shrink, they don't disappear. Is it worth changing your diet (or taking medication) if the most you can achieve is partial plaque shrinkage? Yes! Small regressions in plaque size can produce big benefits; a 1993 study, in fact, demonstrated that a mere 1 percent improvement in arterial size was linked to a 75 percent improvement in cardiac events. And you don't have to wait years for plaques to shrink before realizing the benefits of reducing your blood cholesterol; another 1993 study demonstrated a significant decline in cardiac events within the first 26 weeks of cholesterol-lowering therapy.

In commenting on strict dietary fat restriction, a noted cardiologist wrote that "only a very small minority of patients are willing and capable of following such stringent and austere schedules." I disagree; the major reason that so few patients adhere to this schedule is that so few doctors prescribe it. Instead, national authorities recommend using cholesterol-lowering drugs if the Step Two diet isn't effective. Dietary fat restrictions work; more severe restrictions work better. I offer my patients with heart disease and high cholesterol levels the choice between a 10 percent fat diet and medications. If you make a 20 percent fat diet part of your 15-point program to conquer heart disease before it starts, you won't be faced with such a difficult choice.

Dietary Fats and Human Health

Heart disease is the leading cause of death in the United States, and stroke is in third place. Both are manifestations of atherosclerosis. Dietary cholesterol and saturated fats from land animals and tropical oils promote atherosclerosis by raising blood LDL cholesterol levels. Trans-fatty acids from processed vegetable oils share these properties and add insult to injury by lowering HDL cholesterol levels. Poly-unsaturated vegetable oils are probably neutral. Monounsaturates such as olive oil and possibly canola oil may be protective, probably because they improve blood cholesterol levels and perhaps by acting as anti-oxidants in the arterial wall. Omega-3 oils from marine animals may also be helpful, probably because of their effects on blood clotting mechanisms.

As important as atherosclerosis is, there is more to health. And dietary fats influence many other aspects of human health.

All fats share certain common properties. Some are good; fats are essential for the absorption of vitamins A, D, E, and K. Others are bad; containing 9 calories per gram, all fats are very high in calories. And fats contribute to many problems beyond the cardiovascular system.

Fatty foods promote obesity; in this respect, at least, all fats are created equal, and all are equally harmful.

Fatty foods increase the risk of cancer. Colon cancer is the best example; animal fat is particularly culpable. Diets high in fat also increase the risks of uterine cancer in women, prostate cancer in men, and lung cancer in nonsmokers. The relationship between fat and breast cancer is less clear. It's been hard to confirm a link in American women, possibly because so few are on low-fat diets; in other parts of the world, however, increased fat consumption is associated with an increase in breast cancer.

Heart attacks, strokes, obesity, and cancer — four bad reasons to be good to yourself by reducing your dietary fat. If you need more motivation, consider high blood pressure and gallstones; although high fat consumption isn't a proven cause of either condition, it is a probable contributor to both.

Now that you're motivated to eschew dietary fat, you're ready to learn how to go about it. You'll succeed by setting reasonable goals and by changing your ways slowly but steadily.

Setting Your Goals for Dietary Fat

By now, your mind is probably saturated with fat facts. But it's in a good cause — you've filled your mind with facts so you can keep your arteries open. Three steps remain: deciding how much fat you should eat, finding the fats in food, and learning how to achieve your health goals with a diet that is practical and enjoyable.

If you eat like a typical American, you get 37 percent of your daily calories from fat. It's too much. The National Cholesterol Education Panel and the American Heart Association call for 30 percent. It's better. But 30 percent fat may be too much for you. Consider four things in selecting your personal target: (1) Your blood cholesterol risk ratio (Table 2–3). The higher your cholesterol ratio, the lower your target fat intake should be. (2) Your overall cardiac risk profile (Table 2–11). The higher your score, the lower your target fat intake, even if your blood cholesterol is in the "desirable" range. Cholesterol is only one element in cardiac risk — if you have other risk factors, you should improve your diet as much as possible to help offset those other risks. (3) Your weight and body mass index (Table 2–8). If you want to shed pounds, reduce your fat consumption (and follow the other tips in Chapter 15). (4) Your personal preference. Life should be lovely as well as long, and food is an important source of pleasure. But almost everyone can learn to genuinely enjoy low-fat eating. Make your goals realistic and plan to achieve them gradually so your tastes will have time to change. Leave enough flexibility to allow you to enjoy treats that you find irreplaceable, even if they're laden with "forbidden" fats.

How do these four considerations translate into dietary fat? For healthy people with low cardiac risk scores, thin bodies, and good blood cholesterol levels, 25 or even 30 percent fat is acceptable. For most of us, though, 20 percent is a more healthful target, and it's a target that can be achieved with surprisingly little sacrifice. People who are overweight would do better aiming for 15 percent, as would people with high risk scores or high LDL cholesterol levels. And in my view, patients who already have atherosclerosis should consider reducing their daily fat intake to about 10 percent; it takes some doing, but it's far from draconian, and severe dietary fat restriction has been shown to *reverse* coronary atherosclerosis.

Picking a goal is one thing, eating it is another. There are two ways to estimate the fat content of foods.

First, the percentage of fat in food. This seems easy enough: if your foods all have less than 30 percent fat, your total intake will be less than 30 percent. But there's a trap here. Foods are labeled by *weight;* your daily fat target is calculated on the basis of *calories.* The difference is more than semantic. Consider, for example, "low-fat" 2 percent milk. An 8-ounce serving weighs 250 grams and contains 5 grams of fat; the fat content is indeed just 2 percent by weight. But most of the weight of milk is water, which has no calories. The 5 grams of fat in 2 percent milk contain 45 calories, almost exactly one-third of its total caloric content. Is 2 percent milk low in fat? Compared to whole milk (4 percent fat), perhaps — but it's actually *more* than 30 percent fat.

Fortunately the new food labeling regulations help eliminate the double-talk. Each label lists the food's total calories and the number of calories that come from fat. To find the percentage, just multiply the fat calories by 100, then divide by total calories. For example, whole milk contains 150 calories in 8 ounces; 72 of these calories come from fat, $72 \times 100 = 7200 \div 150 = 48$ — a whopping 48 percent of the calories in whole milk comes from fat.

The new food labels also facilitate a better way to evaluate your fat intake. Each label lists the total fat content of the food in grams of fat. If you know your daily fat allowance, you can see if you can "afford" to eat the fat in front of you. It's an easy method, but there are two provisos. First, the fat content is listed for an average serving size; the average serving is often rather meager, so if you take a larger helping you'll have to account for the extra grams of fat. Second, the labels also interpret the fat contents as a "% of daily value." But this calculation is based on a 2,000 calorie diet with a 30 percent fat intake; if your targets are different (as I hope they are), you'll have to do the math yourself.

To translate your target fat intake into grams of fat per day, use Table 4–3 to estimate your caloric needs. Then use Table 4–4 to determine how many grams of fat you should eat each day. For many people

Table 4–3
TYPICAL DAILY CALORIC INTAKE FOR HEALTHY ADULTS

	Sedentary		Moderately Active		Very Active	
Weight	Men	Women	Men	Women	Men	Women
100	———	1,300	———	1,800	———	2,700
120	1,800	1,560	2,520	2,160	3,600	3,240
140	2,100	1,820	2,940	2,520	4,200	3,780
160	2,400	2,080	3,260	2,880	4,800	4,320
180	2,700	2,340	3,780	3,240	5,400	4,860
200	3,000	———	4,200	———	6,000	———
220	3,300	———	4,620	———	6,600	———

Table 4–4
YOUR TARGET FAT INTAKE

Target Fat %	10%	15%	20%	25%	30%
Calories per Day		Grams of Fat per Day			
1,000	11	17	22	28	33
1,200	14	20	27	33	40
1,500	17	25	33	42	50
1,800	20	30	40	50	60
2,000	22	33	44	56	66
2,500	28	42	56	70	84
3,000	34	50	66	84	100

the concept of gram is quite abstract; to make it concrete, remember that there are about 28 grams in an ounce and 454 in a pound. A teaspoon of sugar weighs about 5 grams; a teaspooon of oil or a pat of butter contains about 5 grams of fat.

Remember that these caloric values assume a stable body weight; if your goals include weight loss, reduce the number of calories in your diet — and lower the fat target you select from Table 4–4.

You'll now have a simple target for your daily fat intake. Remember that it's an average figure — you can eat more fat on some days if you eat less on others. Once you've established your new eating patterns, though, you'll find that you can stay within your target on almost all days without even thinking about it.

You've decided how *much* fat to eat; now, you should determine what *kind* of fat to eat. The key is to reduce your intake of saturated fat. The National Cholesterol Education Panel and American Heart Association suggest that saturated fat be limited to one-third of total fat, but one-sixth sounds better to me. If you agree, just divide your total fat target by 6 to determine your saturated fat target. The new food labels help by listing how many grams of saturated fat there are in each serving. Remember, though, that hydrogenated vegetable oils will affect your body in much the same way as saturated fat from tropical oils and animal sources.

With saturated fat under control, what should you do about the unsaturates? There is more room for debate here, but I suggest a tilt toward the monounsaturates, with olive oil my first choice and canola oil second. In addition, I advocate eating fish at least 2 or 3 times weekly; as a result, the omega-3 polyunsaturates will provide a good proportion of your total dietary fat. Fill in the rest with polyunsaturates from unprocessed vegetable oils.

You need one more target: cholesterol. The average American consumes more than 450 milligrams of cholesterol per day. Our official committees suggest a limit of 300 milligrams for healthy people and 200 milligrams for individuals with high blood cholesterol levels. Ever the purist, I'd rather start with an upper limit of 200 milligrams and go down from there in the presence of a high blood LDL cholesterol level, a high cardiac risk score, or atherosclerosis. The new food labels help with cholesterol, just as they do with fat. Each label lists the food's total cholesterol content in milligrams and tells you what percent of the total daily value it represents. Be sure to take serving size into account, and remember that the percentage you see is based on a generous daily cholesterol target.

Can you get too *little* cholesterol in your diet? No — your body will make the cholesterol it needs (and, unfortunately, much more than it needs if you eat too much saturated fat). Theoretically the ideal amount of cholesterol in the human diet may be as low as zero, but only strict vegetarians can even come close. It's not a bad idea, but it's hardly necessary, especially if you follow the entire 15-point plan to conquer heart disease.

Can you get too little *fat* in your diet? Yes, but it's hard. Very hard — only two fatty acids are essential for health; both are polyunsaturates (linoleic and linolenic acids), and you can get enough of both from small amounts of vegetable oil. A 1994 study found that a diet with only 8 percent fat was both effective and safe, and some oriental cultures maintain excellent health with even less dietary fat. You don't have to go to these extremes to conquer heart disease, but you can reduce your dietary fat to meet your goals without worrying about going too far.

Finding the Fats

It took an unconscionably long time, but at last food labels actually contain useful nutritional information instead of misleading hype. To use them properly, you'll have to read them carefully (Figure 4–2). Skip the large print, concentrating instead on the actual data: the number of calories per serving, the content of the saturated and total fat in grams, and the cholesterol content in milligrams. Be sure to compare the serving size with your appetite. Remember that the percentage listed may not apply to your personal goal. And use the labels to learn about sodium (Chapter 6), fiber (Chapter 8), and vitamins (Chapters 11 and 17).

As helpful as they are, labels may not give you all the facts you need. Small food manufacturers don't have to label their products — nor do giant companies producing small packages. And in restaurants, you're on your own. Use Table 4–5 to find the fats and cholesterol in your favorite foods.

Table 4–5 is far from complete, but it should help you get started. Use it in conjunction with food labels to keep track of your total and saturated fat intake for three typical days. Once you know where you're starting from, you can use the tips in the next few pages to make the changes you need to achieve your goals.

As you look over Table 4–5, you'll see a few things that may surprise you. Granola, for example, hardly lives up to its reputation as a health food; instead, its high fat content places it among the undesirables. Remember to evaluate portion sizes carefully; most Americans, for example, serve more than 3 1/2 ounces, which is used in Table 4–5 for meats, poultry, and fish. Finally, you should recognize that Table 4–5 groups foods into undesirable, acceptable, or desirable strictly on the basis of fat and cholesterol content. You'll need to take other nutritional factors into account when you plan your menu; in general, fat content is a good guide to desirability, but there are exceptions. From the point

FIGURE 4–2: Reading Food Labels

10 steps to get the most from the new labels that have been mandatory since May, 1994.

1. Check the serving size; if your portion is bigger, you'll get more of everything.

2. Check the fat and cholesterol contents. Saturated fat and cholesterol are undesirable — but so are the partially hydrogenated vegetable oils that show up only at the bottom of the label, in the list of ingredients.

3. Check the fiber contents; the more the better.

6. Check the carbohydrate contents. Sugars are less desirable than the "other carbohydrates" — starches and other complex carbohydrates should provide at least 60 percent of your daily calories.

7. Check the protein contents. Only a modest protein intake (15 to 20 percent of calories) is necessary for health.

8. Review the vitamin and mineral contents. Remember, though, that the percentages are calculated on the basis of Recommended Daily Allowances that prevent deficiency diseases; substantially higher amounts of certain vitamins may help fight atherosclerosis.

3. Check the total calories and the calories from fat. To calculate the percent of calories from fat, multiply "calories from fat" by 100; then divide by "calories." (In this example, $10 \times 100 = 100 \div 50 = 20\%$). To conquer heart disease, keep your daily fat intake low, perhaps to 20 percent of your calories. To control your weight, keep your total calories low, too.

4. Check the sodium and potassium contents. A low sodium intake will help reduce your blood pressure; a high potassium intake may help, too.

9. Remember that all the percentages on the label are calculated on the basis of average targets. You may choose to set more stringent standards for yourself (less fat, cholesterol and sodium, more fiber and vitamins).

10. Check the ingredients, looking for partially hydrogenated vegetable oils, sugars, and additives that you may choose to avoid.

Nutrition Facts

Serving Size   1/2 cup (30g/1.1 oz.)
Servings per Container   11

Amount Per Serving	Cereal	Cereal with 1/2 Cup Vitamins A & D Skim Milk
Calories	50	90
Calories from Fat	10	10

	% Daily Value **	
Total Fat 1.0g*	2 %	2 %
Saturated Fat 0g	0 %	0 %
Cholesterol 0mg	0 %	0 %
Sodium 150mg	6 %	9 %
Potassium 350mg	10 %	16 %
Total Carbohydrate 22g	7 %	9 %
Dietary Fiber 15g	60 %	60 %
Sugars 0g		
Other Carbohydrate 7g		
Protein 4g		

Vitamin A	15 %	20 %
Vitamin C	25 %	25 %
Calcium	10 %	25 %
Iron	25 %	25 %
Vitamin D	10 %	25 %
Thiamin	25 %	30 %
Riboflavin	25 %	35 %
Niacin	25 %	25 %
Vitamin B₆	25 %	25 %
Folate	25 %	25 %
Vitamin B₁₂	25 %	35 %
Phosphorus	30 %	40 %
Magnesium	30 %	35 %
Zinc	25 %	25 %
Copper	15 %	15 %

*Amount in cereal. One half cup skim milk contributes an additional 40 calories, 65mg sodium, 6g total carbohydrate (6g sugars), and 4g protein.
**Percent Daily Values are based on a 2,000 calorie diet. Your daily values may be higher or lower depending on your calorie needs.

Calories		2,000	2,500
Total Fat	Less than	65g	80g
Sat. Fat	Less than	20g	25g
Cholesterol	Less than	300mg	300mg
Sodium	Less than	2,400mg	2,400mg
Potassium		3,500mg	3,500mg
Total Carbohydrate		300g	375g
Dietary Fiber		25g	30g

Calories per gram:
Fat 9 • Carbohydrate 4 • Protein 4

Ingredients: Wheat bran, corn bran, wheat flour, salt, baking soda, color added, aspartame, **Vitamins and Minerals:** calcium phosphate, calcium carbonate, sodium ascorbate and ascorbic acid (vitamin C), niacinamide, zinc oxide, iron, pyridoxine hydrochloride (vitamin B₆), riboflavin (vitamin B₂), vitamin A palmitate (protected with BHT), thiamine hydrochloride (vitamin B₁), folic acid, vitamin B₁₂, and vitamin D.
PHENYLKETONURICS: CONTAINS PHENALALANINE

Table 4–5
FINDING THE FATS

High in Saturated Fat and / or Cholesterol, and / or Trans-Fatty Acids; Undesirable

	Portion Size	Total Calories	Total Fat (grams)	Saturated Fat (grams)	% Calories from Fat	Total Cholesterol (milligrams)
Dairy Products						
Whole milk	8 oz.	150	8	5	48	33
Yogurt, plain	6 oz.	105	6	4	47	21
Cottage cheese	4 oz.	117	5	3	39	17
Sour cream	1 oz.	61	6	4	87	12
Cream cheese	1 oz.	99	10	6	90	31
Ricotta cheese (whole milk)	1 oz.	197	15	9	67	58
Ricotta cheese (part-skim milk)	1 oz.	156	9	6	52	25
Cheddar cheese	1 oz.	114	9	6	74	30
Parmesan cheese	1 oz.	129	9	5	59	22
Swiss cheese	1 oz.	107	8	5	65	26
Feta cheese	1 oz.	75	6	4	72	25
Egg yolk	1	63	6	2	80	272
Ice cream (premium)	1 cup	349	24	15	61	88
Ice cream (regular)	1 cup	269	14	9	48	59
Margarine	1 tbsp.	100	11	2	100	0
Meats (cooked)						
Hot dogs (beef)	1	158	14	6	82	31
Bologna (beef)	3 slices	312	28	12	82	58
Salami (beef)	3 slices	262	20	9	71	65
Chuck roast	3½ oz.	350	26	11	67	99
Ground beef	3½ oz.	272	19	7	61	87
Corned beef	3½ oz.	251	19	6	68	98

continued

Table 4–5 continued

High in Saturated Fat and / or Cholesterol, and / or Trans-Fatty Acids; Undesirable

	Portion Size	Total Calories	Total Fat (grams)	Saturated Fat (grams)	% Calories from Fat	Total Cholesterol (milligrams)
Rib roast	3½ oz.	225	12	5	47	80
T-bone steak	3½ oz.	214	10	4	44	80
Liver	3½ oz.	161	5	2	27	389
Lamb chop	3½ oz.	215	9	4	39	215
Bacon	3½ oz.	576	50	18	78	85
Ham	3½ oz.	178	9	3	46	92
Veal cutlet	3½ oz.	271	11	5	37	128
Poultry						
Duck	3½ oz.	201	11	4	50	89
Chicken (with skin)	3½ oz.	253	16	4	56	91
Seafood						
Shrimp	3½ oz.	99	1	trace	10	195
Vegetable Products						
Coconut meat	1 oz.	187	18	16	88	0
Baked Goods						
Croissant	1	235	12	4	46	13
Doughnut	1	210	12	3	51	20
Chocolate chip cookies	1	143	6	2	1	54
Cream pie	1 slice	455	23	15	46	8
Apple pie	1 slice	405	18	5	40	0
Chocolate cake	1 slice	235	8	4	31	37
Pound cake	1 slice	110	5	3	41	64
Waffle	1	245	13	5	48	102
Grain Products						
Granola	1 cup	595	33	6	50	0
Snacks & Sweets						

Pizza	1 slice	290	9	4	28	56
French fries	10 strips	156	8	4	46	9
Potato chips	1 oz.	147	10	3	62	0
Salted crackers	4	50	1	trace	18	4
Chocolate	1 oz.	145	9	5	56	6
Sauces & Dressings						
Mayonnaise	1 tbsp.	99	11	2	100	8
Russian dressing	1 tbsp.	76	8	1	92	4
Hollandaise sauce	1/2 cup	353	34	21	87	94

Moderate to Low in Fat, Saturated Fat, and Cholesterol: Acceptable in Moderation

Dairy						
Low-fat milk (1%)	8 oz.	102	3	2	23	10
Frozen yogurt	1 cup	216	2	0	8	0
Sherbet	1 cup	270	4	2	13	14
Poultry						
Chicken (without skin)	3½ oz.	205	10	3	43	91
Turkey (without skin)	3½ oz.	126	4	1	24	112
Seafood						
Lobster	3½ oz.	98	1	trace	6	72
Cod	3½ oz.	105	1	trace	9	55
Flounder, sole	3½ oz.	99	1	trace	9	58
Grain Products						
Egg noodles	1 cup	160	2	1	11	50
Baked Goods						
Bran muffin	1	125	6	1	43	24
Oatmeal cookie	1	46	3	trace	37	14
Miscellaneous						
Peanut butter	1 oz.	95	8	1	76	0

continued

Table 4–5 continued

	Portion Size	Total Calories	Total Fat (grams)	Saturated Fat (grams)	% Calories from Fat	Total Cholesterol (milligrams)
Moderate to Low in Fat, Saturated Fat, and Cholesterol; Acceptable in Moderation						
Popcorn (oil popped)	1 cup	55	3	trace	49	0
Pretzels	1 oz.	10	trace	trace	0	0
Low-cal French or Italian dressing	1 tbsp.	20	1	trace	45	0
Margarine, soft	1 tbsp.	50	5	1	90	0
Nondairy creamer, light	1 tbsp.	10	1	0	100	0
High in Unsaturated Fats; Acceptable in Moderation						
Walnuts	1 oz.	182	18	2	87	0
Pecans	1 oz.	187	18	2	89	0
Peanuts	1 oz.	164	14	2	76	0
Pistachios	1 oz.	164	14	2	76	0
Sunflower seeds	1 oz.	165	14	1	77	0
Sunflower oil	1 tbsp.	125	14	1	100	0
Safflower oil	1 tbsp.	125	14	1	100	0
Corn oil	1 tbsp.	125	14	2	100	0
Avocado	1	305	30	4	88	0
High in Monounsaturated Fat; Desirable in Moderation						
Olive oil	1 tbsp.	125	14	2	100	0
Canola oil	1 tbsp.	125	14	1	100	0
High in Omega-3 Oils; Desirable in Moderation						
Mackerel	3½ oz.	262	18	4	62	75
Salmon	3½ oz.	216	11	2	46	87
Tuna (fresh)	3½ oz.	184	6	2	31	49

Trout	3½ oz.	105	4	1	26	73
Halibut	3½ oz.	140	3	trace	19	41

Low in Fat and Cholesterol; Desirable

Dairy Products						
Skim milk	8 oz.	86	trace	trace	5	4
Buttermilk	8 oz.	99	2	1	20	9
Low-fat yogurt (plain)	6 oz.	94	trace	trace	3	3
Low-fat cottage cheese	4 oz.	82	1	1	13	5
Egg white	1	16	trace	0	0	0
Egg substitutes	2 oz.	15–60	0–3	0	0–45	0
Frozen yogurt (nonfat)	1 cup	175	0	0	0	0
Baked Goods						
Whole wheat bread	1 slice	70	1	trace	13	0
Bagel	1	200	2	trace	9	0
Pita	½ shell	165	1	trace	5	0
English muffin	1	140	1	trace	6	0
Pancake	1	60	2	trace	30	16
Fig bar	1	52	1	trace	17	5
Grain Products						
Rice	1 cup	225	1	trace	2	0
Spaghetti	1 cup	155	1	trace	6	0
Oatmeal	1 cup	145	2	trace	15	0
Beans						
Garbanzo beans	1 cup	269	4	trace	14	0
Lima beans	1 cup	217	1	trace	3	0
Kidney beans	1 cup	225	1	trace	3	0
Split peas	1 cup	231	1	trace	3	0
Vegetables						
Potato (baked)	1	220	trace	trace	0	0

continued

Table 4–5 continued

	Portion Size	Total Calories	Total Fat (grams)	Saturated Fat (grams)	% Calories from Fat	Total Cholesterol (milligrams)
Low in Fat and Cholesterol; Desirable						
Broccoli	1 spear	50	1	trace	25	0
Carrot	1 wedge	30	trace	trace	0	0
Lettuce	1 wedge	20	trace	trace	0	0
Mushrooms	1 cup	20	trace	trace	0	0
Squash	1 cup	35	1	trace	30	0
Tomato	1	25	trace	trace	0	0
Fruits						
Apple	1	80	trace	trace	0	0
Banana	1	105	1	trace	8	0
Berries	1 cup	80	1	trace	11	0
Dates	10	230	trace	trace	0	0
Melon	1/4	40	trace	trace	0	0
Orange	1	60	trace	trace	0	0
Snacks						
Popcorn (air popped)	1 cup	30	trace	trace	0	0
Graham crackers	2	55	1	trace	9	0
Rye crackers	2	56	1	trace	0	0
Gumdrops	1 oz.	100	trace	trace	0	0
Hard candy	1 oz.	110	trace	trace	0	0
Gelatin	1/2 cup	70	0	0	6	0
Angel food cake	1 slice	160	1	0	0	0
Nonfat mayonnaise, salad dressings, and cheese substitutes	variable	0	0	0	0

Principal source: "Nutritive Value of Foods." U.S. Department of Agriculture.

of view of fat, for example, regular pretzels are a great snack — but they are very *un*desirable in terms of their salt content (Chapter 6). Similarly, gumdrops and hard candy are fat-free, but because they have lots of sugar, they're less than ideal for people who are trying to lose weight. And if Table 4–5 doesn't give all the bad news about food, it doesn't give all the good news either. Some items in the desirable category, for example, are particularly valuable because of their high content of fiber (see Chapter 8) or vitamins (Chapters 11 and 17).

Facing the Fats: Achieving Your Goals

You know how dietary fat and cholesterol promote atherosclerosis and why they are important to health. You understand the differences between saturated and unsaturated fats. You have established personal goals for dietary fat based on your unique needs. You can find the hidden fats in foods. Now it's time to put theory into practice, to put your mouth where your mind is.

Here are some tips for achieving a low-fat diet:

- Change slowly. You eat a thousand meals each year, plus innumerable snacks. Eating habits are deeply ingrained; to avoid kitchen shock, give yourself time to change. Plan to change one item each week; in just a few months, your diet will be much better, and the change will have been painless. Breakfast is a good place to start. Switch from whole milk to 2 percent or 1 percent milk, then skim milk. Change from doughnuts to muffins to bran cereal or from waffles to toast. Add fruits and juices. Before long you'll be ready — and willing — to move on to low-fat lunches.
- Think about food. A low-fat diet is not a punishment, but an opportunity. Read low-fat cookbooks, swap recipes, and be adventurous.
- Give yourself a bit more time in the kitchen. Vegetable-based, low-fat cooking is more time consuming than simply frying up a few burgers. A microwave and food processor will save time; you'll recoup your investment quickly, since vegetables and grains are less expensive than meats and prepared foods.
- Enlist your family in your plans. It will be much easier to change if the other people in your household participate in the effort.
- Plan for the long term — your new style of eating is designed to help you live longer and better; it's not a temporary diet, but a permanent

nutrition program. Measure your progress with a calendar, not a clock.

- Be relaxed. Establish the important principles but give yourself some flexibility in the details; a fatty tidbit here and there won't do you in, but as times goes on, you'll be much less tempted to "cheat."
- Think positively. Expect to succeed, and you will. Expect to enjoy your new style of eating — you will!

If Not Fat, What? Creating a Balanced Diet

To keep the fat out of your arteries and away from your waistline, get the fat out of your diet. To maintain your general health and make eating a pleasure, replace fat with a balanced mix of nutrients. Here are 14 guidelines:

- Eat a variety of foods. There is no perfect food, but you can establish a perfectly wonderful mix of foods.
- Eat fewer animal products and more vegetable products.
- Eat fewer processed foods and more fresh and homemade foods.
- Eat more fiber. You'll help conquer heart disease and many intestinal diseases (Chapter 8).
- Eat more complex carbohydrates and less refined sugar. You'll get many more nutrients, and you'll help control your weight (Chapter 15). Complex carbohydrates should supply about 65 percent of your daily calories.
- Eat protein in moderation. Protein is essential for health, but excess protein adds unnecessary calories and may contribute to calcium loss, osteoporosis, kidney stones, and kidney disease. Protein should provide about 15 percent of your daily calories.
- Eat less sodium and more potassium and calcium. You'll help lower your blood pressure and protect your heart (Chapter 6).
- Eat more grain products, especially whole grains. You'll get fiber, B vitamins, and complex carbohydrates.
- Eat more beans and other legumes. You'll get important vitamins and minerals as well as the soluble fiber that helps fight atherosclerosis (Chapter 8).
- Eat more vegetables, especially those with vitamins A and C. You'll get the fiber, vitamins, and antioxidants you need (Chapter 11).
- Eat more fruits — for the same reasons you eat vegetables.
- Eat more fish; it's a natural way to fight atherosclerosis (Chapter 10).

- If you use alcohol, use it in the way that will protect your heart without harming your health (Chapter 9).
- Adjust your calories to maintain ideal body weight. But remember that fat, fiber, and exercise are even more important than calories (Chapter 15).
- Build a balanced diet around low-fat foods. Eat only low-fat or, better yet, nonfat dairy products. Eat egg yolks only very sparingly. Eat little meat, always trimming away the fat and avoiding prime and other fatty cuts, organ meats, and processed meats. Eat chicken and turkey in moderation, always removing the skin. Use vegetable oils in moderation, favoring olive and canola oils and avoiding hydrogenated vegetable oils and tropical oils.

Thoughts for Food

As a cook, I make a fine doctor. But I do love to eat. Fortunately, my wife understands the great importance of nutrition for health, and she's also a master cook; her experiences and tips are reflected throughout these thoughts for food.

To plan a healthful nutritional program, you have to understand nutrients. But people don't eat nutrients. To plan a good meal, you have to understand food. Happily, the two are entirely compatible: healthful ingredients can be used to make great food.

Good nutrition is essential for good health. But meals are more than nutritional necessities; they should enrich life by providing personal pleasure and interpersonal socialization, interest and variety, and just plain fun.

It's time to put down your calculator and pick up your colander; we're moving from the chem lab to the kitchen — and the dining room.

Poultry

The conversation is so predictable that it's almost a ritual. When I ask my patients to reduce their dietary fat, they invariably reply that they're already "doing fish and chicken." I've learned not to take the answer at face value. For most people, fish and chicken means mostly chicken. Even worse, most people seem to believe that as long as it's chicken, they can cook it any way at all and eat all they want. Right church, wrong pew.

Chicken is flying high in America. In 1950, the average person ate only 8.7 pounds of chicken, but by 1988 chicken consumption had soared to 61.9 pounds per person. As a nation, we now eat more chicken than beef. I'm all for it — but to be a really healthful food, chicken should be cooked and eaten according to simple nutritional guidelines.

Remember that as an animal product, poultry contains saturated fat and cholesterol. Turkey is lowest in fat, earning it a position as the most healthful land-animal food. Chicken is a bit higher in fat but is still an excellent food — if you use it right. The light meat of poultry has less fat than the dark meat; by switching from dark to light, you can save 5 grams of fat in a 3 1/2 ounce serving. You can save even more fat by avoiding the skin. Consider a small chicken breast. If cooked without its skin, it contains only 60 calories. When cooked with its skin, but the skin is removed before it is eaten, it supplies 140 calories. But when cooked and eaten with its skin, it has 200 calories. By removing the skin before cooking, you'll save 140 calories; more important, you'll save more than 15 grams of fat!

It's also very important to cook your chicken properly. Many recipes will allow you to keep poultry tender and moist even if it's cooked without the skin. Instead of frying your chicken, roast, bake, grill, or microwave it. If you do sauté chicken, use broth or wine instead of oil or fat. You can also save fat by using nonstick pans or nonfat or olive oil sprays.

Remember that no matter how you prepare chicken, you must cook it thoroughly. One-third of all the poultry in the United States is contaminated by bacteria that can cause diarrhea in humans. To prevent foul results, follow sound guidelines for cooking and refrigeration; you can get good advice by calling the poultry hotline of the U.S. Department of Agriculture (800-535-4555) during business hours.

You can buy poultry in many forms, ranging from ground meat to hot dogs to sliced meat; because of its lower fat content, turkey is particularly desirable as a substitute for red meat. Remember, though, that smoked turkey is high in sodium. And when you order chicken or turkey at a restaurant, be sure to find out how it's been cooked and what's being served as a sauce or stuffing. Unfortunately, it's very easy to turn a low-fat bird into a high-fat meal.

How much poultry should you eat? The answer, of course, depends on your health (especially your cholesterol, blood pressure, and weight), your goals, and your tastes. Still, from the viewpoint of fat and protein, many people could do well eating less chicken. A standard portion of 3 to 4 ounces (which is about the size of a deck of cards), seems about right. And if you're getting your fish and pasta on schedule, 2 to 4 poultry meals a week will fill out your menu nicely.

Meat

Red meat has gotten a reputation as the bad guy of the American diet. In general, it's a reputation that is well deserved. Meat, of course, is not the only culprit. Still, reducing your meat consumption is an important step in eschewing the fat in your diet.

Meat does contain valuable nutrients, including iron, zinc, vitamins, and protein. But beef, pork, and lamb are all high in saturated fat, cholesterol, and calories; veal has less fat but more cholesterol. All are expensive. Clearly there are many ways to get the good nutrients without the bad constituents of red meat.

You can reduce sharply the fat content of chicken and turkey by simply removing the skin. It's not so easy with beef. Trimming the excess fat away from the outside of meat will help. But seams of fat also run throughout the meat itself, where they cannot be cut away. In fact, it's the fat that gives the meat the taste and texture that people have learned to like. Cattle are kept in pens, stuffed with food, and treated with hormones and antibiotics precisely in order to fatten them up. Adding insult to injury, you'll actually pay more for the fat; except for the costly new "designer beef" and extra-lean ground beef, prime grades of beef are the most expensive because they are the most marbled — they have the most fat.

You don't have to avoid all red meat to be healthy (though it wouldn't hurt). But if you choose to eat meat, you should select it carefully, prepare it properly, and eat it sparingly. Avoid fatty cuts of beef, pork, and lamb. Spare ribs, organ meats (liver, kidney), and processed meats (sausages, hot dogs, cold cuts, bacon) are always on the undesirable list. Break the "prime" and "choice" beef habit; instead of paying more for those high-fat cuts, buy "select," "lean," cuts. Trim all visible fat before cooking. Don't fry or braise meat; instead, roast, grill, broil, or bake it on a rack so that fat can drip away. If you use meat in a stew, be sure to skim off the fat before serving.

Grilling meat may reduce its fat content, but it introduces another hazard — cancer. The very high temperature generated in open-flame cooking produces chemicals (called heterocyclic aromatic amines) that can cause cancer in animals. To reduce your risk, trim the meat carefully to avoid dripping fat that will make the flames flare up. Next, precook the meat in a microwave for two to three minutes before grilling, being sure to discard the juices that accumulate. When you barbecue the meat, use cooler, gray coals and baste carefully to avoid feeding the fire. If flames do flare up, extinguish them quickly by spraying on some water. Similar precautions are reasonable for grilled fish and chicken, but you will also get protection simply by removing their skins before they are eaten.

Buying the leanest meat and cooking it properly will help. So, too, will serving it appropriately. Avoid high-fat gravies and sauces. Remember that catsup and steak sauces are high in sodium. And don't serve seconds.

Best of all, learn that there is life after hamburgers. Meat has always been part of the human diet, but it was a luxury item until the agricultural and industrial revolutions increased its availability and decreased its price. Since then, meat has become a dietary staple while still maintaining its status as a prestige food. We need new ways of thinking about meat, ways that will restore its old role as a dietary supplement instead of a staple. Think of meat as a condiment or side dish instead of a main dish. Make it a small part of your meal, using grains, legumes, and vegetables as your main dish. Reduce the amount of meat you use in casseroles and stews, or eliminate it entirely, using beans or ground turkey instead.

How much meat should you eat? The short answer is the less the better, but the long answer depends on your health, your goals, and your preferences. For most people, 3 to 4 ounces once or twice a week is a reasonable target. For most people, it will take time and effort to reach this goal. Many people will beef about these changes at first, only to discover that they enjoy their new style of eating more than their old.

Don't make the "v word" an issue. The question is not whether to become a vegetarian (I'm not), but how to protect your health while enjoying your food. Think it over and experiment with new ways of cooking and new styles of eating. Discuss it with your family and give it some time. Avoid fiery debate and arrive at a meeting of the minds. Only you can decide what's in your best interests.

Dairy Products and Eggs

Is nothing sacred? After skinning chicken and bashing beef, I'm turning to consider two more icons of the American diet, dairy products and eggs. You'll see, however, that I'm not on a personal vendetta against cows and hens; on the contrary, I'm utterly in favor of low-fat dairy products and egg whites.

The issues, of course, are saturated fat, cholesterol, and, to a lesser extent, salt. Fortunately this is one area in which the food industry is ahead of the average consumer; many low-fat dairy products are already available, just waiting for you to learn how best to use them.

Substitute low-fat milk for whole milk. To ease the transition, start with milk that has 2 percent fat, then move to 1 percent, and finally to skim milk, which is fat-free. You'll save fat and calories without sacrificing calcium, vitamin D, or milk protein.

For cooking, try evaporated skim milk instead of milk or cream. Add 1 tablespoon of cornstarch for each cup of evaporated milk if your recipe calls for heating.

Select nonfat sour cream or make your own sour cream substitute simply by pureeing low-fat cottage cheese in a blender with a touch of lemon juice. If you like your sour cream sour, add several tablespoons of buttermilk or some nonfat plain yogurt. Or use low-fat or nonfat plain yogurt; drain the yogurt through a coffee filter or a double layer of cheesecloth in a strainer in the refrigerator overnight. Discard the water and use the smooth semisolid yogurt in place of sour cream. The low-fat substitute is fine on baked potatoes and excellent as the base for various dips. It's also great for cooking, but if you're using it in a recipe that calls for heating, add 1 tablespoon of cornstarch for each cup of yogurt to prevent it from separating.

Buy nonfat cream cheese or make your own cream cheese substitute. Just drain nonfat yogurt in the refrigerator overnight, then mix in a little olive oil. The chives are up to you; only the cook will know for sure that it's not the real, high-fat spread.

Make your own cream substitute. Puree equal portions of nonfat yogurt and part-skim milk ricotta cheese in a blender until the mix is smooth. You can't heat this "cream," but you can serve it over hot foods. Another cream substitute can be fashioned by adding some nonfat powdered milk to skim milk.

You can even make fake whipped cream. Evaporated skim milk will fill the bill, but this act of low-fat alchemy requires you to place an unopened can of milk in your freezer for a full hour before you whip it. The trick is to keep the temperature low: chill your mixing bowl and beaters before you use them, and if the milk is not whipping well, put the bowl back in the freezer for a few minutes before you resume whipping.

When you're making your own dairy substitutes, you'll be able to control their contents. But commercial substitutes can be tricky. Frozen whipped toppings are high in fat, though newer "lite" varieties are better. Many nondairy creamers are also high in fat, including saturated fat (from tropical oils) in some and trans-fatty acids (from hydrogenated vegetable oils) in others. If you can't get used to low-fat milk or skim milk in your coffee, look for the new "lite" creamers that have less fat — and read their labels carefully, remembering that most list their ingredients for serving sizes of only half an ounce. You can also consider the fat-free nondairy creamers that are now available in most supermarkets.

Use substitutes for butter. Margarine is the easy answer, but remember that it has as much fat and as many calories as butter. The difference is that butter has animal fat, which is composed of saturated fatty acids, while margarine has vegetable oils. The catch is that in order to solidify margarine, manufacturers add hydrogen, creating trans-fatty acids that act like saturated fat. The solution: use liquid or tub margarine instead of stick margarine, and use it sparingly. Nonfat margarine substitutes are now available; they're good on bread but they can't be used for cooking, and they don't fare well in the freezer.

Use nonfat yogurt instead of yogurt made from whole milk. Use nonfat or 1 percent cottage cheese instead of creamed cottage cheese.

Use nonfat or low-fat frozen desserts instead of ice cream. You'll have a fine time testing the many alternatives until you find your favorite. Try frozen yogurt, nonfat ice milk, sherbert, frozen fruit bars, or fat-free ice cream imitations.

Eat only very little cheese. Try the imitation cheese products that are now appearing in dairy departments; they won't fool true cheese-lovers, but they can be useful substitutes for many people. Use part-skim milk ricotta or mozzarella, but use them in moderation because they still contain fat, cholesterol, and sodium. As a substitute for ricotta cheese, use fat-free cottage cheese or try fromage blanc; it's fat-free, but it's expensive and may be hard to find. Or make your own by gently heating buttermilk until it begins to separate; then drain the curd through a coffee filter or through a strainer lined with cheesecloth.

Use many fewer eggs. Don't rely on "low cholesterol," "omega-3," or "range-fed chickens'" eggs. For baking, try substituting 2 egg whites for each egg yolk; if you need extra richness, add a little vegetable oil. Or use frozen or refrigerated egg substitutes; they are also excellent for omelets or scrambling. By using substitutes, it should be easy to limit yourself to no more than 2 or 3 egg yolks per week.

Use less mayonnaise, and stick with "imitation," "lite," or best of all (if you find its taste acceptable), nonfat mayonnaise. You can also make your own substitute from low-fat plain yogurt flavored with a bit of mustard.

Substitution is the key to using low-fat dairy and egg products in a healthful diet. In time, you'll come to enjoy natural low-fat foods that require less preparation. Until then, substitute away. It's chicanery, but it's in a good cause: you'll trick your palate and protect your arteries. And it's really no different from other forms of cooking, all of which require creativity and imagination, if not magic.

You've cut down on meat, dairy products, and even poultry. Replace them with the fantastic five: grains, legumes, vegetables, fruits, and fish.

Grains

Grain products should be one of the five mainstays of your diet. They provide complex carbohydrates, B vitamins, and minerals with very little fat; whole grain foods are also an excellent source of fiber. Aim for 6 or more servings of grain products every day.

Start your day with grains. Bran *cereal* is an ideal breakfast; oat and wheat bran cereals are both excellent, either hot or cold — but be sure to choose brands that are truly high in fiber, and use skim milk or low-fat milk. Beware of granola-type cereals, which are high in fat and calories — another example of a traditional "health" food that does not deserve its reputation. In contrast, whole wheat toast is excellent breakfast food; use small amounts of tub or nonfat margarine for a spread, or try jelly or honey alone. Whole wheat bagels are also excellent; bran muffins are equally good *if* they are baked without hydrogenated oils (see baked goods, below).

Pasta makes a splendid main dish. At lunch or for summer dinners, try cold pasta salads. If you have pasta for dinner as often as we do, you'll enjoy the variety provided by pastas in various shapes; vegetable pastas add to the fun by adding new colors and tastes. Whole wheat pastas will give you a different texture and flavor, as well as some extra fiber. Variety notwithstanding, egg pastas are less desirable because they contain fat and cholesterol, and high-protein pastas are unnecessary since a healthful diet will provide more than enough protein.

Pastas are quick and easy to prepare. A pasta pot with a removable strainer makes cooking even easier. Try gradually reducing the salt in your water; many people learn to enjoy pasta even more if it's cooked in plain water or with savory, oregano, or pepper.

Your family won't complain about "pasta again" if you learn to prepare a variety of sauces. We favor primavera and other vegetable sauces; seafood (such as scallops or salmon) is also splendid over pasta. Chicken, too, can be part of a great sauce. Tomato-based sauces are both traditional and tasty; be aware, though, that commercial tomato sauces are often high in salt. Traditional sauces that you should use very sparingly (if at all) include meat, cheese, and butter sauces.

There are many other ways to add grains to your meal plan. Rice (particularly brown rice), bulgur, couscous, buckwheat, and polenta (yellow cornmeal) are great with any meal. Barley is particularly healthful because it's rich in soluble fiber (see Chapter 8). Begin to think of grain products as main dishes, not side dishes; they're also superb as the base for casseroles. Try cooking your grains with basil, dill, onion powder, or turmeric in place of salt. Leftover grains don't freeze well, but they can be refrigerated for rewarming or for use in soups, casseroles, stuffings, and cold salads.

Breads are wonderful ways to make grains part of your diet. Whole grain breads and rolls are the best for you, but within this category you can find an almost endless variety of tastes, colors, and textures. Bagels and even English muffins can also be delicious when baked from whole grains. For added variety, consider ethnic breads, such as a French baguette or an Italian loaf, a Jewish rye or Syrian pita, a Russian black bread or a Mexican tortilla. I usually eat my bread dry, but my wife prefers to use a little soft margarine; we both enjoy a touch of olive oil instead of a spread from time to time.

Other *baked goods* can also be worthy ways to get grains into your diet, but you'll need to think a bit before you bite into your cookies, cakes, or muffins. Many commercially baked goods are made with eggs and butter; as a result, they contain undesirable amounts of saturated fat and cholesterol. But even "cholesterol-free" baked goods can be problematic. Many are made with palm or coconut oils; despite their vegetable origins, these are saturated fats. And many baked goods are prepared with partially hydrogenated vegetable oils containing trans-fatty acids that can also raise your blood cholesterol levels.

Don't even think about doughnuts, croissants, or Danish pastry. Think carefully about the traditional "healthful" alternative, the muffin. A small bran muffin will give you 2 grams of fiber — but you'll also get 6 grams of fat, 24 milligrams of cholesterol, and 125 calories. Substitute an English muffin, a bagel, or some whole wheat toast, and you'll save all the fat and cholesterol. Remember, though, to go easy on the spread; try jam or honey, and you'll have a satisfying, very low-fat snack.

Many bakeries are starting to offer low-fat muffins, cakes, pies, and pastries. Ask about ingredients, and read labels carefully to find out what you're really getting. Be skeptical, too, of some claims about fiber; remember that "wheat flour" and "unbleached flour" are just refined flour by another name; *whole* wheat (or rye or oat) flour is the real thing.

If you're fond of commercially baked goods, you can always rely on the low-fat standby, angel food cake. Graham crackers, gingersnaps, animal crackers, and fig bars are also healthful. But you can get much more variety by doing some baking yourself. Here are a few tips to add health without sacrificing flavor:

- Use fewer eggs. Try substituting 2 egg whites for each whole egg in your recipe, or use frozen egg substitutes.
- Use less shortening. Most cakes and cookies can be made with just 2 tablespoons of shortening for each cup of flour; muffins and biscuits are fine with half as much, and some yeast breads can be made without any fat. Use vegetable oil in place of melted butter. Use soft (tub) margarine in recipes that require creamed shortening.
- Use less sugar. Try reducing the sugar in your recipes by one-third to one-half; cinnamon, vanilla, or nutmeg can enhance the flavor of baked goods made with less sugar.

- If your baked goods tend to be a bit dry with less fat, try substituting a liquid sweetener for sugar; use 3/4 cup of honey, maple syrup, molasses, or corn syrup in place of each cup of sugar, and decrease the amount of another liquid used in the recipe by a similar amount.
- Use a fruit puree to replace fat in a recipe. Pureed bananas, apricots, prunes, pumpkins, or sweet potatoes add the moisture and texture that you may miss without fat. You can achieve this with apple butter, pear butter (both fat-free despite their names), or even with baby foods such as pureed prunes.
- Use less sodium. One-quarter teaspoon of salt for every cup of flour should suffice for yeast breads; for other baked goods, try reducing the recipe's salt content by half. Use only 1 teaspoon of baking powder per cup of flour in cakes, and 1 1/4 teaspoons per cup of flour in biscuits and muffins.
- Use more fiber. Try substituting whole wheat flour for half the white flour in your recipes.
- Use less chocolate, especially milk chocolate. Replace each ounce of chocolate with 3 tablespoons of cocoa; if you need to replace the lost fat, add 1 tablespoon of canola oil or corn oil for each ounce of chocolate that you've removed.

Each recipe is different, so you'll have to experiment a bit to find the modification that works best for you. With a few creative substitutions, you'll be able to have your cake and conscience, too.

Legumes

Long neglected in the American diet, legumes should be among your dietary staples; they provide complex carbohydrates, soluble fiber, protein, iron, and B vitamins. When you think of them not as legumes, but as beans, peas, and lentils, you'll realize that they are also delicious. Aim for 2 or more servings per day.

It takes some practice to prepare legumes properly. It may even take a little practice to eat them comfortably. You'll learn all about legumes, and other sources of soluble fiber, in Chapter 8.

Vegetables

It may have surprised you to find legumes among the nutritional fantastic five, but it's no surprise that vegetables are a dietary mainstay. Vegetables provide complex carbohydrates and fiber as well as iron, calcium, and many other nutrients. They are loaded with vitamins and are particularly valuable for their beta-carotene and vitamin C contents. Vegetables are naturally low in fat, calories, and sodium. Aim for 3 or more servings per day, including at least one rich in vitamin A (deep green and yellow vegetables) and one rich in Vitamin C (green pepper, cauliflower, asparagus, cabbage, potatoes, tomatoes, spinach) per day. Eat a cabbage-family vegetable at least twice a week.

Vegetables are just as important for their culinary value as for their nutritional role. They add color, texture, and variety to your menu. Cooked or raw, vegetables are delicious.

Don't overcook your fresh vegetables; to maximize their content of vitamins, use only a minimum amount of water, and cook only until they are tender but still crisp. Even better, use a microwave to cook your veggies — you'll preserve nutrients and gain speed and convenience. Vegetables are also excellent when they're stir-fried. But remember to fry wisely; use nonstick pans, nonfat lubricating sprays, or small amounts of vegetable oil. Olive oil comes in a spray allowing you to cover your pan with a very small amount of oil. For seasoning, use lemon juice, pepper, or herbs instead of salt. Substitute butter sprinkles (Molly McButter, Butter Buds) are also good ways to add flavor.

Frozen vegetables are more convenient than fresh vegetables; they are less tasty and more expensive, but they retain most of the nutritional value of fresh produce. Most canned vegetables are lower in vitamins and much higher in salt, making them less desirable. And remember that cream- or butter-based sauces will detract from the nutritional value of any vegetable dish.

Vegetables themselves can be used as fat substitutes in sauces and dips. Experiment with various cooked vegetable purees to add moisture, texture, and thickness to low-fat sauces; you'll also be able to add interesting new flavors. Pureed potatoes or roasted onions are examples.

Salads are a wonderful way to add vegetables to your lunch or dinner. Use salads for a main course or a side dish. Use spinach or Romaine lettuce as a green to get more vitamin A, iron, and fiber. Don't think of a salad as simply lettuce and tomatoes — add peppers, carrots, broccoli, zucchini, or corn. Include legumes such as cooked peas, beans, or garbanzos to give flavor and variety to your salads. For a main-course salad, add some tuna, chicken, or turkey. Be a creative salad-maker.

Be a thoughtful salad-maker. Skip the croutons, olives, and avocados that add unnecessary salt and fat; omit cheese, eggs, and bacon as well.

Dressings also require some thought. You can reduce the fat and calorie content of an oil and vinegar dressing by diluting it with one-third water before you serve it; to compensate for its less intense flavor, try adding herbs or flavored mustard. Avoid creamy dressings unless they are the low-fat or "lite" variety — and use even these sparingly. Fortunately many excellent nonfat dressings are now available.

Although I've never met a vegetable I didn't like, not all vegetables are created equal. Deep green and yellow vegetables and cruciferous (cabbage family) vegetables are valuable for their cancer-fighting properties. Less familiar, perhaps, are the root vegetables, which are being investigated for their possible role in preventing blood clots. Garlic and onions also merit special mention; long used as folk remedies, new scientific data do contain a whiff of evidence that they may in fact help lower blood cholesterol levels, but more studies will be needed to sniff out all the facts (see Chapter 17). On the negative side of the ledger are the saturated fats in palm (and coconut) oils and the unsaturated fats in avocados (technically fruits, but usually found on the vegetable aisles).

Another possible negative consideration is the presence of pesticide residues on produce. Fortunately, this concern is more theoretical than actual. You can minimize your exposure by washing carefully all fruits and vegetables and by selecting organically grown fresh produce.

Even accounting for these concerns, the balance sheet clearly favors adding vegetables to your menu whenever possible. Use them for appetizers, side dishes, and salads. Order extra veggies in restaurants. Use vegetables in soups, and eat them for snacks. Add them to sandwiches. Use them for toppings on pasta. Consider, too, that vegetables can be ideal for main dishes and can be the principal ingredients of wonderful stews and casseroles.

Fruit

Fruit has it all, from nutrients (especially carbohydrates, fiber, beta-carotene, vitamin C, potassium, and iron) to flavor to fun. Few people need to be persuaded that fruit should be a dietary staple, but many may profit from a reminder to eat at least 2 servings (including one rich in vitamin C) per day.

You can enjoy fruit fresh or cooked, frozen or canned, dried or squeezed into juice. Locally grown fruit is inexpensive in season, but transported fruit is available year-round.

It's easy to add fruit to your menu. Fruit juice is a great way to start the day; fruit is also wonderful on your breakfast cereal or as a side dish. At lunch or dinner, fruit can add variety to many salads. Fruit slices are good appetizers, and cold fruit soups are a unique summer treat. Fruit is an ideal snack and a wonderful dessert. It can be served fresh, cooked, or dried, either alone or as a topping over yogurt.

Over the years, patients have given me excuses for almost everything — but I have yet to hear a credible reason for avoiding fruit.

Fish

It's no accident that grains, legumes, vegetables, and fruit head the list of dietary staples. But animal products can also belong on a healthful menu. Fish, in fact, *should* be on your menu. Fish occupies first place among animal products because it contains the omega-3 fatty acids that improve blood cholesterol levels, fight blood clots, and reduce the risk of atherosclerosis. Chapter 10 explains how fish can help conquer heart disease.

Soups

Think of your soup bowl as a nutritional melting pot — soup is an excellent way to add grains, legumes, vegetables, and even fruit to your diet.

Soups present many marvelous opportunities to the health-conscious cook. Noodles, rice, and barley are excellent in soup, as are peas, beans, and lentils. Vegetables, too, can be incorporated into innumerable soups. Vegetable and chicken stocks can be just as tasty as meat-based soups, and they are better for you. Cream-based chowders and soups are not on my menu unless they are prepared with low-fat dairy products. My menu is also free of commercial soups with high sodium content; pepper, mixed spices, and individual herbs provide all the flavor I could ever wish for.

Hot or cold, before a meal or as a main course, alone or accompanied by salad and bread — soup is nutrition with a smile.

Snacks

Three square meals is an American idea ranking close behind motherhood and apple pie. I'm all for moms and for pies (if made with low-fat ingredients), and I love breakfast, lunch, and dinner. But scientists at the

University of Toronto found that men eating 17 snacks a day had better cholesterol levels than men eating the same nutrients in 3 traditional meals. Other researchers at Tufts University found that college students test better after snacking. Don't give up breakfast, lunch, or dinner. But feel free to nibble between meals — as long as your snacks fit into your overall nutrition plan.

My patients frequently complain that they can't find any healthful snack foods. I've recommended dozens throughout this chapter, and I'll list a few here to help you enjoy nutritious noshing.

> Fresh fruit
> Dried fruit
> Raw vegetables, alone or with low-fat dips
> Bread, toast, bagels, bread sticks, rice cakes, matzos
> Melba toast, Ry-Krisp, graham crackers
> Cereals, dry or with skim milk
> Low-salt or unsalted pretzels
> Popcorn (air popped and unsalted)
> Walnuts, unsalted peanuts, almonds, unsalted sunflower seeds
> Fig bars, animal crackers, gingersnaps, vanilla wafers
> Nonfat yogurt and frozen desserts
> Angel food cake
> Homemade baked goods
> Low-fat and low-cholesterol commercial baked goods
> Jelly beans, gumdrops, hard candy

I think you'll agree that it's an appealing list. Choose the ones you like best. None have harmful ingredients but some have valuable nutrients (fruits, vegetables, whole grain baked goods) while others are empty calories (candy).

Remember, too, to avoid traditional snack foods that are not on the list, including chips, doughnuts, salted popcorn and pretzels, cheese, and ice cream. Because of their salt, processed peanuts and seeds are also in the avoid category — but natural nuts and seeds are just fine. If you like peanut butter, make it all-natural, without added salt and fat.

Beware of traditional "health" snacks that are actually high in fat, including commercially baked muffins, granola bars, and carrot cakes. Because of its high fat content (55 percent) and its sugar and calories, you are also better off without chocolate, especially milk chocolate, which adds dairy fat to its natural cocoa butter. But you can make your own brownies and chocolate cakes using powdered cocoa, egg whites, and vegetable oils; you won't save many calories, but you'll save fat while satisfying your sweet tooth.

Desserts

No problem here; just choose from fresh fruit, dried fruit, homemade baked goods, low-fat commercially baked cakes, nonfat yogurt with fruit or other toppings, and low-fat frozen desserts. You'll stay within your daily dietary fat allotment, but you'll have to exercise a little restraint if calories are a concern.

Caffeinated Beverages

Coffee and tea have been popular the world over for centuries. Without abandoning these traditional sources of caffeine, twentieth-century America has added another, cola drinks. Popular wisdom holds that since caffeine is so popular, it must be harmful. Indeed, most heart-healthy diets ban or restrict caffeine. I disagree; Chapter 17 explains why.

Alcohol

Nutritionists dismiss alcohol as nothing more than a source of empty calories. Doctors disparage alcohol as a major health hazard. The critics have a point. But if it's used correctly, alcohol can be an asset in the fight against atherosclerosis. Chapter 9 explores the pros and cons of alcohol in detail.

Shopping

Unless you're actually down on the farm, careful shopping is the first step toward healthful eating. Pick a market with a good selection of fresh fruits and vegetables; many now offer salad bars featuring precut veggies that can save you lots of time.

Make a shopping list and stick to it, allowing yourself to browse only in the produce section. Don't shop when you are hungry or harried.

Above all, read labels. Don't stop with the big print or the calorie content. Learn to understand the fat, saturated fat, cholesterol, dietary fiber, carbohydrate, sugar, and sodium contents of the foods you eat most often. Remember to evaluate the listed portion sizes to see if they are realistic. Last but not least, check expiration dates to be sure your food is fresh.

If you're interested in foods that are not labeled, ask about their contents. Clerks at the bakery or deli counters may not have the information handy, but the manager can get the facts for you by the time you next return to shop. Meanwhile, look up your foods in the tables in this chapter or in reference books.

Buy what you like, as long as you know what's in it for you.

Eating Out

When you do your own meal planning, shopping, and cooking you have control over your diet. When you eat out, however, you relinquish some of that control. Still, you can learn ways to enjoy good nutrition away from home — without being an unwelcome guest or a cantankerous customer.

First, establish your goals. Unless you have medical problems that require strict adherence to a diet, you can be a bit more flexible away from home. I'm not suggesting that you regress all the way to hollandaise and sirloin; particularly if you eat out often, it is important to maintain the good habits you've been working so hard to establish. But you can be more adaptable away from home. Eventually, I predict, you'll be so happy with your new style of eating that you'll want to stick with it for reasons of taste and preference as well as health.

Healthful eating at a friend's house depends greatly on the circumstances. Your close friends and relatives will surely know your preferences; if not, a discreet phone call can ensure that the menu will contain at least some of your type of food. At informal, family-style gatherings you can always ask for a healthful substitute, but formal dinners are a problem. I've learned to eat a rather generous snack before I leave home, as much because of my appetite as my nutritional values. It is usually possible to load up on a salad, vegetables, and breads; if rice or pasta is on the menu, you're assured of a filling meal. If it's socially uncomfortable for you to decline a serving of food you'd rather not eat, accept a small portion, cut into it and have a taste or two, and leave the rest — while voicing praise for the items you really do like.

As people understand the importance of good nutrition, it's getting easier and easier to eat at their homes. Restaurateurs, too, are catching on, so you should be able to eat well at eateries.

Choose a restaurant that offers healthful foods. You do not have to restrict yourself to counterculture vegetarian food shops. Most restaurants offer enough choices to give you tasty and nutritious options; if yours doesn't, find a new restaurant.

Finding the right restaurant won't do you any good if you don't order wisely. To order well, you need to know how the food is prepared. Many menus are starting to specify the choices that are low in fat, cholesterol, salt, and calories. If the menu doesn't have this information, ask your server. You don't need a full recipe; just ask about ingredients such as butter, cream, and eggs.

Avoid temptations even before you order. Ask to have your bread served without butter. If your table has a bowl of pickles, chips, or salted nuts, ask to have it removed. Similarly, ask to have leftovers cleared promptly at the end of your meal so you won't be tempted to eat more than you really want — or to polish off your companion's food.

When the menu arrives, be adventuresome. While maintaining your guidelines, take advantage of the chef's skill to experience new recipes and varieties of healthful foods. Restaurants offer a wonderful opportunity to get your quota of fish, which can be difficult (and expensive) to make at home. Most menus offer poultry dishes; stick with chicken or turkey, and remember to remove the skin. Order food that is baked, steamed, broiled, or poached rather than fried. Pasta or rice dishes are excellent choices, but remember to consider the sauce. Don't order fish, chicken, or pastas that have cream or cheese sauces; if you can't find a sauce you want, ask to have your food prepared plain, with the sauce on the side.

Don't undo your careful selection of a main dish by surrounding it with poor choices. Look for vegetable- or pasta-based appetizers. Choose vegetable- or chicken-based soups instead of cream soups or meat soups. Order vegetables, potatoes, rice, or pasta for your side dishes; needless to say, salad is also an excellent choice. But remember to select only healthful sauces, toppings, and dressings; if you have any reservations, ask to have them served on the side. And you can always supplement your meal with bread or rolls to fill you up, as long as you go easy on the spreads.

Desserts, of course, represent a special hazard. Fruit is a reliable choice, but you'll have to hold the whipped cream or rich sauce. Frozen yogurt hasn't yet cracked the restaurant scene, but sorbet has. And you can always skip dessert until you get home — or to a frozen-yogurt shop.

Ethnic restaurants can give you a great chance to experience new foods; because they may be unfamiliar, however, you may have to order with extra care.

Italian restaurants are obvious favorites. Minestrone or pasta and bean soups, pasta dishes of all sorts, and Italian bread are good choices — but order your sauces with care (marinara and primavera are good bets), and hold the Parmesan cheese and garlic butter. Ask to have your food prepared with a reduced amount of oil. Beware of the salt in tomato sauces, the fat in meat sauces, the cheese in lasagna and ravioli, and everything in Alfredo sauce (which has been aptly called a heart attack on a plate).

Mexican restaurants will allow you to enjoy beans, rice, and chicken dishes. Skip the guacamole, nachos, fried tortillas, cheese, and beef.

At Indian restaurants, you can experiment with tandoori chicken, seafood, chicken or vegetarian curries, and dal (lentils). Avoid the lamb, coconut dishes, and fried breads. Remember that butter is butter, even if it's called ghee.

Chinese restaurants present a challenge. The food in rural China is healthful, indeed, averaging 15 percent fat, 15 percent protein, and 70 percent carbohydrates. Even in urban China, the average diet contains only 25 percent fat. But in America, Chinese restaurants feature foods high in fat, calories, and salt. A few examples: an egg roll has 11 grams of fat, 190 calories, and 462 milligrams of sodium; a very small, one-cup portion of stir-fried vegetables has 5 grams of fat, 187 calories, and 538 milligrams of sodium; and 1 cup of fried rice has 13 grams of fat, 371 calories, and 674 milligrams of sodium. The solution: order lots of white rice, ask to have your vegetables steamed instead of fried, ask to have your seafood or chicken dishes steamed or stir-fried with only small amounts of oil, and order food prepared without MSG. In short, eat like the Chinese really do: start with lots of rice, adding only small amounts of the "main" dish; if you use chopsticks to pick up the entree, you'll automatically drain away lots of the salt- and fat-rich sauce.

You can use similar care at Greek, Thai, Japanese, and Middle Eastern restaurants. French food still has me stymied, but you can enjoy new treats at almost any other ethnic establishment. Your greatest nutritional problems, in fact, won't come from exotic but from quintessentially

American establishments: steak houses, fast-food restaurants, sub shops, pizza parlors, and delis.

At any restaurant, be it American or ethnic, spend a moment or two thinking about food safety. Look around to be sure the restaurant, and its employees, are clean. Be sure that cold food is served cold and hot food hot. Don't hesitate to send back any food that looks, smells, or tastes spoiled. If you have any food allergies, be sure to ask about hidden ingredients before you order.

The typical American eats one of every five meals away from home. You can be typically inclined toward eating out as long as you don't fall into the typical traps of bad nutrition.

Cheating

Healthful, low-fat nutrition does require planning, practice, and persistence. In a surprisingly short time, though, it will become automatic, and you'll actually prefer bran to bacon. But until then, can you allow yourself to "cheat?"

The short answer is yes. Unlike nicotine, fat is not addicting; you can indulge in a fatty morsel from time to time without risking all your progress. But new research does raise some worry about cheating. In 1993, Dr. George Miller of London's Medical Research Council reported that a single high-fat meal could activate the blood clotting system within 6 to 7 hours, and a 1994 study from Sweden reported similar results. Remember that blood clotting is the third step in the process that blocks coronary arteries and causes heart attacks. Remember, too, that heart attacks are most common early in the morning; although further research will be necessary to confirm a link, it is tempting to speculate that last night's steak is a cause of this morning's trip to the coronary care unit.

Cheat if you must, but cheat in moderation. Better yet, build plenty of alternatives into your nutritional repertoire so you can enjoy flexibility without guilt. Best of all, follow all 15 points of this book's plan to conquer heart disease — if you have open arteries, you won't have to worry about always closing your lips to "forbidden" foods.

Chapter 5

Exercise —
The Best-Kept Secret
in Cardiology

CAN YOU RUN AWAY from heart disease? Yes — and you can also walk, swim, bike, or dance away from America's leading killer. Exercise is the perfect complement to diet in the fight against atherosclerosis. More than 2,400 years ago Hippocrates explained that "eating alone will not keep a man well, he must also take exercise. For food and exercise, while possessing opposite qualities, yet work together to produce health." In fact, exercise is an indispensable part of your comprehensive program to conquer heart disease and enhance health.

Exercise is a natural function of the human body; our bodies are engineered for physical work, and they work best when they are used naturally. Remember that our earliest human ancestors lived as hunter-gatherers; to obtain the food needed to sustain life, primitive humans were constantly on the move. We would do well to recapture some of that physical activity for today's world, to say nothing of the fiber and nutrients that we've removed from the modern diet.

Even when people turned to an agricultural lifestyle about 10,000 years ago, physical labor was the rule. And so it remained over the millennia; as recently as the nineteenth century, in fact, 30 percent of all the energy used for agriculture and manufacturing in the United States was derived from human muscle power.

All that changed with the industrial revolution. We've replaced hoes with tractors, hammers with welding torches, and washtubs with washing machines. The results have been marvelous; modern technology has enabled us to create a society of unprecedented affluence and convenience. Freed from physical work, humans have used mental work to carry science and technology to new heights. But progress has its price. Environmental pollution is one example, mental stress another.

Often overlooked is the price we pay for sedentary living. Modern technology enables us to live very nicely without breaking into a sweat. But America has become the land of the couch potato. Our idea of exercise is to watch sports on TV, with remote controls adding insult to injury. And injury is what we get for our sedentary ways — not the muscular aches and pains that may result from physical activity, but the heart attacks, strokes, hypertension, diabetes, and obesity that result from the lack of exercise. Disuse of the body is abuse of the body.

America can do better. You don't have to push a plow or scrub clothes by hand to regain the exercise we've lost. Instead, use some of the leisure time technology has given you to add recreational exercise to your life; you'll be rewarded with enjoyment and vigor as well as health.

How Exercise Protects Your Heart

Exercise provides many benefits to the cardiovascular system: it fights atherosclerosis directly, it improves other cardiac risk factors, it strengthens the heart itself, and it improves the circulation.

Exercise fights atherosclerosis at all three levels: the blood cholesterol, the arterial walls, and the blood clotting system. Regular aerobic exercise is the best way to raise blood levels of HDL ("good") cholesterol; in this respect, exercise is the ideal companion to a low-fat diet, since diet can reduce LDL ("bad") cholesterol but cannot boost HDL to protective levels. As an extra plus, exercise will help reduce the amounts of LDL and triglycerides in the blood.

Exercise fights atherosclerosis by protecting the blood vessel walls. Aerobic exercise lowers blood pressure, thus reducing the stress on arteries and preventing the vascular injury that allows LDL cholesterol to begin forming fatty plaques.

Finally, exercise helps prevent the blood clotting mechanism from forming the clots that are the final step in causing most heart attacks. People who exercise have lower levels of fibrinogen, the major clotting protein that is itself associated with heart attack risk. Exercise decreases the stickiness of blood platelets, thus making it harder for clots to block arteries. Exercise also boosts the activity of natural clot-busting enzymes in the blood. Last but not least, regular exercise makes the blood less viscous or thick, so it can flow through vessels more easily.

In addition to fighting atherosclerosis directly, exercise helps by reducing the other modifiable heart attack risk factors. Regular aerobic exercise improves blood cholesterol levels, fights hypertension, lessens the risk of diabetes, controls obesity, and dissipates mental stress. Look back at Table 2–11, and you'll see how these changes could improve your cardiac risk score. Tobacco abuse is the only modifiable risk factor that is not directly improved by exercise — but people who become physically fit develop a sense of mastery and self-confidence that often helps them control smoking and other bad habits.

Exercise improves the heart itself. Muscles grow stronger with repetitive use, and the heart muscle is no exception. Regular aerobic exercise strengthens the muscle of the left ventricle, the heart's main pumping chamber. Because the fit heart can pump more blood with each beat, it can slow down and still meet all the body's needs for blood and oxygen. Exercise also makes the heart muscle more efficient, so it needs less oxygen for itself. In animals, at least, regular exercise actually stimulates the formation of collateral coronary arteries, increasing blood supply to the heart even if blockages are present; we don't know if the human heart also develops collaterals because of exercise, but it's an intriguing possibility.

The third way that exercise protects the heart is by improving the circulation. Exercise training makes it easier for muscles to extract oxygen from blood. It also increases the number of capillaries, the tiny blood vessels that actually deliver oxygen to and remove wastes from tissues. As a result of these improvements in the circulation, the heart doesn't have to work as hard to pump blood to the tissues.

Regular exercise fights atherosclerosis and reduces cardiac risk factors, greatly reducing the risk of heart attacks. But exercise does more than fight disease: it also enhances health. It bolsters cardiac function and aids the circulation. At rest, the heart pumps about 5 quarts of blood per minute; during exercise it should be able to pump more than 20 quarts per minute. The fit heart can pump much more blood, enabling people who exercise regularly to achieve extraordinary levels of activity. And the fit heart can sustain peak work for much longer, greatly enhancing human endurance.

Exercise and Health

A healthy heart won't do you much good if the rest of your body is sick. Because the 15-point program to conquer heart disease restores the best elements of natural living, it combats many other diseases as well. Exercise is no exception.

Regular exercise helps prevent and treat metabolic diseases. Diabetes is an excellent example. Exercise enhances tissue sensitivity to insulin, the hormone that allows sugar to move from the blood into the body's cells. Because it lowers blood sugar levels, exercise is an important — but often neglected — adjunct to the therapy of diabetes, while also protecting diabetics from heart attacks and strokes. And new research from the 1990s has demonstrated that regular exercise can actually help prevent diabetes, particularly in people who are at high risk for the disease because it's in their families.

Exercise is indispensable for the control of another metabolic disease, obesity. Regular aerobic exercise burns up body fat. Chapter 15 explains why diets invariably fail unless exercise is a full partner in the weight control effort.

Muscles need exercise to keep them healthy; without work, muscles "retire," becoming weak and scrawny as muscle fibers shrink in a process called atrophy. In fact, exercise is the *only* way to strengthen muscles; despite their widespread use by athletes, protein and amino acid supplements are worthless for muscles and may even contribute to medical problems such as kidney disease and osteoporosis. Exercise helps muscles in three ways: aerobic exercises build endurance, resistance exercises develop strength, and stretching exercises promote flexibility. Even if your goals don't include competitive sports, a balanced exercise program will help you look better, feel better, and enjoy improved function in daily life and a lower risk of common musculoskeletal problems such as low back pain.

Physical activity also keeps bones strong. Osteoporosis, or thin bones, is a major problem in America today; it causes 113 million fractures in the United States annually, including many debilitating hip and spine fractures. Because they lose calcium from their bones after menopause, women are particularly vulnerable. Bones that are put to work retain their calcium; weight-bearing exercise helps prevent osteoporosis, even in elderly women.

Heart disease is the leading cause of death in the United States; cancer is in second place — and exercise can actually reduce the risk of certain cancers. Colon cancer will be diagnosed in 150,000 Americans this year, and about 60,000 will die from the disease. Doctors can now detect colon cancer early, when it is curable. You can do even better by preventing the disease. A low-fat, high-fiber diet will help — and so will regular exercise. At least seven studies have demonstrated that people who are sedentary are 1.3 to 1.6 times more likely to develop colon cancer than are people who exercise. Exercise fights colon cancer by facilitating the rapid elimination of toxins from the intestinal tract.

Quite another mechanism is involved in preventing female reproductive cancers. By reducing estrogen levels, exercise reduces the risk of cancers of the breast and female reproductive tract by up to 50 percent, particularly in women who begin regular exercise early in their reproductive years. About 175,000 American women will be diagnosed with breast cancer this year, and 45,000 will be killed by the disease; cancers of the uterus and cervix will be diagnosed in 70,000 women. Exercise might have helped save many thousands of female cancer victims.

Exercise helps the mind as well as the body. Chapter 14 details the way exercise counters stress and depression.

Exercise in the Treatment of Atherosclerosis

The ultimate test of any technique used to conquer heart disease is its ability to treat patients who already have the disease. How does exercise meet this test?

Very well.

Our own efforts in this regard date back to 1978, when a cardiac rehabilitation program was added to the Harvard Cardiovascular Health Center. Since then, we've used aerobic exercise — along with diet and stress reduction — to treat several thousand patients with coronary artery disease. Nor is our program unique; hundreds of similar programs are now in full tilt across the United States and around the world.

Almost all cardiac rehabilitation programs report similar, very heartening results. Patients who exercise regularly improve dramatically. They exhibit great increases in their capacities to exercise without developing signals of cardiac distress such as shortness of breath or the chest pain of angina. Their blood pressures decline. Their HDL cholesterol levels rise and their LDLs fall. They require less medication. They lose weight and their spirits, work performance, and sexual function all improve. Patients with atherosclerotic blockages of their leg arteries improve as well, often regaining the ability to walk without experiencing debilitating leg cramps.

By now, even the skeptics agree that exercise does wonders for the functional capacities of patients with coronary artery disease. The $64 million question, though, has been more difficult to answer: does exercise actually reduce heart attacks and prolong the lives of people who have already had at least one heart attack?

It's been hard to resolve this question because a scientific answer depends on randomized trials in which heart attack victims agree voluntarily to be arbitrarily assigned to receive standard medical care or the same excellent care plus exercise. As you can imagine, these studies are difficult, time consuming, and expensive. Dozens have now been completed; almost all report improved survival in the patients who exercise, but few have included enough patients to permit a statistically valid conclusion.

The debate was settled in 1988 and 1989 when two groups of scientists headed by Drs. Gerald O'Connor and Neil Oldridge analyzed the question by combining the results of previous separate trials. This technique, called meta-analysis, permitted the evaluation of more than 4,000 heart attack survivors who were enrolled in exercise rehabilitation programs. The result: exercise produced a 25 percent reduction in the rate of heart attacks and in the overall death rate.

Cardiac rehabilitation programs have demonstrated that exercise is effective even in patients who already have atherosclerosis. They have also taught us that exercise is safe, even in heart patients. A survey of hundreds of programs found only one fatality for every 783,979 hours of exercise in these high-risk patients. Heart patients, of course, require special screening, instruction, and monitoring to exercise safely — but after they graduate from rehabilitation programs, they go on exercising at home, much as you should. More than a dozen of our patients, in fact, have gone on to run marathons without any problems.

We have learned how to make exercise safe and effective for patients with heart disease, and I'll show you how similar guidelines can protect you during exercise. But don't wait until you have cardiac disease — if you make aerobic exercise a regular part of your 15-point program to conquer heart disease, you won't ever need a fancy cardiac rehabilitation program.

Exercise and Aging

Atherosclerosis is traditionally considered to be an inevitable part of the aging process. I disagree; in my view, it's a man-made disease, an unnecessary product of the bodily abuse and disuse that are so common in industrialized societies. Unlike atherosclerosis, however, aging *is* an inevitable, natural process. Can exercise modify aging itself?

Take a 35-year-old man and place him at complete bed rest for 3 weeks. Then perform a detailed series of physiologic studies. You'll find that your subject's heart can pump less blood than it could just 3 weeks earlier. His lungs can take up less oxygen. His muscle mass is lower, as is his bone calcium content. His blood is more viscous, or thick and sticky. His body fat, blood sugar, and cholesterol are higher, as is his blood pressure. What's happened? By all these parameters your subject has aged 10 years during just a few weeks of complete inactivity.

Don't feel guilty about your "experiment" — your subject will recover his youthful numbers with just a few weeks of exercise. The weakness and fatigue that accompany prolonged inactivity will also melt away. But you should feel guilty if you do this experiment on yourself: physical inactivity produces physiological changes that mimic the aging process.

Older people have more cardiovascular risk factors, including higher blood pressures, higher LDL, and lower HDL cholesterol levels. Average blood sugars rise by about 6 points per decade, explaining the much higher prevalence of Type II diabetes in the elderly. Body fat increases with age, averaging 44 percent in 65-year-old women but only 25 percent in 25-year-olds. The net result is a progressive increase in atherosclerosis and heart disease and a progressive decline in the heart's pumping capacity. For example, the heart of an average, healthy 25-year-old can pump two and a half quarts of oxygen per minute, while a healthy 65-year-old can pump only one and a half quarts. Even worse, the senior citizen's heart will continue to weaken; by age 80, it may be able to pump no more than one quart of oxygen per minute, a level insufficient to support even modest daily activities without fatigue and breathlessness.

Jonathan Swift said that "every man desires to live long, but no man would be old." You *can* live long without feeling old. As part of the 15-point program to conquer heart disease, exercise will help keep your heart and circulation healthy. It will also retard all of the "changes of aging" that are actually produced by inactivity rather than longevity. Consider the healthy 25-year-old whose heart can pump two and a half quarts of oxygen. He is free of disease, but is he entirely healthy? A 25-year-old *athlete's* heart can pump *more than twice* as much oxygen per minute. And with regular exercise it will retain that edge over the years.

Studies from Johns Hopkins, Tufts, and the University of Toronto have amply confirmed that older people who exercise have much stronger hearts and much lower risk factor profiles. It's new data, but the explanation is very old indeed; Hippocrates, the father of medicine in ancient Greece, taught, "That which is used develops; that which is not used wastes away." Exercise can't turn back the clock, but it can make all the measurements seem that way. An active 70-year-old can have the functional capacity of a healthy but sedentary 50-year-old. Perhaps because of the sedentary values of our modern world, we turn to another ancient authority, the Roman poet Cicero, for a summary: "Exercise and temperance will preserve something of our youthful vigor, even into old age."

It is never too late to start; Cicero, again: "No one is so old that he does not think he could live another year." Ask Albert Gordon, who ran his first marathon at age 80. Ask Kenneth Beer, who was winning Super Seniors tennis championships at age 87. Ask John Fleck, who swam and race-walked in the 1991 Senior Olympics at age 99. Or ask Herman Johannesen, who continued cross-country skiing until age 111.

You don't have to be a competitive athlete to benefit from exercise in maturity. Modest exercise increased the bone density of 60-year-old women studied in Toronto. And weight lifting greatly improved the muscular function in 87- to 96-year-old (!) nursing home patients in Boston.

It's also never too *early* to start. Emulating their parents, I suppose, the youth of America are woefully sedentary; only 36 percent exercise regularly, and a mere 32 percent are able to pass minimal fitness tests. It's one of the reasons that a Michigan study of elementary school children detected one or more atherosclerosis risk factors in an astounding 98 percent, including elevated cholesterol levels in 41 percent and hypertension in 28 percent.

Atherosclerosis begins in childhood — if we let it. The fight against heart disease should begin in childhood and continue throughout life. Make exercise part of your program; as the poet John Gay pointed out 300 years ago, "Exercise thy lasting youth defends."

Sloth versus Exercise: Burdens and Benefits

Sedentary living places a devastating strain on America's health.

More than 60 percent of the adult population does not get enough exercise; since sedentary living multiplies the risk of heart attack by a factor of 1.9, the lack of exercise accounts for 205,000 heart attack deaths in the United States each year.

More than 63 million Americans have hypertension; regular exercise could reduce that number by 30 to 50 percent.

Stroke is the third leading cause of death in America, claiming 150,000 lives each year. By fighting atherosclerosis, hypertension, and blood clotting, exercise could prevent many of these deaths, to say nothing of the suffering experienced by the 350,000 Americans who survive strokes each year. In fact, sedentary people are nearly 3 times more likely to suffer strokes than are fit people.

Cardiovascular disease is the most important consequence of sedentary living, but it's far from the only problem. Consider that 24 million Americans have osteoporosis, 12 million have diabetes, and 34 million are obese. Add the 150,000 cases of colon cancer, the 175,000 cases of breast cancer, and the 70,000 reproductive tract cancers that strike Americans every year. Factor in the anxiety and depression that afflict millions more. Exercise could reduce all of these tragically high numbers.

Hundreds of thousands of deaths, suffering in the millions — it's mind-boggling. When the numbers are so very large, it can be hard to see how they apply to you. Fortunately, Dr. Willard Manning and his colleagues have done the math for you. Their 1991 book, *The Costs of Poor Health Habits,* calculates that every mile you *don't* walk will shorten your life by 21 minutes. Keep it in mind and look at your watch the next time you put your feet up on the couch.

Sloth is costly in dollars as well as in suffering and premature death. Dr. Manning calculates that each mile not walked will cost you $.12 in medical expenses and $.22 in lost wages. And the financial burden is shared by all of society; over a lifetime, each sedentary person will run up a tab of $1,955 for the rest of us to pay. All in all, the lack of exercise drains $5.7 billion from the American economy every year.

Fortunately, all the burdens of sedentary living can be counterbalanced by the benefits of exercise. The bottom line is longevity. Studies have shown that regular exercise can reduce all-cause mortality by more than 25 percent and increase average life expectancy by about 2 years. Using Dr. Ralph Paffenbarger's Harvard alumni data, I calculate that if you exercise optimally you'll gain about 2 hours of life expectancy for each hour of exercise.

Health and longevity are the bottom line of exercise, but they don't tell the whole story. Exercise is fun; you'll enjoy life more and have lots more energy if you are physically fit. Exercise is a treatment you'll learn to love.

For all its benefits, exercise is far from perfect. Not all forms of exercise are equally beneficial, and even the most beneficial forms of exercise can have untoward consequences. To plan an exercise program with maximal benefits and minimal risks, you'll need more information.

What Type of Exercise Is Best?

When it comes to conquering heart disease, only one type of exercise will do the trick: it's *aerobic exercise.* When you exercise aerobically, you'll be using your large muscle groups in a rhythmic repetitive fashion for prolonged periods of time. You'll be working hard enough to raise your heart rate to between 70 and 85 percent of its maximum; you'll break into a sweat, but you won't feel winded or breathless. After you get into shape, you'll find yourself both relaxed and energized by aerobics. You'll be able to choose among many activities, including brisk walking, jogging, biking, swimming, aerobic dance, stair climbing or rowing machines, cross-country skiing on snow or machines, and racquet sports. You'll be able to work out alone or with a companion, gaining solitude or socialization as you see fit. Best of all, you'll be protecting your heart and circulation by pumping up your HDL cholesterol, lowering your blood pressure, lowering your blood sugar, reducing your blood's tendency to form clots, and burning away body fat.

Aerobic exercise sounds great — and it is. But while your heart and blood vessels are crucial to your health, they're not the only things that count in life. To enrich your life, consider adding other forms of exercise to construct a balanced program for your whole body.

Flexibility exercises are very important for muscles, ligaments, and joints. Without them, in fact, aerobic exercise might make your muscles tight and stiff. Flexibility exercises will prevent that; they'll keep you limber and graceful, improving your body mechanics and posture and reducing your risk of sprains and strains. You can improve your flexibility with dynamic stretching exercises based on calisthenics or static stretches based on yoga; the former are ideal for the warm-ups and cooldowns that should accompany aerobics, and the latter are excellent for reducing mental tension. Flexibility exercises should be part of your exercise program.

Exercises for strength are a bit more controversial. To understand why — and to be able to use them properly — you'll need to understand a little muscle physiology.

Physiologists divide muscular activity into two categories. One is called isotonic, or dynamic, exercise; it's already familiar to you because it's the basis of all aerobic exercise. When muscles exercise isotonically, their fibers shorten, moving joints through their range of motion to propel you along the jogging trail or through the water. In isotonics, muscles contract, but they don't develop increased tension. The blood vessels in muscles widen, increasing blood flow and lowering blood pressure. To provide the increased blood flow, the heart speeds up and pumps more blood — it's the reason why aerobic conditioning improves cardiovascular function.

The other form of muscular work is called isometric, or static, exercise. Examples include lifting a heavy weight or pushing hard against an immobile object. In isometrics, muscle fibers do not shorten, but muscle tension increases. As a result, the muscles' blood vessels narrow, causing your blood pressure to rise. Your heart will work harder, but instead of pumping more blood at a lower pressure, it will be pumping against a high pressure without increasing its rate. It's like having high blood pressure — and, in fact, repetitive isometric exercise will result in thickening and stiffness of the left ventricle, just like the effects of hypertension.

Isometrics sound bad — but they're not all bad. Weight lifters use isometrics to increase strength, bodybuilders use them for bulk, and competitive athletes use them for power and peak performance. The rest of us can use them to keep our muscles strong — if we use them appropriately. The trick is to avoid high-resistance isometrics. Instead of grunting and straining hard a few times, do high-repetition, low-resistance work; you'll build muscle strength without taxing your circulation. You can do high-rep, low-resistance isometrics with free weights, Nautilus-type machines, or even with the weight of your own body in calisthenics.

High-resistance isometrics should be avoided by anyone with high blood pressure, heart disease, or other circulatory problems. Low-resistance isometrics are safe for the circulation; they don't contribute to the fight against atherosclerosis, but they can be a nice supplement to a balanced fitness program. The choice is yours — but don't let strength training cut into your aerobic exercise quota. Although many health clubs tout high-rep circuit training as an aerobic exercise, it is actually a poor substitute for true aerobics.

Speed training is the fourth type of exercise. Physiologists call it anaerobic training because muscles are working so hard that they outpace the heart's ability to deliver oxygen. Athletes call it sprinting or interval training; they depend on it to prepare for peak performance. Cardiologists call it trouble, since it pushes the heart to its maximum.

You can think of speed training as the saturated fat of exercise. It's OK for healthy people if it's used in moderation with appropriate planning, but it has no role in fighting atherosclerosis or enhancing health.

What type of exercise is best for you? Aerobics are the key for your heart, your circulation, and your metabolism. Flexibility exercise is important to keep you in shape for aerobics. Strength training is a nice supplement for your muscles if you do it right. Speed training is the form of exercise you can forget as fast as you'd like.

How Much Exercise Is Best?

Call it misinformation or call it wishful thinking: most doctors who answer this question reply with the old guideline of 20 minutes, 3 times a week. They're selling you short.

It is true that every little bit of exercise helps. And in fact, 60 minutes of aerobics per week will help quite a bit. But an hour a week should be your *minimum* goal; 3 to 4 hours a week is an *optimal* goal for conquering heart disease.

Chapter 2 explained the basis for this recommendation, citing Dr. Ralph Paffenbarger's Harvard Alumni Study. That study compared the protective benefits of various amounts of exercise. As little as 500 calories of exercise per week — about an hour's worth of aerobics — did reduce the risk of heart attacks and cardiac deaths. But protection increased steadily with increased exercise. Maximal benefits were achieved by 2,000–3,000 calories of exercise per week, or about 3 to 4 hours of vigorous aerobics; beyond that, additional exercise produced neither help nor harm.

Many other studies provide similar data: a little exercise is good, but more is better — up to a point. The reason for the plateau is not clear, but I have a theory that may explain it. Remember that exercise fights atherosclerosis at all three stages, improving the blood cholesterol, protecting the arterial wall, and modulating the blood clotting system. Among these many protective mechanisms, raising the HDL cholesterol is perhaps the most important. Even a little exercise will raise the HDL; studies from California, for example, show that walking just 8 miles a week will boost HDL levels by a small but significant amount over several months. But larger amounts of exercise will boost the HDL more — up to a point. Runners, for example, will boost their HDL levels higher with every mile they run up to an average of 40 miles per week; additional training may improve their racing times, but it won't increase their HDLs further, nor will it further reduce their cardiac risk.

Setting Your Exercise Goals

You established your goals for dietary fat on the basis of your cardiac risk factors, your body weight, and your habits and preferences. Use the same strategy to set your exercise goals. The higher your cardiac risk score (Table 2–11) and the higher your body mass index (Table 2–8), the more you need aerobic exercise. For risk reduction and longevity, set 1 hour of aerobics per week as a minimal goal, with 30 minutes a day a much more desirable target. For weight reduction, though, you may choose to build to higher levels, perhaps even to an hour a day;

these higher levels may also become the goals for people who exercise for athletic competition and for people who get mentally hooked on exercise for its own sake.

You won't do very well if you try to go from a 40 percent fat diet to a 20 percent fat diet overnight. With exercise, too, you'll need to achieve your goals gradually. In fact, people who need exercise the most because they are out of shape (Table 2–6) or overweight will need the most time to build up to their optimal exercise levels.

Even the most stringent dietary fat restriction won't do you any good if it only lasts a day. Exercise, too, should be a regular part of your lifestyle; make permanence one of your exercise goals.

You won't succeed in restricting your dietary fat if you try to force yourself to eat foods you don't like. With exercise, too, it's wise to pick something that's enjoyable, convenient, and natural. But once you get started, you'll benefit greatly from exploring new options that add variety to your program — whether it's in a diet program or an exercise plan.

You'll have to work extra hard to restrict your dietary fat if you go it alone. Your exercise goals, too, will be more easily attained if you enlist the support of your family and friends.

You'll find it easier to achieve a diet that will fight atherosclerosis if you learn about nutrition and think about food. To help you use exercise to conquer heart disease, this chapter will provide practical advice about exercise.

It's hard to go too far with dietary fat restriction, but it's surely possible to harm your health with an extreme diet. Exercise, too, can have its complications. Before getting started on your exercise program, you should understand the potential hazards of exercise so you can take precautions to prevent them.

Medical Complications of Exercise

Exercise does have risks. Many people make the mistake of using these risks as a rationalization for remaining sedentary. Don't fall into this trap; the *lack* of exercise is far more hazardous than is exercise itself. Still, you should understand the downside of exercise so you can make your program safe and effective.

Cardiac Complications

Let's start with the bad news: exercise can precipitate sudden cardiac death. Now the good news: it's rare. But in man-bites-dog fashion, exercise-induced deaths get all the publicity. People who die during sleep make the obituary page, but people who die playing ball make the front page.

Exercise-induced deaths fall into two distinct groups.

In young athletes, the culprits are usually congenital heart diseases or primary disorders of the heart muscle. Pete Maravich, for example, died during a pick-up basketball game because he was born with abnormally hooked-up coronary arteries; in contrast, Hank Gathers died on the court because he had a thickened, abnormal heart muscle, or cardiomyopathy. Boston Celtic star Reggie Lewis died at age 27 because of myocarditis, an inflammation of the heart muscle. Although rare, these tragedies remind us that exercise is a serious business. Young athletes should protect themselves by following simple precautions. A competent physical examination should precede competition; athletes with heart murmurs should be considered for further testing, including EKGs and echocardiograms (Chapter 18); so, too, should athletes whose families have histories of premature or exercise-induced deaths. Above all, athletes must learn to listen to their bodies, promptly reporting dizziness, fainting, chest pain, palpitations, undue breathlessness, or other unusual occurrences during exercise. And, like all of us, young athletes should avoid strenuous exercise during the flu and other viral infections (as mentioned in Chapter 1).

In older people, sudden death during exercise usually results from atherosclerosis and heart attacks. Running guru Jim Fixx is a tragic example; another, closer to home, is my marathoning buddy Jim Spertner. Both were highly conditioned athletes who died in their early 50s while jogging. But both had risk factors, including former tobacco abuse and strong family histories of early cardiac deaths. Both had been sedentary and overweight for most of their lives. As a person who shares all these traits, I share your worries about exercise-induced heart problems. But I won't share another factor common to Fixx, Spertner, and most other middle-aged people who die during exercise: they experienced chest discomfort during exercise but failed to get medical attention. The best way to protect your heart during exercise is to fight atherosclerosis before it occurs; the second best way is to listen to your body.

We know that heart attacks and sudden cardiac deaths are more common in the early morning hours. Should you avoid exercise in the morning? It's a good question, with a good answer: exercise is equally safe at any time of day if it's done right. The best evidence comes from Dr. Paul Murray's 1993 study of nearly 300 cardiac rehabilitation patients who were monitored during a total of more than 252,000 hours of exercise. About half exercised regularly at 7:30 A.M., the rest at 3:00 P.M. Even in these patients with atherosclerosis, exercise was equally safe in the morning and afternoon. It's reassuring news, particularly since early morning exercise is most convenient for many people. But if you work out in the morning, remember to delay breakfast until afterward — you should never exercise within 2 hours of eating. And as I speculated in Chapter 4, a fatty dinner, rather than morning exercise, may be the reason heart attacks peak early in the day.

What symptoms should alert you to the possibility that exercise is overstressing your heart? They are the same symptoms of angina or heart attacks that we should always heed, but they're a little harder to hear during exercise because of the "background noise" of heavy breathing that's a normal part of exercise. Still, listen for chest pressure, tightness, or pain. Be alert for disproportionate shortness of breath, fatigue, or sweating. Take note of dizziness, lightheadedness, fainting, or an irregular or unduly rapid heartbeat. Even "indigestion" warrants your attention if it comes on during exercise. Most often, these symptoms are not actually signs of heart trouble, but you should not take a chance. Instead, stop exercising at once and report them to your doctor. Remember what we teach medical students: chest pain is the most common symptom of heart trouble, denial the second most common.

Exercise-induced cardiac death is rare. Dr. Paul Thompson, for example, studied runners in Rhode Island, finding one death per 396,000 hours of jogging. Similarly, Dr. Kenneth Cooper's famed Institute of Aerobics Research has reported no deaths in more than 375,000 hours of exercise, including 1.2 million miles of jogging and walking.

To protect yourself during exercise, get an appropriate checkup before you exercise, and listen to your body during exercise. Above all, get into shape gradually, then stay in shape. Studying all the sudden deaths in Seattle, Dr. David Siscovick found that the greatest risks occur in people who stress themselves with strenuous exercise without first working themselves into shape. Such "weekend warriors" are 56 times more likely to die during an hour of exercise than they are during a sedentary hour. People who exercise regularly also increase their risk during peak exertion, but to a much smaller degree — and their overall risk of sudden death is actually *60 percent lower* than in people who never work out at all. Much the same is true of nonfatal heart attacks. Two 1993 studies found that sedentary people are about 100 times more likely to suffer heart attacks in an hour of strenuous exercise than in an hour of rest — but people who exercise regularly are largely protected from exercise-induced heart attacks. And that's the bottom line: regular exercise will actually *reduce* your risk of heart attacks and sudden cardiac death.

Other Complications of Exercise

Musculoskeletal problems are by far the most common adverse effects of exercise. Most can be prevented by careful warm-ups and stretching, good equipment and technique, appropriate pacing, and common sense. Many others can be nipped in the bud by early recognition and self-treatment. You'll find guidelines for the proper care of your muscles, joints, and ligaments later in this chapter.

Exercise can cause problems with the body's internal organs. Chief among these is exercise-induced asthma; it's actually quite common, but it can often be prevented by avoiding strenuous sports in cold, dry air. If prevention fails, exercise-induced asthma usually responds extremely well to simple prescription inhalers. People who cough or wheeze during exercise should check with their doctors, since treatment will generally allow them to remain fully active. Less often, exercise can produce heartburn or diarrhea. Intestinal or urinary tract bleeding are rare but dramatic exercise-induced symptoms; although they are usually not serious, they surely warrant a competent medical evaluation. Women who exercise very strenuously can develop menstrual irregularities, but this problem resolves with diminished exercise and weight gain.

Medical Evaluations Prior to Exercise

You didn't have to see a nutritionist before starting your low-fat diet. Do you have to see a doctor before you begin an exercise program?

You won't need a special pre-exercise physical if you've been getting appropriate routine medical care. In general, this should include a comprehensive checkup every 5 years between ages 20 and 35, every 2 years between 35 and 50, and every year thereafter. You should have your blood pressure, blood cholesterol profile, and blood sugar tested at regular intervals (see Chapter 2); I generally check them during each comprehensive physical exam. Healthy adults should also have at least one baseline electrocardiogram (see Chapter 18). If you've passed all of these tests and if you feel well, you don't need an extra checkup prior to exercise. If, on the other hand, you have abnormal test results or abnormal symptoms, you should see your doctor before you start an exercise program. It's good advice, too, for people who are very sedentary, very overweight, elderly, or who have high risk factor profiles (Table 2–11).

Should you have a stress test (Chapter 18) prior to exercise? The theory is appealing: if you exercise in a hospital lab with an EKG monitor hooked up and medical personnel at attendance, you'll be able to detect heart problems so that they won't occur when you're out jogging on the roads. Appealing or not, stress tests have not proved beneficial for pre-exercise screening. The best evidence comes from a 1991 study of 3,617 men aged 35 to 59 who were at high risk for heart disease because of high cholesterol levels. Even in these high-risk people, annual stress tests were not able to predict exercise-induced cardiac problems before they occurred. The good news, though, is that such problems were rare, occurring in only 2 percent of subjects during 7 years of exercise.

Eighty-three percent of doctors who run marathons don't put themselves through routine stress tests. I'm among that majority. But a majority of doctors recommend pre-exercise stress tests for their patients. Until recently, I was among this group as well, even publishing this advice in medical textbooks. With the latest information, though, I no longer recommend *routine* screening stress tests prior to exercise. But pre-exercise stress tests are still mandatory for people with cardiac symptoms or suspected heart disease; all cardiac rehabilitation patients, for example, must have a stress test before they enter a supervised exercise program and another before they graduate to independent exercise. Exercise tests can also be useful for people who need a detailed exercise prescription and for those needing the motivation of charting their progress with serial tests.

If you are unsure about your health or insecure about exercise, check with a cardiologist or internist who is knowledgeable about exercise and heart disease. Don't begin vigorous exercise with lingering uncertainties — but don't let uncertainties deter you from actually getting on with it. Enlist exercise in your fight against atherosclerosis.

Your Exercise Program

You began eliminating the obvious fat from your diet even while you began to learn the details about nutrition and atherosclerosis. You should begin to use your body even as you learn how to construct a complete exercise program. Make exercise a part of your daily life. Get off the bus a stop or two early, and walk the rest of the way. Pull into the first parking space you see instead of circling around to minimize your walking. Take the stairs instead of the elevator, especially going up. Walk to the neighborhood store — and back, if your bundles aren't too heavy. Consider using a hand mower or hedge clipper instead of a power model. Catch up with a friend during a stroll instead of with a phone call. Take your kids for a bike ride instead of a car ride. It may not add up to enough exercise to conquer heart disease, but it will help get you started.

To construct a formal exercise program consider three types of exercise: aerobic, flexibility, and strength.

Aerobic Exercise

Aerobics will be the key to your program — but before you get started, plan to warm up and cool down.

Give yourself a full 10 minutes to warm up prior to exercise. It's very important to raise your heart rate gradually instead of starting out in high gear. Use walking or calisthenics to warm up. Best of all, incorporate stretching exercises into a warm-up routine; you'll warm up your muscles and ligaments as well as your heart, reducing your risk of injury. Similarly, give yourself at least 5 minutes to cool down after you complete your aerobics; first walk, then stretch to protect your limb muscles and your heart muscle.

Consider three elements in planning your aerobic exercise program:

1. *Frequency:* If you are out of shape, begin by exercising only 3 times a week or every other day; you'll avoid injury by giving out-of-shape muscles a full 48 hours to recover from the unaccustomed stress of exercise. As you improve, you can increase to 5 times a week, then — if you choose — to daily workouts. Competitive athletes, in fact, often

work out twice a day. But even "jocks" should follow a rule that should guide all of us: alternate easy and hard exercise sessions to give your muscles a chance to recover.

2. *Duration:* Once again, your plans will depend on your starting point. If you're a beginner, aim for 10 minutes per session at first. As you improve, extend each aerobic workout, but do so gradually; be persistent but not impatient — you're building a lifetime of exercise, a marathon rather than a sprint. As a rule of thumb, add 10 percent every week; it may not seem like much, but before long you'll be at a full 30 minutes of aerobics. If your goals call for even more exercise, build from there — but continue going slowly, and consider dividing your exercise into two daily sessions if your schedule permits.

3. *Intensity:* This is the only tricky part of your plan for aerobic exercise. If you are accustomed to exercise, you can simply work out at a comfortable pace, gradually increasing your intensity as you improve further. But if exercise is new to you, you'll need to be more careful; extra care is particularly important for people over 40 and for those with atherosclerosis risk factors.

Your goal for aerobic intensity is to work out hard enough to reap gain but not so hard as to cause pain. As a rule, exercising at 70 to 85 percent of your maximum is ideal. If you're out of shape, older, overweight, or working to correct cardiac risk factors, start at the low end or even below it, perhaps at 50 to 60 percent of maximum. No matter where you start, build up within your target range as you improve.

You can gauge intensity in one of three ways: subjectively, with an exercise chart, or by measuring your heart rate.

The subjective method is the easiest but least precise. After you warm up thoroughly, exercise hard enough to work up a sweat but never so hard that you're breathless. It's the "talking pace" — you should have enough wind in reserve to be able to carry on a limited conversation while you are exercising. With experience, you can learn to estimate your exercise intensity with remarkable accuracy. Our cardiac rehabilitation patients learn to rate themselves on the Borg Scale, which ranges from a score of 2 ("very, very easy") to 20 ("very, very hard"); we check them with cardiac monitors and find that subjective ratings are quite reliable.

A second way to judge aerobic intensity is to look up your activity on a chart that provides intensity values. Table 5–1 is an example. If you're out of shape, start at modest levels, perhaps 5 calories per minute. As

Table 5-1
INTENSITY OF EXERCISE

Intensity Level	Daily Activities	Recreational Activities
1 calorie per minute	Complete rest	
2 to 2½ calories per minute	Standing Desk work Driving an automobile Typing (electric)	Strolling (1 mile per hour) Playing cards Sewing, knitting
2½ to 4 calories per minute	Auto repair Radio, TV repair Janitorial work Typing (manual) Bartending Riding lawn mower	Level walking (2 miles per hour) Level bicycling (5 miles per hour) Billiards, bowling Shuffleboard Woodworking (light) Driving a powerboat Golf (using a power cart) Canoeing (2½ miles per hour) Horseback riding (walk) Playing various musical instruments
4 to 5 calories per minute	Bricklaying, plastering Pushing a wheelbarrow (100-lb load) Machine assembly Driving a tractor-trailer in traffic Welding (moderate load) Cleaning windows Housework Pushing light power mower	Walking (3 miles per hour) Cycling (6 miles per hour) Horseshoe pitching Volleyball (6-man, noncompetitive) Golf (pulling bag cart) Archery Sailing (handling small boat) Fly-fishing (standing with waders) Horseback riding (sitting while trotting) Badminton (social doubles) Energetically playing various musical instruments
5 to 6 calories per minute	Painting, masonry Paperhanging Light carpentry Raking leaves Hoeing	Walking (3.5 miles per hour) Cycling (8 miles per hour) Ping-Pong Golf (carrying clubs) Dancing (fox-trot) Badminton (singles) Tennis (doubles) Vigorous calisthenics
6 to 7 calories per minute	Digging in garden Shoveling light earth Average sexual activity	Walking (4 miles per hour) Cycling (10 miles per hour) Canoeing (10 miles per hour) Horseback riding (posting while trotting) Stream fishing (walking in light current in waders) Ice- or roller-skating (9 miles per hour)

continued

Table 5-1 *continued*

Intensity Level	Daily Activities	Recreational Activities
7 to 8 calories per minute	Shoveling (10-lb load 10 times per minute) Splitting wood Snow shoveling Hand lawn-mowing	Walking (5 miles per hour) Cycling (11 miles per hour) Badminton (competitive) Tennis (singles) Square dancing Downhill skiing (light) Cross-country skiing (2^1/$_2$ miles per hour in loose snow) Waterskiing
8 to 10 calories per minute	Digging ditches Carrying 80 lbs. Sawing hardwood	Jogging (5 miles per hour) Cycling (12 miles per hour) Horseback riding (gallop) Downhill skiing (vigorous) Basketball Mountain climbing Ice hockey Canoeing (5 miles per hour) Touch football Paddleball
10 to 11 calories per minute	Shoveling (14-lb. load 10 times per minute)	Running (5^1/$_2$ miles per hour) Cycling (13 miles per hour) Cross-country skiing (4 miles per hour in loose snow) Squash (social) Handball (social) Fencing Basketball (vigorous)
Above 11 calories per minute	Shoveling (16-lb. load 10 times per minute)	Running 7 miles per hour = 12 calories per minute Running 8 miles per hour = 13 calories per minute Running 9 miles per hour = 15 calories per minute Running 10 miles per hour = 17 calories per minute Cross-country skiing (5+ miles per hour in loose snow) Handball (competitive) Squash (competitive)

Source: Modified from Simon, H.B.
"Exercise, Health and Sports Medicine." In *Scientific American Medicine* (New York: Scientific American, 1994).

Table 5–2
CALORIES BURNED IN EACH MILE
OF WALKING OR JOGGING

Body Weight (pounds)	Calories
100	67
110	74
120	83
130	89
140	95
150	100
160	108
170	115
180	121
190	128
200	135
210	141
220	148

you improve, build up to activities that burn about 8 calories per minute. If you maintain this level, you can burn up your 2,000 calories per week in about 35 minutes a day. If you choose to increase your intensity to 10 calories per minute, and your body tells you it's OK to do so, you'll save 10 minutes a day — or you'll be able to burn a full 3,000 calories per week in about 40 minutes a day.

The figures in Table 5–1 apply to people weighing 150 pounds; people who weigh less will burn fewer calories, while people who are heavier will use more energy to move them along. Table 5–2 illustrates the effect of body weight on the energy used in walking or jogging. Your pace, style, and efficiency don't have much influence on how many calories you burn per mile; walkers will consume nearly as many calories per mile as top-flight runners, but of course they'll take much longer to cover each mile.

The third way to evaluate how hard you're exercising is the most accurate, but it's also the most difficult. Still, it's the "gold standard" because it uses your actual heart rate; our patients with atherosclerosis all learn this method, and you can, too.

The first step is to learn how to take your pulse. You can use the carotid artery in your neck or the radial artery in your wrist. Practice

Table 5-3
YOUR TARGET HEART RATE FOR AEROBIC EXERCISE

Age	Maximum Heart Rate	Target Range Beats per Minute		10-Second Pulse Count	
		Low (70% max.)	High (85%)	Low	High
20	200	140	170	23	28
25	200	140	170	23	28
30	194	136	165	22	27
35	188	132	160	22	26
40	182	128	155	21	26
45	176	124	150	20	25
50	171	119	145	20	24
55	165	115	140	19	23
60	149	111	135	18	23
65	153	107	130	17	22

while you are resting comfortably; because your heart rate will be slower at rest, taking your pulse will be easier. After you've mastered the technique, begin checking your pulse during exercise. Count the beats during 10 seconds, than multiply times 6 to find your heart rate.

Once you know how to count your heart rate, you can adjust your exercise intensity to keep your heart rate in the target range of 70 to 85 percent of maximum. If you've had a stress test, you'll have been told your maximum rate and you can determine your target range with precision. But most healthy people don't need stress tests; they can simply subtract their age in years from 220 to find their predicted maximum, then calculate the 70 to 85 percent target range. Even easier: look it up in Table 5-3.

Start at the low end, then build up as you improve. You'll be amazed at how much more you'll be able to do without exceeding your maximum heart rate. Your pulse count is a reliable and simple way to be sure you're exercising at a safe, effective aerobic intensity, but like most rules, it has an exception. Swimmers should deduct 10 beats per minute from their target heart rates because the diving reflex, a cardiovascular response to immersion in water, automatically slows the heart by about 10 beats per minute.

Options for Aerobic Exercise

After you learned the theory of the low-fat diet, you turned to the task of shopping, cooking, and — at last — eating as you should. Now that you've mastered the principles of aerobics, you can decide how to put theory into practice. As with foods, you'll be able to choose from a large menu of effective and enjoyable aerobic activities. As with diet, your choices will depend on personal preference, experience, and convenience. As with eating, you'll be best served exploring many options so you can build variety, flexibility, and balance into your program.

Walking is an ideal basis for aerobics. It's natural and easy, requiring no instruction and little equipment. It's adaptable to all climates, allowing you to enjoy nature when it's nice out or to be comfortable in a shopping mall when it's nasty. It can be a solitary activity or an opportunity for companionship. And walking is nearly injury-free. As Charles Dickens put it, "Walk and be happy, walk and be healthy."

The only trick to walking is to walk, not stroll. Push yourself into your aerobic range and keep yourself there. Wear athletic clothing and expect to sweat. And don't forget to wear high-quality walking shoes, the only equipment that you really need to walk away from atherosclerosis.

Jogging and running have all the advantages of walking but add one big plus and an equally big minus. Both relate to the fact that running is more intense than walking. On the plus side, you'll be able to push yourself harder, getting a better workout in less time. On the minus side, you'll be subjecting your body to substantial impact. Walkers have one foot on the ground at all times, but runners are airborne during part of each stride; the faster you run, the greater your "flight time" — and the harder your impact on landing. On average, a runner's legs absorb 100 tons of impact force in each mile.

Impact notwithstanding, jogging and running can be safe as well as enjoyable. The trick is to pay extra attention to the details, such as good shoes, soft running surfaces, and diligent warm-up and stretching activities. Above all, runners must listen to their legs and backs as well as their hearts and lungs; responding to early complaints will prevent major injuries.

If you're just getting started, walk before you jog and jog before you run. People with arthritis and those who are overweight or older will do well to stick with walking, but others can build up to the extra intensity of running. The Old Testament says it all: "They shall run and not grow weary" (Isaiah 40:31).

Swimming and aquatic exercises are the least traumatic of all aerobic activities: the water absorbs 90 percent of the force of gravity, providing cushioning and protection. Another advantage is that swimming uses the whole body, so it conditions the arms and back as well as the legs. It's also the only aerobic exercise that develops flexibility, obviating the need for supplementing stretching exercises. But swimming has disadvantages as well. To walk or jog your way to a healthy heart, you need only good shoes and a safe street, but to swim you need water. You also need a lifeguard for safety, and you need to know how to swim. Finally, swimming is somewhat less desirable than land exercise in the fight against atherosclerosis since it is less effective in reducing body fat. Because it's not a weight-bearing exercise, swimming is also less effective in preventing osteoporosis.

Swimming is highly recommended for people with arthritis or other musculoskeletal problems. Even people who can't swim can benefit from water exercises known as aqua-dynamics. For more intensity, just put on a flotation vest and "run" in water — your muscles and joints will thank you, and so will your heart.

Biking is another excellent aerobic activity. It can be gentle or intense, solitary or shared. Because of the bike's mechanical advantage, bikers can cover much greater distances than walkers or even runners — in fact, they have to cover greater distances in order to get a full aerobic workout. Biking is low in impact, but accidents and traumatic injuries are a real hazard. Another disadvantage is that biking is weather-dependent. But within these limitations, biking is a splendid aerobic option. Involving only a little skill and a little caution, biking requires only two bits of equipment: a bike and helmet. It won't do you much good to have a healthy heart if you have a cracked skull.

Walkers, runners, swimmers, and bikers typically measure their accomplishments in terms of distances instead of time or calories. Table 5–4 compares the distances typically required to burn 2,000 calories in each sport.

Aerobic dance is the fifth major option for aerobics. It has the advantage of using all the body's major muscle groups, and it adds the stimulation of music and the challenge of mastering new steps and routines. Aerobic dance is usually a group activity; as such it has the advantages

Table 5-4
TYPICAL DISTANCES REQUIRED TO BURN 2,000 CALORIES

Activity	Distance
Swimming	5 miles
Walking	20 miles
Running	20 miles
Cross-country skiing	20 miles
Skating	60 miles
Biking	100 miles

of instruction, companionship, and the motivation that a fixed schedule provides. Group activities, though, allow less room for flexibility; fortunately, videotapes can bring aerobics right into your home. Aerobic dance is splendid for the cardiovascular system, but because it's a moderately high-impact activity, musculoskeletal injuries are a risk. To minimize injuries, wear good aerobic shoes, and try to use a forgiving dance floor instead of a hard surface. Low-impact aerobics is another option that's as friendly to feet as to hearts.

These five aerobic options are only the most common entrees on your menu of exercises that fight atherosclerosis. *Ice-skating* and *cross-country skiing*, for example, are ideal aerobic sports for winter; *roller-blading* can fill out the year aerobically. Although it's a bit esoteric and inconvenient, *rowing* is a splendid option for warmer climates. Vigorous singles *racquet sports* and full-court *basketball* are competitive sports that contribute to cardiac health as well as fun. Beware, though, of relying on either of America's favorite sports; *baseball* and *golf* are great for recreation, but they're just not intense enough for aerobics. Golfers, though, can get modest cardiovascular benefit from walking the course, especially if they carry their own bags.

Like so many other aspects of modern life, aerobic exercise is increasingly entering the realm of high technology. *Exercise machines*, though, aren't labor-saving gadgets. Instead, they allow users to labor against atherosclerosis in the convenience and privacy of their homes or with the companionship and support of health clubs.

Like the human body itself, exercise machines are subject to a major drawback: disuse. Americans invest more than $2 billion annually in exercise machines; these machines will pay for themselves in health many times over, but *only* if they are used regularly. The stationary bike is a prime example. Purchased with the best of intentions, the average bike is used for a lifetime total of only 87 miles. The exercise bike is a splendid device for cardiovascular fitness; too often, though, it's composed of two pedals, one wheel, and no riders.

Go beyond good intentions: use an exercise machine for good health. Listen to music to help keep you motivated, or keep up with the world by watching TV or listening to the news; you can even do your daily reading on an exercise bike, gaining time as well as health. Or read with your ears while you pedal with your feet. Listening to books on tape is a great way to motivate exercise — particularly if you resist the temptation to finish the tape in your car or den, so you'll have to get on your bike or treadmill to find out how the story ends.

Many types of machines are available; all are convenient, take little skill, produce few injuries, and are adaptable to the aerobic needs of beginners or competitive athletes. Beware of budget models, which are usually flimsy and are often difficult to calibrate for proper use. In most cases, sturdy and reliable models are available for $200–$400. You can spend much more on high-tech models, but their sophisticated electronic programs and monitors are worthwhile only if you need bells and whistles to keep you interested and motivated.

Stationary bikes are the workhorses of cardiac rehabilitation programs, health clubs, and home fitness programs. They are compact, durable, quiet, and relatively inexpensive. Most will exercise only leg muscles, but some have handlebars that are rigged for simultaneous arm exercise. Most models use a flywheel for resistance; a heavy wheel will give you a smoother ride. Some bikes use air paddles for resistance; you'll get a pleasant breeze that may encourage you to keep pedaling. Look for a sturdy bike with an adjustable, comfortable seat, smooth pedaling action, and controls that allow you to select the proper resistance level each day. Warm up at very low resistance, then work out at a resistance and speed that put you into your aerobic range; finally, cool down at low resistance.

Cross-country skiing machines have the advantage of working your arms and back as well as your legs. Because they produce little impact, they cause few injuries. Many people find them more challenging than bikes, an asset if motivation is a problem. They do require a bit of balance and coordination, though, and they take up more space than bikes; they are also more expensive. In general, skiing machines that use cables and flywheels provide smoother skiing than those using pistons.

Rowing machines provide many of the same advantages of skiing machines; they work the upper and lower bodies and produce no impact. They can, however, trigger muscle spasms in people who are prone to back problems. Like skiing machines, rowers tend to be more expensive and less compact than bikes. Cable and flywheel models are preferable to piston models.

Treadmills provide the advantages of walking and jogging in the convenience of an indoor setting. Because good treadmills are quite expensive and require substantial floor space, they are better suited to your health club than your home.

Stair climbers have surged in popularity since their introduction in 1985. Stair climbing is an excellent way to condition your heart and your legs — which is why competitive athletes run stadium steps and dancers do step-aerobics. Climbing machines allow high-intensity aerobic exercise with low impact; some climbers allow simultaneous arm and leg exercise. Club models are quite expensive, but sturdy and reliable home models can now be purchased for little more than the cost of a stationary bike. Look for a stair climber with large pedals and a sturdy frame. Both the handrails and the step height should be adjustable to match your size and stride. And, like all exercise machines, a good climber should have resistance controls that are precise and easy to set.

Exercises for Flexibility

Aerobic exercise is an essential part of the fight against atherosclerosis. Flexibility exercise is not—but stretching exercises are important to keep your muscles fit for aerobics. They will also help reduce stress, an asset for your heart and head as well as your torso and limbs.

Stretch before and after aerobics, as part of your warm-up and cooldown routines. Stretch when you wake up to start your day smoothly; stretch before bed to relax tense muscles. Stretch early and often, but stretch properly — if you stretch to the point of pain, you can cause muscle pulls instead of preventing them.

Table 5–5
EXERCISES FOR FLEXIBILITY

Achilles stretch	Leg spread
Calf stretch	William's exercise for the back
Hamstring stretches	Cat's back stretch
Hip stretch	Shoulder stretch
Groin stretch	Neck stretch

Plan a routine that fits your body's needs, concentrating on your stiffest joints and on the muscles you'll be using most for aerobics. Consult a trainer or yoga teacher or read a fitness book for details. Most routines will incorporate the flexibility exercises listed in Table 5–5.

Exercising for Strength

Aerobics will build a strong heart; resistance exercises will not. High-resistance isometrics, in fact, can overtax the cardiovascular system and should be avoided by people with hypertension and heart disease. But low-resistance, high-repetition exercises can enhance muscular endurance and strength without stressing your heart. They are a nice asset for general fitness and health, even though they don't fight atherosclerosis.

There are three ways to do low-resistance strength exercises: you can use the weight of your body in calisthenics, you can use free weights (dumbbells or barbells), or you can use resistance machines (Nautilus and others). If you choose to exercise for strength, though, remember a principle that applies equally to all three techniques: you are better off lifting a 10-pound weight 10 times than a 100-pound weight once.

You'll need hands-on instruction at a club to use resistance machines properly. If you choose to work out for strength at home, you can select from the exercises listed in Table 5–6. As with all forms of exercise, go slowly and listen to your body. The American College of Sports Medicine recommends doing 8 to 12 repetitions for each of your larger muscle groups twice a week; you should be able to accomplish this in about 15 minutes. I'm all for adding strength exercises to your exercise schedule — unless, of course, they cut into the aerobics that you need to conquer heart disease.

Table 5–6
EXERCISES FOR STRENGTH

Calisthenics	Weights
Windmills	Lateral raise
Body twists	Curls
Knee-ups	Press
Push-ups	Front and rear leg raises
Leg raises	
Bent-knee sit-ups	

Preventing Injuries

Put your muscles to work against atherosclerosis. But take care of your muscles and joints so they can do the job for your heart.

The cardiovascular benefits of exercise depend on steady, repetitive exercise. Muscles, too, thrive with this type of use. But overstress, either in the form of a sudden, excessive force or chronic overuse, can cause injury. Most injuries can be prevented by appropriate warm-ups and cool-downs, good equipment, and proper technique. Flexibility exercises are also very helpful; if muscle imbalance is present, strength exercises that correct the problem can prevent injury.

If you are starting out healthy, you can take excellent care of your heart without a cardiologist. If you listen to your body, you can treat most exercise-related strains and sprains without an orthopedist. Use the 5-step PRICE program for early treatment:

Protection. Use special exercise gear or equipment to protect any area of your body that is especially vulnerable to injury.

Rest. This is the key. Don't deny pain, stiffness, or weakness. If you have an injury, rest the damaged muscles or joints until they recover. But if you've built a balanced program, you'll usually be able to substitute another heart-friendly aerobic activity while an injured muscle recovers.

Ice. Ice packs are the best way to fight inflammation early on. If you sustain an injury, apply ice for about 10 minutes as soon as possible. Repeat the treatment 4 times a day for the first 2 days.

Compression. An elastic bandage will fight inflammation while providing support and comfort. It should be snug and firm, but never so tight that it cuts off circulation.

Elevation. Use gravity to reduce inflammation and swelling by draining fluid away. Use pillows or cushions to prop up your injured limb as often as possible in the early stages of an injury.

Consider taking aspirin or ibuprofen to reduce inflammation and pain; read the directions carefully to be sure you are using these non-prescription drugs safely, and never use them on your own if you've had ulcers, bleeding problems, or other serious medical conditions.

If you are successful in identifying injury early and treating it promptly, you may then be able to take care of your own rehabilitation program. After the acute injury has settled down, begin your rehab by applying heat 3 or 4 times a day. Add range-of-motion exercises, ideally right after you remove the heating pad. Progress to weight bearing, then gradually resume your aerobic program. Until recovery is complete, it's a good idea to apply an ice pack to the injured area after you exercise.

Don't let injuries deter you from exercising to fight atherosclerosis. You can prevent or treat most problems yourself. But don't be stubborn: if necessary, consult a doctor, physical therapist, sports podiatrist, or trainer for help. Take all the help you can get so you can go on helping your heart with aerobic conditioning.

Building a Balanced Program

To fight atherosclerosis with diet, you need balanced nutrition instead of simple fat restriction. To conquer heart disease with exercise, you need a balanced fitness program. Chapter 4 helped you learn your way around the kitchen; here are 20 tips to help you find your way around the gym:

1. Make physical activity part of your daily life. Put your body to work as much as possible; household chores, stairs, and walking for transportation will not substitute for aerobics, but every little bit will help.
2. Make aerobics a priority. It's more time consuming than the other elements of your 15-point program, but it's an essential part of the fight against atherosclerosis. You won't *find* the time to exercise, but you can *make* the time you need. Once you're in shape, your added vigor and efficiency will compensate for the time you invest in exercise. And in the end, you'll regain all that time by living longer as well as better.
3. Be sure your heart and muscles are healthy before you begin a vigor-

ous exercise program. In most cases routine medical evaluation will suffice, but if you have cardiac risk factors or suspicious symptoms, consult with your doctor about special evaluations. Even if medical problems are discovered, you'll probably be able to exercise, but you will need special precautions and guidelines.

4. Choose the exercises that are best for you. Consider your body build, health, preferences, athletic experience, family and professional needs, and finances. Try various activities and schedules until you find a program you can really enjoy.

5. Set realistic goals. Your ultimate objective is to conquer heart disease, an entirely achievable goal. But don't set your exercise goals unreasonably high; disappointment and frustration will be your only reward. Don't set your goals too low, either; your physical capacity will improve remarkably with patience and persistence.

6. Aim for slow but steady progress. Shakespeare explained it all: "Too swift arrives as tardy as too slow" (*Romeo and Juliet*).

7. Keep a fitness log. Record your exercise level, your weight, and the way you feel. You'll be amazed to see how much you improve in just a few months.

8. Exercise regularly. It's easier to gain weight than to lose it, and it's easier to become deconditioned than to get into shape. Maintain your gains with regular exercise.

9. Be flexible about exercise. You can be regular without being rigid. Don't feel guilty if you have to miss a few sessions because of other commitments; in fact, you *should* skip exercise if you are injured or ill. But don't go too far in this direction either; flexibility is one thing, laziness another.

10. Adjust your schedule to the weather. Don't push yourself in the heat and humidity — or in the cold or rain.

11. Build variety into your exercise. Variety will keep you interested and mentally fresh. You'll also be able to exercise indoors when the weather is harsh, or to use your arms if a leg is sore.

12. Eat and drink appropriately. Don't eat at all in the 2 hours before you exercise. But drink plenty of water before, during, and after exercise, particularly in warmer weather.

13. Dress appropriately, aiming for comfort, convenience, and protection rather than style.

14. Use good equipment, especially good shoes. Invest the time, as well as the money, you need to make a good choice; you'll save in the long run.

15. Exercise safely. Walk or jog facing the traffic; bike with the traffic, but

in either direction, avoid busy roads. Wear a helmet for biking. Wear reflectorized gear after dark. Beware of cars, dogs, and humans.

16. Exercise with companions. You can get lots of practical help from more experienced partners, and you can share encouragement and reinforce motivation with people of all fitness levels.

17. Get instruction. It's never too late to learn a new skill.

18. Consider entering competition. A healthy heart is a long-term goal. A fun run can give you a short-term goal for added motivation and fun.

19. Make exercise part of a healthful lifestyle. You can't fight atherosclerosis optimally unless you exercise, but you can't do it with exercise alone. Use the self-confidence and discipline you gain from mastering your body to improve your diet, stop smoking, and make the other changes you need to protect your heart.

20. Listen to your body. The cardiac symptoms summarized on pages 150–152 are, of course, of paramount importance. But don't overlook early distress signals from your muscles and joints (pain, swelling, stiffness), lungs (coughing, wheezing, breathlessness), intestinal tract (nausea, heartburn, diarrhea, bleeding), urinary tract (bleeding), reproductive system (menstrual irregularities), or nervous system (headaches). Most often, the sounds of your body will be harmonious, but if there are discordant tones, face the music early so you can keep yourself humming along toward a healthy heart.

The Secret Is Out

Most people know that exercise is good for them, but few learned it from their doctor.

The medical facts are no secret. In *1953* Professor J. N. Morris reported that the physically active conductors on double-decked London buses had far fewer heart attacks than the physically sedentary bus drivers. In the ensuing 40 years, more than 110 medical studies have used much more sophisticated techniques to reevaluate Dr. Morris's observation, and nearly all have confirmed the fact that exercise fights atherosclerosis, both in healthy people and in patients who already have the disease. These studies, moreover, prove that exercising regularly is just as important as controlling hypertension, lowering elevated blood cholesterol levels, and giving up cigarettes.

With all these facts, why do a mere 8 percent of primary care physicians rate themselves as successful in helping their patients establish programs? For that matter, why is the subject glossed over in most of the medical textbooks that doctors rely on? Why did the American College of Cardiology delay an official endorsement of aerobic exercise until 1990? Why did the National Cholesterol Education Program wait until 1993 to list sedentary living as a cardiac risk factor?

Why is exercise the best-kept secret in cardiology? I'm not sure, but I can guess. I suspect three factors. The first is American medicine's love affair with technology; doctors are trained to value fancy new advances rather than the basics. Second, doctors are much better at taking care of patients than they are at teaching patients to care for themselves; most would rather prescribe medicines than promote lifestyle changes. Finally, doctors may neglect to promote exercise because they neglect to exercise themselves; one survey found that only 27 percent of physicians exercise for even 1 hour a week — and the survey was done in California! The same physicians who gobble doughnuts at cardiac grand rounds are "too busy" to "find" time to exercise.

Physicians, heal thyself. Listen to the wisdom of Edward Stanley, the Earl of Derby, who wrote in 1873, "Those who think they have not time for bodily exercise will sooner or later have to find time for illness."

Chapter 6

Blood Pressure: Minerals Make a Difference

IN THE LAST THREE CHAPTERS, you've learned how to control smoking, cholesterol, and lack of exercise, three of the five major heart attack risk factors. Now it's time to consider the fourth major risk factor, high blood pressure.

Don't skip this chapter, even if you have a "normal" blood pressure. Everyone should pay heed to blood pressure. For one thing, blood pressure increases with age, at least in industrialized societies; even if your blood pressure is where you want it now, it is likely to rise unless you take steps to keep it down. For another thing, the concept of "normal" has little meaning for blood pressure and health. The lower your blood pressure, the lower your risk of illness, particularly heart disease and stroke. People with hypertension, of course, need to work the hardest at blood pressure control — but all of us can benefit from the simple lifestyle changes that will lower blood pressure and keep it down over the years.

Dietary minerals are the key to blood pressure control. By reducing one and increasing others, you can unearth something even more valuable than gold: good health.

Blood Pressure in America

The figures are staggering. One of every 4 American adults has high blood pressure; among people older than 60, the figure is 1 in 2. More than 2 million Americans develop hypertension every year. And in addition to the 50 million adults with hypertension, another 30 million have borderline blood pressure readings.

If high blood pressure is so common, can it really be a disease? The answer is yes, twice over, in fact. Hypertension is an important disease for each person with the condition; high blood pressure greatly increases the risk of heart attack, heart failure, stroke, visual loss, kidney failure, and premature death — if that's not a disease, what is? And hypertension is also an important disease for American society, a byproduct of the poor diet, obesity, lack of exercise, alcohol abuse, and mental stress that characterize modern life. In most cases, hypertension is a man-made disease; in all cases, it's a tremendous health burden for individuals and for society. The most common of all cardiovascular diseases, hypertension has reached epidemic proportions in America.

All the complications of hypertension can be prevented by early treatment. First, though, high blood pressure must be detected; unfortunately 46 percent of hypertensive Americans don't even know they have the problem. Once a diagnosis of hypertension has been established, excellent treatments are available; unfortunately 56 percent of hypertensive Americans are not being treated, and 75 percent are not achieving optimal results from treatment. And even this inadequate level of treatment is tremendously expensive. More than 20 million Americans take blood pressure medication, at an average cost of more than a dollar a day. In all, we spend more than $7 billion a year for the medical management of hypertension. It's money well spent — but we could do much, much better. Simple lifestyle changes could go a long way toward controlling hypertension without medications.

Chapter 2 explained how you should check your blood pressure and what your blood pressure goals should be. In this chapter, we'll explore ways to achieve those goals.

High Blood Pressure and Heart Disease

Hypertension is a major cause of heart disease. People with high blood pressure are 2.1 times more likely to suffer heart attacks than people with normal blood pressures; in all, hypertension accounts for 195,000 heart attack deaths in the United States each year.

High blood pressure does not affect blood cholesterol levels, nor does it activate the blood clotting system. How, then, does it contribute to atherosclerosis? By producing damage to the arterial wall itself. Elevated blood pressure injures the intima, the innermost layer of the arterial wall. Damage to the delicate inner membrane of endothelial cells opens the gates to LDL cholesterol. LDL enters the damaged blood vessel wall, undergoes oxidation, and initiates the process of plaque formation that eventually blocks arteries, causing heart attacks.

In addition to causing atherosclerosis of the coronary arteries, hypertension damages the heart muscle itself. The heart's main pumping chamber, the left ventricle, has to work extra hard to propel blood against the resistance of high blood pressure. Over the years the left ventricle becomes enlarged, thick, and stiff. Eventually it stretches, thins, and weakens. The result: congestive heart failure. The symptoms: weakness, fatigue, shortness of breath, and swelling of the legs and abdomen. The outcome: premature death.

Hypertension is bad news for the heart. But there is good news, too. Lowering blood pressure protects the heart; a reduction of only 3 points, for example, reduces the likelihood of suffering a heart attack by 5 percent.

High Blood Pressure, Atherosclerosis, and Health

Hypertension stresses every artery in the body. It's no surprise that it causes many problems beyond the heart itself.

The arteries of the brain and nervous system are particularly vulnerable to the effects of high blood pressure. Five hundred thousand Americans are felled by strokes each year; two-thirds of all stroke victims have hypertension. Like the risk of heart attacks, the risk of strokes increases in direct proportion to the increase in blood pressure; even Stage 1 hypertension (160/95, for example) quadruples the risk of stroke. Stroke is the third leading cause of death in America. In all, hypertension accounts for 50,000 stroke deaths every year.

Heart disease and strokes are the most lethal consequences of hypertension, but they don't tell the whole story. High blood pressure damages the eyes. Doctors can see this simply by looking at the back of the eye through an instrument called an ophthalmoscope; high blood pressure produces narrowing and thickening of the arteries, resulting eventually in hemorrhages, visual loss, and even blindness. The kidneys, too, are subject to arterial damage if high blood pressure goes undetected and untreated. Abnormal results of blood tests called BUN and creatinine are the early markers of hypertension; kidney failure is the final consequence.

As bad as these problems are, they used to be much worse. Stroke deaths have declined by more than 30 percent in the past 10 years alone; since 1950, stroke deaths in America have been reduced by two-thirds. Kidney failure has declined just as dramatically. Control of hypertension is a major reason for progress in both areas. Reducing blood pressure merely 3 points, for example, will reduce the risk of stroke by 8 percent; the overall death rate will decline by 4 percent. A 3-point reduction in blood pressure is easy to achieve without medications; in fact, you can do much better.

Sodium: The Mineral That Matters Most

Sodium may not be familiar to you as a mineral, but it's surely familiar to you as a compound: sodium chloride — salt. If you're like most Americans, in fact, salt is far too familiar to you.

Salt is a natural compound. More than that, it's an essential part of the natural world, providing the environment that's essential for all marine life.

Sodium is an essential part of the animal world. More than that, it's an indispensable part of the human body, regulating the fluid balance of cells and plasma that is essential for life.

Although it's entirely natural and absolutely essential for life in the sea and on land, large amounts of salt are not a natural part of the human diet. Because it's so indispensable, the human body has a remarkable capacity to conserve salt. Only tiny amounts of dietary salt are required to maintain the body's fluids. Extra dietary salt doesn't contribute at all to health — but it contributes a great deal to hypertension.

Salt and Body Fluids

Dietary salt is absorbed from the intestinal tract, always bringing water along with it. Salt enters the blood, where it is the major mineral constituent of the plasma and fluids that bathe the body's cells. Without enough salt, these fluids lose their water volume; dehydration is the result. But the body can work hard to prevent this; when salt is plentiful it's excreted in urine and sweat, but when dehydration is a threat, the kidneys and sweat glands retain salt to a remarkable degree. Water always follows salt; that's why your urine is voluminous and clear when you are well hydrated but scant and concentrated when you're dry. To be sure the body's balance of sodium and water are just right, an elaborate series of control mechanisms in the blood vessels and brain signal the kidneys to retain or excrete sodium as needed; they also control the sensation of thirst so you'll provide water in amounts that match the body's sodium supply.

Salt and Blood Pressure

With such effective control mechanisms why worry about salt? Just eat and drink what you like; your thirst mechanism, kidneys, and sweat glands will keep your body fluids in balance.

It's quite true that you don't need a nutritionist or doctor to regulate your body's fluids; just give it enough salt and water, and it will do the rest. Under normal circumstances, the body can adjust to a daily water intake ranging from one quart to many quarts; two-thirds of the human body is water, but an average intake of two quarts per day (including the half-quart present in a day's solid food) is plenty. Under normal circumstances the body can adjust to a salt intake ranging from a pinch to many spoonfuls. The kidneys can rise to the challenge of a high salt intake, excreting the excess so the body doesn't become bloated. Unfortunately, though, blood pressure rises along the way.

Sodium and Blood Pressure

Despite intensive study, physiologists are not sure exactly how excess dietary sodium contributes to hypertension. The excess salt and water are promptly excreted, but it seems likely that the blood volume is expanded, at least to a subtle degree, in the process. When pipes are overfilled with water, resistance increases; a pump must work harder to propel the water, and pressure in the system rises. The human circulation is, of course, much more complex than a simple hydraulic system, but the analogy may help explain why high levels of dietary sodium contribute to hypertension.

The observation that salty foods raise blood pressure is far from new. Nearly 4,700 years ago the Emperor of China, Huang Ti, wrote, "If too much salt is used in food, the pulse hardens." Emperor Huang's Americanized descendants should keep that in mind when they add soy sauce or MSG (mono*sodium* glutamate) to food.

Ancient wisdom notwithstanding, the role of salt in producing hypertension has been controversial among American blood pressure experts. Some patients respond dramatically to changes in dietary salt, raising their blood pressure when their sodium intake rises and lowering their blood pressure when dietary salt is restricted, but other patients don't demonstrate this relationship. New studies, however, have gone a long way toward resolving the debate; by comparing salt intake with blood pressure levels around the world, they demonstrate that dietary sodium *is* a major cause of hypertension.

It's an important issue, warranting a quick look at several representative studies. The famous INTERSALT Study is an international effort that has been tracking the blood pressures of 10,079 men and women in 52 centers from 32 countries in North and South America, Europe, Africa, and Asia (north, south, east, and west). In addition to having their blood pressure measured with meticulous technique, subjects were weighed and measured so their body mass index could be calculated. Dietary sodium, potassium, and alcohol intakes were evaluated; to double-check dietary minerals, urine samples were collected and analyzed for sodium and potassium. It has been an enormous amount of work, but the results are clear: dietary sodium is directly related to blood pressure, even after other factors that raise blood pressure (obesity, low dietary potassium, and alcohol consumption) are considered. And the relationship is very strong: in centers where the average sodium intake was low, only 1.7 percent of subjects had high blood pressure, but where sodium intake was high, 13.4 percent were hypertensive.

A second example: the series of three papers by Drs. Law, Frost, and Wald published in 1991 in the *British Medical Journal*. Using the technique of meta-analysis, these investigators combined the findings of studies in 24 communities from around the world; in all, dietary sodium and blood pressure were evaluated in more than 47,000 people. The results were striking. In both industrialized and underdeveloped countries, dietary salt is directly related to blood pressure; for each 2,400 milligrams of sodium in the daily diet, blood pressure increases by about 10 points. The effect of dietary sodium is strongest in the elderly and in people with hypertension; in other words, eating salt increases blood pressure the most in precisely the people who are most vulnerable to heart attacks and strokes. Fortunately, the effects of dietary salt were reversible: Dr. Law and his colleagues found that even a modest reduction in dietary sodium lowers the blood pressure substantially in as little as 5 weeks.

By now, many other studies have confirmed these observations. Increasing dietary salt increases blood pressure; reducing sodium intake lowers blood pressure.

When it comes to blood pressure, salt is a four-letter word.

Salt in the American Diet

America is the land of hypertensives; our national addiction to salt is one reason for this sorry fact.

The average American consumes more than 4,000 milligrams of sodium per day; that's the equivalent of more than 2 teaspoons of table salt, perhaps 10 times more than the body needs to keep its fluids in balance.

It wasn't always that way. Salt was a scarcity for primitive humans. They got along quite well on minimal amounts of dietary sodium; when they found salt, in fact, they used it for barter instead of eating it. Because it was rare, salt became valuable; it was mined from the earth and recovered from evaporated sea water, but it remained too expensive for ordinary people. With the technological advances of industrial revolution, however, salt became plentiful and inexpensive. It did find a valuable role as a food preservative, but pickled and salted foods have long since outlived their benefits. No longer used for currency or as a food preservative, salt is currently added to foods strictly for flavor. For health, however, salt's transfiguration from valuable to victual has been far from tasty. Salting your food is assaulting your blood pressure.

Even today, people in many isolated societies around the world consume very, very little salt; examples include the Yonomano Indians of Brazil, the Bushmen of Kalahari, and the Solomon Islanders. Hypertension is virtually nonexistent in these people, and blood pressure does not rise with age as it does in all salt-using industrialized societies; not coincidentally, heart attacks and strokes are also rare in these "primitives."

America does not lead the world in salt consumption, but we come close. Where do we get our 4,000 milligrams of daily sodium? Only 10 percent derives from the natural salt content of our food. Another 15 percent tumbles from our salt shakers. An astounding 75 percent of our dietary salt is added to our food during the manufacturing process; just 10 potato chips, for example, contain more sodium than 25 pounds of potatoes.

The human body has evolved mechanisms enabling it to function best with low amounts of dietary sodium. The human mind has developed ways of adding salt to foods that are naturally low in salt. Faced with a choice between nature and industry, we're currently gobbling up processed foods. But we can overcome our acquired taste for salt. By weaning ourselves from junk food, we'll save lots of fat and calories as well as salt; by returning to natural foods, we'll benefit from additional vitamins and fiber. By matching human behavior to human evolution, we'll conquer heart disease.

Setting Your Goals for Dietary Sodium

There is no Recommended Daily Allowance for sodium; instead of setting a *minimum* amount required for health, national authorities now offer targets for *maximum* sodium intake. The Joint National Committee on Detection, Evaluation, and Treatment of High Blood Pressure calls for an average daily sodium intake of less than 2,300 milligrams; the National Academy of Sciences proposes a 2,000 milligram maximum, about 50 percent of the current average.

How much sodium should you eat? The less the better. Remember that blood pressure is continuously related to dietary sodium; the lower your sodium intake, the lower your blood pressure. There is no "normal" or "safe" blood pressure; the lower your blood pressure, the lower your risk of heart attack and stroke. The more you cut your sodium intake, the more you'll fight atherosclerosis.

Set your goals according to your needs. Check your blood pressure, and use Table 2–4 to interpret it. Unless your blood pressure is optimal, reduce your dietary sodium (among other things) to help bring it down.

Remember, too, that as important as blood pressure is, it's only one factor in atherosclerosis. Check your overall cardiac risk score (Table 2–11); if it's high, reduce your dietary sodium to help improve the blood pressure component of risk. In general, 2,000 milligrams is a reasonable goal, but if you are at risk 1,500 milligrams might be better.

Set your goals according to your tastes and preferences. Some people find it easy to give up salty foods; for others it's difficult. But remember that salt is an acquired taste; if you make changes slowly but progressively, you'll acquire a genuine liking for *low*-salt foods.

Where's the Sodium?

Salt is the most obvious — and important — source of sodium, but there are others; baking powder, baking soda, and MSG are examples of high-sodium products. Remember, too, that salt has just as much sodium even if it's called sea salt, brine, garlic salt, onion salt, or seasoned salt.

At long last, the new food labels make it easy for you to find out exactly how much sodium you're eating. Labels now state the actual sodium content per portion, and tell you what that represents as a "% of daily value." The Food and Drug Administration's daily value for sodium is 2,400 milligrams; your target may well be lower; if so, you'll have to recalculate the percentage figure. It's also important to evaluate portion size with care.

Table 6–1 lists the sodium content of representative foods. Tally up your intake on each of three average days; if you are exceeding your target level, take steps to achieve your goals.

Shaking the Habit

Because we've been conditioned to "like" salt, change can be difficult. Here are some grains of advice to help you succeed.

1. Change gradually. Low-sodium foods may seen bland and unappetizing at first, but you'll actually grow to like them if you wean yourself off salt slowly. Before long, you'll actually be tasting *food* — it's good!
2. Begin by omitting salt from your table, then from your cooking. Learn to use other seasonings to enhance the flavor of your foods. Salt substitutes containing potassium chloride are fine, but beware of "low-sodium" salt that is only sodium chloride diluted to make the sodium

Table 6-1
SODIUM CONTENT OF SELECTED FOODS

Food	Serving Size	Sodium content (milligrams)
Grain Products		
Pasta	$^1/_2$ cup	less than 5
Rice	$^1/_2$ cup	less than 5
Cooked cereal	$^1/_2$ cup	less than 5
Bread	1 slice	110–175
Cake and pastry	1 slice	100–400
Muffins and biscuits	1	170–390
Pancakes (from mix)	1	150
Ready-to-eat cereals	1 oz.	100-360
Vegetables		
Fresh (cooked without salt)	$^1/_2$ cup	most less than 50
Frozen (without sauce)	$^1/_2$ cup	most less than 70
Frozen (with sauce)	$^1/_2$ cup	140–460
Canned	$^1/_2$ cup	140–500
Canned (with sauce)	$^1/_2$ cup	150–900
Legumes		
Dried beans, peas, lentils (cooked without salt)	1 cup	less than 5
Baked beans, canned	1 cup	600–900
Nuts		
Peanuts, cashews, almonds, walnuts, pistachios (fresh or roasted, unsalted)	$^1/_2$ cup	less than 10
Salted nuts	$^1/_2$ cup	300–600
Fruits		
Fresh, frozen, or canned	$^1/_2$ cup	less than 10
Meat, Poultry, Fish		
Fresh meat	3 oz.	less than 90
Ham	3 oz.	1,100
Bacon	2 slices	275
Corned beef	3 oz.	800
Chipped beef	3 oz.	3,600
Hamburger (fast-food restaurant)	3 oz.	450
Hot dog	1	700
Bologna	1 slice	220
Salami	1 slice	250
Poultry		
Fresh poultry	3 oz.	less than 90
Turkey roll	3 oz.	500
Frozen turkey or chicken dinner	1 dinner	1,000–2,000
Fish		
Fresh fish	3 oz.	less than 90
Tuna, canned	3 oz.	300
Salmon, canned	3 oz.	300–440
Sardines, canned	3 oz.	550
Shrimp, canned	3 oz.	2,000
Herring, smoked	3 oz.	5,200

continued

Table 6–1 *continued*

Food	Serving Size	Sodium content (milligrams)
Dairy Products		
Egg	1	60
Egg substitute, frozen	1/4 cup	120
Milk	1 cup	120–160
Yogurt	1 cup	120–160
Unsalted butter or margarine	1 tsp.	2
Salted butter or margarine	1 tsp.	115
Natural cheeses	1/2 oz.	110–450
Cottage cheese	1/2 cup	450
Processed cheese	2 oz.	700–900
Cheese spread	2 oz.	700–900
Juices and Soups		
Fruit juice, fresh, frozen, or canned	1 cup	less than 10
Tomato juice, canned	1 cup	800
Vegetable juice, canned	1 cup	800
Canned, condensed, and dehydrated soups	1 cup	600–1,200
Condiments and Dressings		
Oil and vinegar	1 tbsp.	less than 5
Prepared salad dressing	1 tbsp.	80–250
Catsup	1 tbsp.	150
Meat tenderizer	1 tbsp.	1,750
Mustard	1 tbsp.	65
Barbecue sauce	1 tbsp.	130
Soy sauce	1 tbsp.	1,000
Teriyaki sauce	1 tbsp.	690
Worcestershire sauce	1 tbsp.	69
Tomato sauce	1 cup	1,500
Tomato paste	1 cup	77
Snack and Convenience Foods		
Pizza	1 slice	500–1,000
TV dinner	10 oz.	1,000–2,000
Candy	1 oz.	less than 25
Peanut butter	1 tbsp.	26
Pickle	2 oz.	700
Olives	2	385
Pretzels	1 oz.	450
Potato chips	1 oz.	250
Crackers, plain	1 cracker	30–60
Crackers, cheese flavor	1 oz.	300
Popcorn, air popped	1 oz.	1
Popcorn, buttered and salted	1 oz.	550
Beverages		
Coffee, tea	1 cup	2
Carbonated beverages	8 oz.	less than 40
Wine	4 oz.	12
Beer	12 oz.	25

Principal source: "Nutritive Value of Foods." *U.S. Department of Agriculture.*

less concentrated. Experiment with pepper, herbs, lemon juice, and other sodium-free seasonings.

3. Avoid fast foods, convenience foods, processed snacks, and other junk foods. Chips, pretzels, pickles, salted crackers, and salted popcorn are particularly high in sodium.

4. Beware of condiments. Catsup, some prepared mustards, soy sauce, and teriyaki sauce are all high in sodium, as are various commercial dressings. Tomato sauce is loaded with sodium; tomato paste is not.

5. Avoid cured or processed meats; hot dogs, bacon, luncheon meats, and smoked poultry are all very high in sodium; one small portion of chipped beef has enough sodium for three days. Fresh meats are low in sodium (but high in saturated fat and cholesterol).

6. Read food labels and ask about the salt and the sodium-rich sauces in restaurants, too.

7. Choose fresh foods over processed foods whenever you can. Be particularly careful to evaluate canned foods. Canned soup, canned tomato and vegetable juices, and canned fish are usually very high in sodium. So, too, are most dried soups and bouillons. Although many frozen foods have less sodium than canned foods, frozen dinners and pizzas are typically very high in sodium.

8. Eat lots of fresh fruits and vegetables. You'll avoid sodium and get vitamins and fiber that can help conquer heart disease. You'll also get potassium, which may help lower your blood pressure.

Potassium: Good News for Blood Pressure

In many ways, potassium occupies an opposite role from sodium in the human body. High concentrates of sodium are present in plasma and in the fluids that surround the body's cells; only low concentrates of potassium are found in those same fluids. Inside cells, the situation is reversed, with potassium present in high concentration, sodium in small amounts. A large intake of potassium in the diet promotes the excretion of a large amount of sodium in the urine.

In many ways, potassium and sodium occupy opposite positions in food. Lots of sodium is present in processed foods, but little is found in natural foods. Potassium is abundant in many natural foods.

Potassium and sodium occupy opposite positions in the American diet. We eat far too much sodium, but not enough potassium.

Potassium and sodium also fill opposite roles in the regulation of blood pressure. High dietary sodium raises blood pressure; high dietary potassium tends to lower blood pressure.

Potassium and Blood Pressure

In a sense, Dr. W. T. L. Addison is the Huang Ti of potassium. The emperor of China implicated sodium as a cause of hypertension in 2697 B.C., but Dr. Addison's medical studies showing that potassium could reduce blood pressure weren't published until 1928. Within just a few years, Drs. Priddle, McQuarrie, and others confirmed those observations, culminating in Dr. Kemper's famous rice diet of the 1940s.

Independent studies from the United States, Japan, Belgium, Kenya, Zaire, England, Scotland, St. Lucia, and China have all agreed that high intakes of dietary potassium are associated with lower blood pressure readings. The INTERSALT Study is an example (see page 176); it found that high potassium levels predicted low blood pressure readings even after considering body mass index, dietary sodium, and alcohol consumption.

With all this data, why isn't potassium considered as important as sodium for the regulation of blood pressure? The answer resides in the results of treatment trials. Numerous studies have shown that sodium restriction will lower blood pressure, both in normal people and in hypertensive subjects. In contrast, trials of potassium supplements have been less conclusive. Since 1980 at least 22 trials have been conducted; most suggest that supplementary potassium tends to lower blood pressure in normals and hypertensives, but few have demonstrated statistically conclusive results. In 1991 and 1992, however, independent meta-analyses combined data from earlier trials and concluded that potassium supplements *can* help lower blood pressure.

Where do we stand with regard to potassium and blood pressure? I don't think there is enough proof to justify the routine use of prescription potassium supplements. But there is plenty of evidence that high intake of dietary potassium from natural sources is very helpful.

It's back to nature, once again. Eat lots of potassium-rich foods to help lower your blood pressure and conquer heart disease.

Setting Your Goals for Potassium

How much potassium should be in your diet? The body can conserve potassium much as it can sodium, and there is no Recommended Daily

Table 6–2
POTASSIUM CONTENT OF SELECTED FOODS

Food	Serving Size	Potassium (milligrams)
Fruits		
Apple	1 medium	159
Apricots	1 large	100
Banana	1 large	740
Cantaloupe	$1/4$ melon	250
Dates	1 cup	1,150
Orange	1 medium	270
Peach	1 medium	170
Raisins	1 oz.	210
Vegetables		
Asparagus	4 spears	186
Lima beans	1 cup	740
Beets	1 cup	530
Broccoli	1 spear	491
Carrots	1 medium	233
Mushrooms	1 cup	259
Potato	1 medium	844
Spinach	1 cup	307
Squash, winter	1 cup	896
Tomato	1 medium	255
Dairy Products		
Milk	1 cup	370
Yogurt	8 oz.	442
Fish, Poultry, Meat		
Cod	$3^{1}/_{2}$ oz.	336
Tuna	$3^{1}/_{2}$ oz.	301
Chicken	$3^{1}/_{2}$ oz.	200
Hamburger	$3^{1}/_{2}$ oz.	298
Grain Products		
All-Bran cereal	1 oz.	350

Allowance for potassium. The Food and Nutrition Board of the National Academy of Sciences recommends at least 2,000 milligrams of potassium a day and adds that it's perfectly safe to consume three-times-higher amounts. I'd add only one proviso: patients with kidney disease need medical supervision of their dietary potassium, as do patients taking potassium-retaining diuretics and certain other medications.

Natural foods are the best source of potassium; have a look at Table 6–2, and add lots of potassium to your diet. Naturally.

Calcium: Another Mineral That Can Help

Familiar as the mineral that's essential to keep bones strong, calcium is often overlooked as a mineral that may help keep blood vessels soft. Fortunately, the two roles are not contradictory; by consuming an adequate amount of calcium, you can help keep your bone density up and your blood pressure down.

Calcium in the Body

The calcium in food is absorbed by the intestinal tract; vitamin D is essential for this process. After entering the blood, calcium is bound to proteins for transport throughout the body. Most of the calcium is deposited in bones; in fact, the calcium in bones constitutes nearly 25 percent of the body's weight. Because bones are being remodeled continuously, they need a constant supply of calcium; insufficient calcium is a major contributor to osteoporosis and fractures, particularly in postmenopausal women. But too much of a good thing can be harmful; the body prevents blood calcium levels from getting too high by excreting excess calcium in the urine.

Calcium does far more than build strong bones and teeth. In fact, it has an important role in blood clotting, nerve function, and muscle contraction.

Because it's so important to health, the blood calcium is closely regulated by the body's control mechanisms. Two hormones play a critical role; parathormone raises the blood calcium level, while calcitonin lowers it. Because these hormones are so efficient, you don't have to worry about your blood calcium concentration; just be sure to take in enough calcium, and your body will do the rest.

Calcium and Blood Pressure

Blood pressure rises when arteries narrow, increasing resistance to the flow of blood. Arteries narrow when muscle cells in their outer layers contract. Calcium has a major role in regulating muscle contraction, relaxing the muscles in arteries. Hence, it's not surprising that calcium may have a role in regulating blood pressure.

More surprising, perhaps, is the fact that the relationship between calcium and blood pressure was largely overlooked until recently. It's a new area of investigation, and many questions remain unanswered.

Still, there is enough data to recommend a high intake of calcium to fight atherosclerosis by keeping your blood pressure down.

More than 30 studies from around the world have evaluated dietary calcium and blood pressure. Most, but not all, have reported that people who eat lots of calcium-rich foods have lower blood pressures and a reduced risk of developing hypertension. For example, a study in Puerto Rico found that milk drinkers are half as likely to have high blood pressure as are people eating low-calcium diets. Similarly, the large U.S. Nurses' Health Study, which has taught us so much about diet and atherosclerosis, found that low dietary calcium was associated with a 22 percent increase in the risk of hypertension. Although most studies have been conducted in adults, one interesting investigation found that calcium may even affect blood pressure in infancy; babies had lower blood pressures at 1, 6, and 12 months of age if their mothers had calcium-rich diets.

Collectively these population studies suggest strongly that high-calcium diets are associated with lower blood pressure readings. As in the case of potassium, however, trials of supplementary calcium have produced contradictory results. At least 25 trials have been performed; almost all have used calcium supplements in pills rather than foods. Better results have been noted in patients with hypertension than in people whose blood pressure was normal to begin with. And a 1991 study of pregnant women found that calcium supplements reduced their risk of developing hypertension by about 30 percent. But not all the studies found such good results, and even when calcium supplements reduced blood pressure the effect was modest.

Until more data are available, the bottom line for calcium and blood pressure is similar to the potassium story: high-calcium foods should be encouraged to control blood pressure and reduce the risk of atherosclerosis, but calcium supplements do not appear necessary for hypertension. But there is an important difference between potassium and calcium: calcium supplements can be very beneficial for reasons beyond blood pressure and atherosclerosis.

Setting Your Goals for Calcium
Unlike sodium and potassium, there *are* Recommended Daily Allowances for calcium. The National Academy of Science suggests an intake of 1,200 milligrams per day for all healthy adults; many other authori-

Table 6-3
CALCIUM CONTENT OF SELECTED FOODS

Food	Serving Size	Calcium (milligrams)
Dairy Products		
Milk	1 cup	292
Skim milk	1 cup	302
Yogurt	1 cup	415
Low-fat yogurt	1 cup	452
Cottage cheese	1 cup	138
American cheese	1 oz.	174
Swiss cheese	1 oz.	272
Feta cheese	1 oz.	140
Vegetables		
Broccoli, cooked	1 cup	205
Spinach, cooked	1 cup	245
Fish		
Salmon, canned	3½ oz.	237
Sardines, canned	3½ oz.	240
Crab	1 cup	140
Oysters	1 cup	111
Other Foods		
Tofu (bean curd)		
Firm	1 cup	516
Regular	1 cup	260

ties, though, raise the target for postmenopausal women to 1,500 milligrams, and in their 1994 report, the expert committee of the National Institutes of Health also recommended 1,500 milligrams a day for older children and young adults of both sexes.

How are we doing with dietary calcium? Not well at all: American women average only 565 milligrams per day, while men consume an average of 975 milligrams.

Dairy products are the best dietary source of calcium; to reduce the risk of atherosclerosis, though, you should choose nonfat or lowfat varieties. Remember, too, that dairy products can be high in sodium (Table 6-1). Fish are high in calcium and can help fight atherosclerosis in their own right (Chapter 10). The vegetable world can also supply calcium, particularly in broccoli, spinach, and soybean products such as tofu.

Table 6-3 lists the calcium content of some foods. Keep track of your diet for 3 average days to see if you're achieving your goal of

1,200–1,500 milligrams per day. If not, cultivate a taste for skim milk and broccoli!

Broccoli and tofu notwithstanding, it can be hard to get enough calcium from dietary sources. If you don't reach your calcium target with foods, consider calcium supplements, which are widely available without a prescription. Most supplements are composed of calcium carbonate; some are synthetic, while others are made from oyster shells or bones. Calcium supplements are available in pill form and as chewable antacid tablets (Tums and other brands), which are particularly convenient. Find the least expensive, most palatable supplement, but be sure it meets the standards set by the U.S. Pharmacopoeia, a nonprofit testing lab. And be sure you get at least 400 units of vitamin D per day from fish, fortified dairy products, or supplements so you can absorb the calcium your body needs.

The major concern about calcium supplements is the risk of kidney stones. A 1993 study of 45,619 men, however, found that a higher intake of calcium actually *decreased* the risk of symptomatic kidney stones. This report published in the *New England Journal of Medicine* shatters another old medical belief about calcium — but provides welcome reassurance for all of us.

A high intake of calcium, either from foods or from supplements, is important to maintain strong bones and prevent osteoporosis. Although it's still inconclusive, there is some early data suggesting that calcium supplementation may even reduce the risk of colon cancer. And among the many good reasons to be sure you're getting enough calcium is its role in maintaining a healthy blood pressure. A mineral with many roles, calcium can help fight atherosclerosis.

Magnesium: Every Little Bit Helps

Magnesium is the fourth mineral that's involved in maintaining a normal blood pressure. We know the least about its role, but we should learn more.

An essential nutrient, magnesium has an important role in many of the body's processes, including blood clotting, bone formation, and protein synthesis. Like calcium, it is also important for muscle metabolism and function.

Magnesium has many similarities to calcium, and interest in its role in blood pressure began in much the same way, with the observation that people who drink hard water have less hypertension and lower heart disease death rates. At least 5 studies have evaluated the link between dietary magnesium and blood pressure; 4 of the 5 linked high magnesium consumption to lower blood pressures.

Intrigued by these observations, doctors have studied the use of magnesium supplements to treat hypertension. At least 9 clinical trials have been conducted. The results have been disappointing, with little fall in blood pressure and frequent complaints of diarrhea.

At present, magnesium supplements do not appear to be beneficial for hypertension. But magnesium supplements are finding an exciting role in the treatment of patients with atherosclerosis. New studies from the 1990s have shown that intravenous magnesium injections are very helpful to patients with heart attacks and to those undergoing open heart surgery. It's not known just how magnesium helps in these serious situations; it does not appear to work by changing the blood pressure, but it does reduce the occurrence of dangerous disturbances of the heart rhythm. Lab experiments suggest that magnesium may protect the heart from oxidative damage; Chapter 11 discusses the role of antioxidants in conquering heart disease.

Although magnesium supplements help heart attack victims, they are not necessary for healthy people. Still, it's important to get enough magnesium from your diet. The Recommended Daily Allowance is 280 milligrams for women and 350 milligrams for men. The best sources of magnesium are whole grains, legumes, leafy green vegetables, seafood, soybeans, nuts, apricots, and bananas; happily they are all foods that can help fight atherosclerosis in many ways.

Beyond Minerals: Controlling Blood Pressure Without Medications

You can go a long way toward controlling your blood pressure by adjusting your intake of 4 minerals. Of greatest importance is the reduction of dietary sodium. Important, too, is a high intake of potassium, calcium, and probably magnesium.

Reducing your blood pressure is central to the fight against atherosclerosis. Because blood pressure is so complex, you can't rely on minerals alone to do the job. Fortunately, many elements of your 15-point plan to conquer heart disease will help with your blood pressure. Weight reduction (Chapter 15) and exercise (Chapter 5) are of prime importance. Stress reduction (Chapter 14) can be very helpful. Smoking cessation (Chapter 3) is essential, as is avoiding alcohol abuse (Chapter 9). There is even evidence that reduction in saturated fat (Chapter 4) and increases in dietary fiber (Chapter 8) can help. Although the evidence is less secure, fish (Chapter 10) and antioxidant vitamins (Chapter 11) may also help control blood pressure as they fight atherosclerosis in other ways.

Like the fight against atherosclerosis itself, controlling blood pressure involves many factors. Doctors can play a critical role in treating hypertension, just as they do in other cardiovascular diseases. But if you're faithful with a comprehensive lifestyle program, you'll be able to do an even better job on your own.

Chapter 7

Aspirin:
An Old Medication
with New Uses

I T'S DISCUSSED at erudite medical meetings and promoted on TV. It's the subject of scholarly papers in medical journals and full-page ads in popular magazines. It's available in every pharmacy in the country and in every supermarket and convenience store. Fifteen thousand tons of it are produced in the United States each year. It's found in nearly every medicine chest in America. It's so widely used as a home remedy that it's hard to realize it's one of the most effective medications to prevent heart attacks. It's aspirin.

An Old Medication

Although aspirin was not the first medicine used to treat human disease, it is much older than most drugs still in use today. Dr. Arthur Hollman, consulting cardiologist at London's University College Hospital, provides a fascinating account of aspirin's early history. Hippocrates is credited with chewing aspirin-containing willow bark to relieve fever, but the active ingredient in aspirin was first administered to patients by the Reverend Edward Stone in 1763. As with so many other great discoveries, aspirin was an accident. Reverend Stone was using quinine to treat malaria, but he found it difficult to obtain the drug, which was extracted from expensive cinchona bark. Whether inspired by God or man, Reverend Stone noticed that the bark of the indigenous willow tree had a bitter taste similar to that of imported cinchona bark. He used powdered bark from the willow, a *salicaceae* species, to treat malaria. It didn't work. Willow bark doesn't have quinine, but it does contain salicin, which is converted by the body into salicylic acid, the active ingredient in aspirin.

Salicin was purified in 1830 by Dr. Thomas Maclagan, who used it to treat rheumatic fever, still an excellent use for aspirin. Despite its efficacy, the drug wasn't widely used until 1874, when a synthetic process increased its availability. Within just a few years, salicylic acid became the main treatment for fever and the rheumatic diseases.

The modern era of aspirin began in 1899. Thwarted from administering salicylic acid to his father because of his stomach irritation, Felix Hoffman synthesized acetylsalicylic acid; his employer, the Bayer Company, gave it the name it still bears today. The rest is history.

New Uses for Aspirin

For all its efficacy in so many diseases, it took a half century for aspirin to find a role in the treatment of heart disease — and another quarter century for doctors to begin accepting that role. Another modern cardiologist, Dr. James Dalen, gets my thanks for alerting me to the early studies of aspirin and coronary artery disease. The pioneer in this new use of aspirin was not a Greek physician, an English minister, or a German chemist, but a California general practitioner, Dr. Lawrence L. Craven.

Like other general practitioners of his day, Dr. Craven took care of many types of patients. He noticed that his tonsillectomy patients experienced increased bleeding if they used aspirin for pain. Recognizing that aspirin seemed to interfere with blood clotting, Dr. Craven reasoned that the drug might help prevent heart attacks.

From today's scientific perspective, we can applaud Dr. Craven's keen observations of aspirin's effect on clotting and his insightful speculation that it might prevent the formation of coronary artery clots. From today's perspective, though, we might question Dr. Craven's next act: as early as 1948, he began to advise all his male patients between the ages of 40 and 65 to take aspirin daily. But if we question a broad therapeutic recommendation based on speculation rather than data, we must nevertheless register clear approval for Dr. Craven's third step: he set out to collect data to evaluate his theory.

Between 1948 and 1956, Dr. Craven kept track of about 8,000 patients who had been taking aspirin under his direction. After using higher doses initially, he had reduced the dose to 1 aspirin daily and was considering a further reduction to 5 tablets per week. But 1 a day seemed to be working well enough: none of Dr. Craven's 8,000 male patients developed heart attacks while taking aspirin. Dr. Craven also reported on 18 patients who were started on aspirin after recovering from heart attacks; not one suffered a second attack. Finally, Dr. Craven noted that no patient in the entire group experienced a major stroke, though he expressed concern that aspirin might increase the risk of brain hemorrhages.

Time has proven that Dr. Craven was amazingly prescient in his theory about aspirin's mode of action, his use of aspirin for atherosclerosis, his aspirin dosage, and even his concern about side effects. Lawrence Craven was also ahead of his time in realizing that his observations alone were not sufficient to prove aspirin's role in preventing heart attacks. In his 1956 paper he anticipated the need for controlled clinical trials; he wondered "will experimental and clinical research in its slow but steady progress eventually test the observations here presented? Only the future can tell whether they are finally to be substantiated or refuted." Dr. Craven died a year later, unaware of the developments in statistics and research methodology that would eventually test his observations. He was also unaware that it would take more than three decades to validate his work.

How Aspirin Prevents Heart Attacks

It has taken years of study. It has required the efforts of innumerable scientists. It has cost hundreds of thousands of dollars. But research has eventually confirmed Dr. Craven's hunch: aspirin protects the heart by inhibiting blood clotting.

Remember from Chapter 1 that atherosclerosis is a three-stage process. It starts in the blood with high levels of LDL cholesterol. The next stage occurs in the wall of the coronary artery: LDL cholesterol enters through injured endothelial cells and undergoes oxidative damage, thus initiating the complex series of inflammatory events that lead to the formation of atherosclerotic plaques. As the process continues, the plaques gradually enlarge, eventually impeding the flow of blood through the artery's narrowed channel. Aspirin does not appear to influence any of these steps. But it does influence the final stage that leads to heart attacks, the formation of blood clots on the atherosclerotic plaques. In most heart attacks, it is a blood clot that finally blocks the artery, depriving heart muscle of vital oxygen, thus causing the death and destruction of heart cells and tissues.

Blood clotting is itself a complex process. Clotting is initiated by platelets, tiny cell fragments that are present in huge numbers in the blood. Platelets are produced in the bone marrow; they survive in the blood for about 10 days before being destroyed. Because they are so short-lived, platelets must be produced by the bone marrow and released into the blood on a continuous basis.

Aspirin inhibits the tendency of platelets to stick to injured vascular surfaces, where they initiate clotting. Only tiny amounts of aspirin are needed to inhibit platelet function; as a result, only small doses of the drug are used to fight heart attacks. Aspirin's effect on platelets is permanent; as a result, the drug does not have to be taken every 3 or 4 hours to inhibit clotting (but frequent aspirin doses are needed to treat fever or pain). The bone marrow cranks out new platelets on a continuous basis; as a result, aspirin has to be taken at least 3 times a week to maintain its effect by inhibiting new platelets.

Platelets are just the initiators of a complex clotting cascade that involves many blood proteins. Interestingly, an elevated level of one of these proteins, fibrinogen, is a marker for increased heart attack risk. Aspirin does not affect fibrinogen levels, but two other elements of your 15-point program to conquer heart disease do: exercise and weight loss reduce blood fibrinogen levels. Aerobic exercise also increases the body's ability to break up newly formed clots, thus reopening blocked arteries. And another strategy in the fight against atherosclerosis also reduces clotting, since the omega-3 fatty acids in fish oil inhibit platelet function.

Aspirin, of course, is not the only drug that inhibits blood clotting. Doctors can administer various anticoagulants to treat heart attack victims. In the early stages of heart attacks, clot-busting enzymes can open blocked coronary arteries. An injectable anticoagulant, heparin, can keep arteries open. And some heart patients receive Coumadin pills at home for long-term anticoagulation. But even compared with these prescription anticoagulants, the drug that does the best job of preventing coronary artery clots is the nonprescription drug you can use yourself to fight atherosclerosis: aspirin.

Aspirin's Role in Preventing Heart Attacks

When Dr. Lawrence Craven began using aspirin to prevent heart attacks nearly 50 years ago, he recommended the drug to middle-aged and older men without known heart disease. Should healthy men take aspirin prophylactically in the 1990s?

The best answer comes from the U.S. Physicians' Health Study, which began in 1982. In this trial, 22,071 male physicians between the ages of 40 and 84 agreed to take either aspirin or placebos, inert tablets formulated to look exactly like aspirin. Half the subjects were randomly assigned to take one aspirin tablet every other day, while the others took the dummy pills; neither the physician-subjects nor the physician-investigators knew which group took the real thing

The code was broken after 5 years. The results: the men taking aspirin had 44 percent fewer heart attacks, a highly significant reduction. Aspirin was particularly effective in preventing early morning heart attacks, which were reduced by nearly 60 percent.

Not all the men taking aspirin in the U.S. Physicians' Study enjoyed equal protection; instead, benefit was confined to men above age 50. In addition, although aspirin reduced both fatal and nonfatal heart attacks, it was not effective in preventing the first symptoms of angina that developed in 331 men during the trial. Taken together, these facts suggest that aspirin does not reduce the formation of new atherosclerotic plaques, but it does prevent clots from blocking arteries already partially narrowed by old plaques.

Nothing is perfect; the men taking aspirin in this large and careful trial did experience some side effects, with mild stomach irritation heading the list. Aspirin was also linked with a number of bleeding problems, but most were minor. More worrisome were the 13 cases of brain hemorrhages in the aspirin takers (right again, Dr. Craven); however, since

6 similar episodes occurred in the men taking placebos, a statistical analysis concludes that the risk of brain hemorrhage was not significantly increased by aspirin use.

The results of the U.S. Physicians' Health Study were first published in 1988. In that same year, the findings of a similar trial in British physicians became available. The British Aspirin Trial, which involved only 5,139 subjects, did not find any benefit for prophylactic aspirin. Does this mean you have to be an American to benefit from aspirin? Not at all. In fact, the British trial used a dose substantially greater than the 325 milligrams every other day used in the American study. It's one reason that only low doses of aspirin are recommended for the prevention of heart attacks. And even if the question of dose is set aside, a combined analysis of the two trials demonstrates that aspirin reduces the risk of heart attack by 33 percent in men above 50 on both sides of the Atlantic.

Like Dr. Craven's 8,000 patients, the subjects in the U.S. and British physicians' aspirin trials were men — not because of a lack of women doctors, but because women are chronically underrepresented in clinical studies. What is known about the value of prophylactic aspirin in women?

A randomized, controlled clinical trial similar to the Physicians' Study will be needed to answer this important question; such a trial has been initiated, but the results won't be available for several years. Until then, the best answer comes from the Nurses' Health Study, in which 87,678 American women aged 34 to 65 were questioned about their aspirin use and their history of heart disease. In all, women who took 1 to 6 aspirin tablets in an average week experienced 25 percent fewer heart attacks compared with women who took no aspirin; the best protection — nearly 40 percent — occurred in women older than 50. Women who averaged more than 7 aspirins per week were not protected, regardless of their age. Aspirin did not appear to affect the risk of stroke in women.

Admitting the need for more data, the situation for women seems similar to that for men: low-dose aspirin reduces the risk of first heart attacks in people who are at highest risk, at least in those older than 50. Aspirin is of even greater benefit for people who have already had heart attacks. If you are fighting atherosclerosis before you develop the disease, you'll need a few more facts to help you decide if aspirin is right for you. If you already have heart disease, your need is greater and your decision is easier.

Aspirin in the Treatment of Atherosclerosis

The ultimate test of any technique used to conquer heart disease is its ability to treat patients who already have the disease. Smoking cessation, dietary fat restriction, and exercise have passed the test. How does aspirin measure up?

Very well indeed. So well, in fact, that it's the only medication I recommend for *all* patients with coronary artery disease (unless, of course, they cannot tolerate aspirin). In many cases, aspirin is the only drug that heart patients take on a regular basis.

The first randomized trial of aspirin's ability to prevent recurrent heart attacks was begun in 1971. It found that 1 aspirin per day reduced recurrent heart attacks by 25 percent, but because only 1,239 subjects were studied, the results did not meet the demanding standards of statistical significance. Since then, however, many additional studies have examined the question. The subjects have included angina patients with impending heart attacks (so-called unstable angina), patients with silent ischemia (painless angina), patients in the acute stages of new heart attacks, patients with evidence of old heart attacks, and patients undergoing coronary artery bypass operations and angioplasties. The subjects have been women and men, young and old. The preparations used have ranged from plain aspirin to buffered aspirin, coated aspirin, and even Alka-Seltzer. The aspirin dose used most often in these studies was 1 tablet, 325 milligrams, per day, but doses as low as 75 milligrams per day have also been studied.

Needless to say, the fine print varies from trial to trial. But the big picture is indisputable: aspirin provides significant protection from recurrent heart attacks in patients with atherosclerosis. In a 1994 meta-analysis of 174 studies, Dr. Richard Peto of Oxford University placed the overall protection at about 25 percent; he estimated that appropriate aspirin use could prevent 20,000 deaths in the United States each year.

Except for those with aspirin allergies, active bleeding, or a need for other anticoagulants, every patient with coronary artery disease should be taking low-dose aspirin to prevent recurrent attacks. Unfortunately only 1 of 3 patients who should be taking aspirin is actually doing so.

As in so many other areas, Americans are overlooking the obvious, failing to take advantage of this simple, inexpensive, effective way to fight atherosclerosis.

Aspirin, Stroke, and Atherosclerosis

Atherosclerosis is a systemic disease. Although its ultimate cause is human behavior, it acts through the body's metabolism, potentially affecting every artery in the body. The most important vascular targets of atherosclerosis are the coronary arteries. Following close behind are the arteries of the brain; the leg arteries are third in importance. Aspirin can help fight atherosclerosis in these locations, too.

Aspirin is very effective in reducing the risk of stroke in patients who have had transient ischemic attacks, or TIAs. The relationship between TIAs and stroke is very similar to the relationship between angina and heart attacks. In TIAs, the brain is temporarily deprived of blood flow and oxygen, but because flow returns quickly, cell death does not occur. Whereas the typical symptom of angina is chest pain, TIAs can have a wide range of neurologic symptoms, including disturbances of vision, speech, or consciousness, weakness of an arm or leg, or changes in sensation. The symptoms last from minutes to hours; although patients recover fully, they are at high risk for suffering full-blown strokes with brain cell death and permanent disability.

Most patients with TIAs have atherosclerotic plaques blocking arteries in their necks or brain. By preventing clots from forming on these plaques, aspirin reduces the risk of complete blockages and strokes. Most patients who receive aspirin for TIAs are given 1 tablet, 325 milligrams, per day, but studies have shown that lower doses — even as little as 30 milligrams daily — are equally effective.

Aspirin is also effective in preventing strokes caused by heart disease. Patients with atrial fibrillation have irregular heart rhythms because their atria, the heart's smaller pumping chambers, do not contract normally. Clots can form in the left atrium; strokes result if the clots break away and travel to the brain. Aspirin is effective in preventing these clots, at least in patients younger than 75, but new research indicates that a prescription anticoagulant, Coumadin, is even more effective. Clearly all patients at risk for stroke should use aspirin or other anticoagulants only under a doctor's care.

Although less serious than heart attacks and strokes, atherosclerosis of the arteries that supply blood to the legs is a major problem. Like the heart muscle, leg muscles need more oxygen when they're working hard; like the heart muscle, leg muscles that are deprived of oxygen signal their distress with pain. Patients with blockages of their leg arteries get cramps when they walk. In advanced cases, they can hardly walk at all, and if atherosclerosis progresses farther, they may develop pain at rest, then gangrene.

Surgery can restore the flow of blood to the legs by bypassing blocked arteries. But aspirin can also help; in the U.S. Physicians' Health Study, men taking 1 aspirin tablet every other day had a 50 percent reduction in their need for vascular surgery.

Diabetics are at particularly high risk for developing atherosclerosis. But they are also at risk for eye hemorrhages. Aspirin should help their hearts — but will it harm their eyes? A 1992 study of 3,711 men and women with diabetes provides the answer: aspirin reduced the risk of heart attack without increasing the incidence of eye problems.

Aspirin and Health

Low-dose aspirin prophylaxis has proved helpful to fight atherosclerosis regardless of whether the plaques involve arteries of the heart, brain, or legs. Can low-dose aspirin help prevent medical problems unrelated to atherosclerosis?

Aspirin acts by inhibiting an important class of chemicals called prostaglandins. Prostaglandins are found throughout the human body, which is why aspirin has so many effects. Prostaglandins are present in platelets and arteries, enabling aspirin to fight atherosclerosis. Prostaglandins have a key role in producing pain and fever, again explaining why aspirin is so effective in treating these common problems. And prostaglandins also account for some of aspirin's potential adverse effects, including stomach irritation and kidney disorders.

Prostaglandins are present in intestinal cells, and exciting new research suggests that low-dose aspirin may help prevent colon cancer. As least 5 studies have found that low-dose aspirin use is associated with an approximate 50 percent reduction in colon cancer. Although some of the studies are small, a 1991 study in the *New England Journal of Medicine* evaluated 662,424 men and women; over a 6-year period, aspirin use was associated with a 40 percent lower risk of dying from colon cancer. And a 1993 report extended the observation to cancers of the esophagus, stomach, and rectum; taking aspirin at least 16 times a month was associated with a significantly lower death rate from each of these malignancies. Laboratory experiments using indomethacin and piroxicam back up the studies of aspirin and human cancer; both of these aspirin-like drugs are effective in preventing intestinal cancers in animals. Before you rely on aspirin to protect you from intestinal cancer, though, you should realize that not all the studies agree. A 1993 analysis of the U.S. Physicians' Health Study did not confirm that aspirin reduces the risk of colon cancer, perhaps because it was a relatively short-term study. A 1994 study from Atlanta, however, supported a link between aspirin use and protection from cancers of the colon and rectum.

It's far too early to recommend aspirin for the prevention of cancer; even so, keep these intriguing observations in mind when you decide if low-dose aspirin should be part of your fight against atherosclerosis.

Low-dose aspirin may have other benefits. In the U.S. Physicians' Health Study, for example, it reduced the occurrence of migraine headaches. Other studies suggest that as little as 50 milligrams a day may reduce the risk of hypertension during high-risk pregnancies. Like the cancer study, these evaluations are preliminary, but they emphasize the need for further research into the effects of low-dose aspirin.

Aspirin and Illness

Low-dose aspirin is finding new uses as a preventive treatment designed to maintain health. High-dose aspirin has long been a mainstay of treatment for many patients who are sick.

Aspirin is familiar to all of us as an effective treatment for pain and fever. It is also an excellent anti-inflammatory medication, finding many uses in patients with arthritis, tendinitis, and other inflammatory conditions. Despite the availability of many new aspirin-like medications (ibuprofen and the prescription nonsteroidal anti-inflammatory drugs), aspirin remains the benchmark drug for the therapy of inflammation, fever, and pain.

Therapeutic doses of aspirin are much higher than preventive doses. Most adults who require aspirin therapy start with two 325 milligram tablets every 4 to 6 hours and move up as needed; most preventive regimens use no more than 325 milligrams per day, with some going as low as one-quarter of that dose. Paradoxically, perhaps, high doses of aspirin are much *less* effective for heart attack prevention than are low doses.

If you are using low-dose aspirin to fight atherosclerosis, you may still develop conditions that would normally call for higher doses of aspirin or other nonsteroidal anti-inflammatory drugs. How should you respond to this need without compromising the preventive benefits of aspirin?

For treatment of pain or fever, the answer is easy: use acetaminophen (Tylenol and many other brands). Acetaminophen doesn't inhibit prostaglandins, nor does it affect platelets and arteries. You can continue taking low-dose aspirin while using therapeutic doses of acetaminophen. But if you require medication for inflammation, you have few options; use therapeutic doses of aspirin while you must, resuming low-dose prevention when you can.

Less is better, at least with regard to aspirin and atherosclerosis.

The Other Side of the Tablet: Adverse Effects of Aspirin

Like all medications, aspirin has potential toxicities; like all medications, it must be used with care; like most medications, the side effects of aspirin are greater when the dose is higher. When it comes to the adverse effects of aspirin, less is better.

Low-dose aspirin is safe; most people can use it without experiencing any problems. The most frequent adverse effect of low-dose aspirin is stomach irritation, but it's usually mild and responds to antacids. Less common, but more worrisome, is bleeding. Even low doses of aspirin reduce blood clotting — that's exactly how it fights atherosclerosis. A little extra care while shaving is the only precaution most people will need, but all aspirin users may have to settle for black-and-blue marks from time to time. However, nobody with an active bleeding problem should take aspirin, and everybody who takes aspirin should stop the drug at least a week before undergoing surgery. The greatest concern about low-dose aspirin is the risk of brain hemorrhages, but large trials, such as the U.S. Physicians' Health Study, provide reassurance that low-dose aspirin doesn't actually increase the risk of bleeding into the brain. Finally, even small amounts of aspirin can trigger asthma in people who are allergic to the drug; true aspirin allergies, though, are rare.

High-dose aspirin is another matter. While still generally safe, therapeutic doses of aspirin can cause stomach inflammation, ulcers, and intestinal bleeding. Ringing in the ears is another dose-dependent side effect of aspirin. Prolonged use of high-dose aspirin has also been associated with interstitial nephritis, an uncommon kidney disorder. And children with chicken pox or the flu may develop a serious liver problem (Reye's syndrome) if they take aspirin, which is why most pediatricians prefer acetaminophen for fever or pain in kids.

These potential side effects may make aspirin sound hazardous to your health. Indeed, they should remind you to treat aspirin as a medication worthy of respect, but they should not scare you away from using the drug properly. Americans purchase about 30 billion aspirin tablets annually. That amounts to 100 pills per person per year. Despite all the aspirin that's consumed, serious side effects are really quite infrequent, even though many people are taking it for the wrong reasons in the wrong doses. Despite all the aspirin that's consumed, many people who could benefit from aspirin are not taking it at all.

If you choose to take aspirin, use it properly and take it with care.

Aspirin for Atherosclerosis: Preparations and Doses

It's not as simple as it used to be; nowadays, aspirin comes in many sizes and shapes.

Aspirin contains just one active ingredient, acetylsalicylic acid; all forms of aspirin will fight atherosclerosis equally well (but don't make the mistake of relying on aspirin substitutes such as acetaminophen). Aspirin preparations, however, do differ in their propensity to cause stomach irritation. Ordinary aspirin is fine if it sits well with you, but if it upsets your stomach, try taking it with milk, meals, or antacids — or switch to a buffered or coated aspirin preparation. Like most cardiologists, I generally recommend enteric coated aspirin (Ecotrin and other brands); it is the least likely to cause stomach irritation, and its slower rate of absorption may be an asset for low-dose aspirin regimens.

It's easy to suggest enteric coated tablets to aspirin users but harder to be sure what dose is best. Aspirin comes in many sizes: normal strength (325 milligrams), extra-strength (500 milligrams), half-strength (162 milligrams), and quarter-strength (81 milligrams, the amount in "baby aspirin").

It's hard to recommend a single dose to fight atherosclerosis because many different doses have been effective. The key is to use a low dose of aspirin; a single 325-milligram tablet per day is the *top* dose, but even lower amounts will do the job. A 1994 study, in fact, found that as little as *3 to 10 milligrams* of aspirin can inhibit platelet-induced clotting without producing any irritation of the stomach lining. Aspirin doses as low as 30 milligrams per day have been found to protect against strokes, but more study will be needed to see if these very low doses also provide chemical protection against heart attacks. Even now, however, there is general agreement that 81 milligrams per day is an effective dose for preventing heart attacks.

I generally recommend the dose schedules which have been best studied. For patients with known coronary heart disease, I suggest one full-strength (325 milligrams) enteric-coated aspirin tablet per day. To fight atherosclerosis before it appears, I suggest the same 325-milligram tablet every other day — but if it's hard to stick to an alternate-day schedule, I'm equally happy with a Monday-Wednesday-Friday program or with a half- or quarter-strength tablet every day.

Is Low-Dose Aspirin Right for You?

If aspirin had no adverse effects, everyone could take it. If everyone cared for his or her heart with a comprehensive program to fight atherosclerosis, no one would need it. Since neither is the case, you'll have to decide if aspirin is right for you.

If you are allergic to aspirin or if you have active bleeding problems or ulcers the decision is easy: don't take aspirin.

If you are healthy, the decision depends on your risk of atherosclerosis and your ability to use aspirin without adverse consequences. Most people can tolerate low-dose aspirin; in my view, people who are at risk for atherosclerosis should use it.

In America of the 1990s, unfortunately, just being a 50-year-old man or a postmenopausal woman means you are at risk for a heart attack and that you're a candidate for low-dose aspirin. But age alone does not tell the whole story; much younger people may be at high risk. To find out where you stand, review your overall heart attack risk score (Table 2–11). If your risk is moderate, think seriously about aspirin; if you are in a high-risk group, take low-dose aspirin so you won't have to call me in the morning.

Low-dose aspirin can be an important tool in the fight against atherosclerosis. But it's not a quick fix; even 44 percent protection against heart attacks is not good enough when your health is at stake. Consider making aspirin part of your 15-point program — but don't neglect the other steps you need to conquer heart disease.

Chapter 8

Dietary Fiber: The Power of Positive Eating

CAN ROUGHAGE in your diet keep your arteries smooth? It's a long way from your stomach to your coronary arteries; still, putting some oat bran in the former can help keep atherosclerotic plaques out of the latter.

Atherosclerosis is not part of the normal human condition, but fiber is part of the normal human diet — or, at least, it should be. Our primitive human ancestors consumed more than 50 grams of dietary fiber per day. Even today, the typical diet in developing countries provides more than 50 grams per day. Industrialized societies pride themselves on being more refined, and so is the food they eat. Average Americans include only 11 grams of fiber in their daily fare. We should be eating much more, perhaps three times more.

Where did all the fiber go? It's another case of the human mind getting ahead of human nature. In this case, blame lies not with the chemist who first added hydrogen to healthfully unsaturated vegetable oils, but to the miller who first separated the wheat from the chaff — and then threw out the bran. Refined flour is only part of the problem. In addition to abandoning whole grains, the Western diet has turned from vegetables, fruits, and legumes — all of which contain lots of fiber — to foods made from animal products, which have no fiber. We process foods to refine flavor and texture. The result, in fact, is a lack of culinary variety — and a variety of new diseases.

Atherosclerosis is one of those diseases.

What Is Dietary Fiber?

Your mother called it roughage, and her mother called it bulk. Food manufacturers call it crude fiber and nutritionists call it dietary fiber. Chemists call it a nonstarch polysaccharide polymer composed of at least 20 sugar residues; that's certainly a mouthful, but instead of filling up with words — fancy or plain — fill up with fiber. By any name, it's good for your health.

Despite all the formidable (and unappetizing!) terminology, dietary fiber is really quite straightforward. Like starch, fiber is a complex carbohydrate made of dozens, even hundreds, of sugar molecules linked together into large branched chains. Unlike starch, however, dietary fiber resists the action of human digestive enzymes. Because it cannot be broken down in the intestinal tract, fiber is not absorbed into the body; instead, it passes unchanged into the stools, bringing water along with it. Since it's not absorbed, dietary fiber has no caloric value, and it doesn't provide the body with any nutrients. Perhaps because it has no "nutritional value," fiber was thought to be expendable. Nothing could be farther from the truth: caloric value, no; health value, yes.

Dietary fiber is found only in plant cells; no animal products contain any fiber. Dietary fiber forms the structural backbone of plant stems, leaves, and seeds. And, although we speak of it as a single entity, there are actually many types of fiber, just as there are many types of plants.

The Types of Fiber

Table 8–1 lists the major types of fiber; it's really not important for you to figure out the difference between a pectin and a lignin, but it is important for you to understand the two major types of fiber, soluble and insoluble.

Soluble fiber is well named: it dissolves in water, but since it can't be absorbed by humans, it remains in the intestinal tract. Soluble fiber delays stomach emptying, producing a feeling of fullness after eating fiber-rich foods; in the lower intestinal tract, its gel-like consistency makes the stools softer and easier to pass. Soluble fiber improves bowel function, but it has several properties that also make it an important ally in the fight against atherosclerosis. First, it improves sugar metabolism, reducing blood insulin levels. Second, most types of soluble fiber lower blood

Table 8–1
DIETARY FIBER: CHEMICAL TYPES AND
REPRESENTATIVE FOOD SOURCES

Fiber	Chemical Structures	Food Sources
Soluble	Gums	Oats, beans, legumes, guar
Soluble	Pectin	Apples, citrus fruits, soybeans, cauliflower, squash, cabbage, carrots, green beans, potatoes
Soluble	Mucilage	Psyllium
Soluble and insoluble	Hemicellulose	Barley, wheat bran, and whole grains, brussels sprouts, beetroot
Insoluble	Lignin	Green beans, strawberries, peaches, pears, radishes
Insoluble	Cellulose	Root vegetables, cabbage, wheat and corn, peas, beans, broccoli, peppers, apples

cholesterol levels. Oats, beans and other legumes, barley, and seeds are excellent dietary sources of soluble fiber.

Insoluble fiber does not dissolve in water, but it draws water into the intestinal tract, making the stools bulkier and promoting prompt elimination of fecal material. Insoluble fiber does not affect blood sugar or cholesterol, but it does protect against many intestinal disorders. Wheat bran, whole grain products, and most vegetables are excellent sources of insoluble fiber.

Soluble fiber helps fight atherosclerosis; insoluble fiber fights intestinal diseases. Both are important for health, but the average American diet is woefully deficient in both.

Dietary Fiber and Heart Disease

The Old Testament reports that Daniel and his peers looked and felt healthier when they switched from a diet of rich food and wine to vegetables and water. It wasn't a controlled clinical trial, but it has more than a kernel of truth. Contemporary clinical observation certainly supports a change from rich foods to vegetables, fruits, and grains (but not the abandonment of wine; see Chapter 9).

Professor J. N. Morris, the same British epidemiologist who first documented the protective effects of exercise in 1953, was among the first to demonstrate the link between dietary fiber and heart disease. Studying London transportation workers, he reported in 1977 that high-fiber diets reduced the risk of coronary artery disease, even after taking other risk factors into account. Since then, this observation has been confirmed in more than 20 industrialized countries from around the world. For example, a 20-year study of 1,001 middle-aged men living in Ireland and Boston found that a high intake of fiber decreased the risk of heart disease by 43 percent. Similarly, a 1987 American study suggested that merely increasing dietary fiber from 12 to 18 grams per day could decease the risk of coronary artery disease by 25 percent. A higher, and perhaps more realistic, standard was set by a 1982 Dutch study; it found that men eating the least amount of fiber had 4 times more heart disease than men eating the most fiber, and set the protective target at 37 grams per day.

Dietary fiber fights atherosclerosis in several ways. The ability of soluble fiber to lower blood cholesterol levels is the most important; not to be overlooked, though, is the role of fiber in controlling other cardiac risk factors, such as high blood pressure, diabetes, and obesity.

Dietary Fiber and Blood Cholesterol: Oat Bran Redux

Drs. deGroot, Lugken, and Pikaar deserve credit for the first observation that soluble fiber lowers blood cholesterol; in 1963, they reported that adding rolled oats to the diet could reduce blood cholesterol levels by 11 percent in just 3 weeks. For unknown reasons, though, oats were kept on the back burner for nearly 20 years; doctors didn't rediscover the benefits of oat products until the 1980s.

Between 1984 and 1988, a series of feeding experiments on healthy people with high cholesterol levels demonstrated that oat bran reduced blood cholesterol; in these studies, daily dietary supplements of 50 to 100 grams of oat bran reduced blood cholesterol levels by up to 23 percent.

Ever eager for a quick fix, the American public began a love affair with oats. By 1990, American oat production had doubled, reaching 100 million bushels annually; whereas horses made oats the gasoline of the nineteenth century, humans were making oats the food fad of the twentieth. Oat bran was everywhere: in cereals, muffins, breads, and even cupcakes.

After boiling along for 5 or 6 years, the oat bran craze cooled off abruptly in 1990, when a study from Harvard disputed oat bran's ability to lower cholesterol levels. This study found that wheat had the same effect on cholesterol as oats; it calculated that eating oat products didn't lower cholesterol because of soluble fiber, but because people who were filled up with oats stayed away from fatty foods. Exit oat bran.

But oats wouldn't roll over. The Harvard study was careful and competent, but it involved only 20 subjects — and they were all healthy young women with normal blood cholesterol levels. Like other cholesterol-lowering programs, soluble dietary fiber works best when it's needed most, when blood cholesterol levels are higher to begin with. Doctors and nutritionists continued to study oat products. The population groups, dosages, and protocols varied, but the results were amazingly uniform: oat bran *does* lower blood cholesterol levels.

A 1992 meta-analysis of 20 trials demonstrated that oat bran works. It works best when it is eaten in large amounts, and it's especially effective in people with high LDL cholesterols. On average, 3 grams of soluble fiber per day, the amount contained in 50 grams (about 2 ounces) of oat bran, will reduce blood cholesterol levels by about 15 percent. That may not sound like much, but it should translate to a 30 to 40 percent reduction in the risk of a heart attack. More good news: cholesterol levels fall within a matter of weeks after starting oat bran, and they stay down for years if dietary intake stays up. And a 1993 study assures us that oat bran will further lower blood cholesterol levels even in people already eating low-fat diets.

Now that we know oats work, scientists are trying to determine how they work. The essential factor in oat products is, in fact, the bran. More specifically, it's a chemical called beta-glucan, which appears to bind cholesterol-rich bile salts in the intestinal tract, preventing the body from reabsorbing cholesterol into the bloodstream. Two prescription medications, cholestyramine and colestipol, can do the same thing (see Chapter 18) — but they are vastly more expensive than oat bran. And say what you will about oats, you'll love the way they taste after you've tried cholestyramine!

Beta-glucan is a soluble fiber. If it lowers blood cholesterol levels, so should other forms of soluble fiber — and they do.

Beans and other legumes rival oat bran's ability to lower blood cholesterol levels. At least 15 studies have investigated various legumes; whether fresh, dried, or canned, beans lower cholesterol levels, both in normal people and in those with high blood cholesterol levels. On average, 100 grams (about 3 ounces) of beans per day will reduce the blood cholesterol by about 15 percent.

Almost any form of soluble fiber will reduce blood cholesterol levels if sufficient amounts are incorporated into the diet. Barley, prunes, and sugar beets have all passed the test, as have diets supplemented with mixed fruits and vegetables. Rice bran, though, is only minimally effective.

Soluble fiber lowers cholesterol when it's eaten in foods; can it do the job if it's consumed by itself as a dietary supplement? Indeed it can. The best results have been obtained with psyllium, a fiber-rich natural grain from the Indian subcontinent. At least 17 trials have evaluated psyllium supplements, finding that they work about as well as oat bran. On average, about 10 grams of psyllium per day will lower cholesterol by up to 15 percent within 2 to 4 months. With a 50-year track record as a bulk laxative, psyllium has also proven safe; rare individuals exhibit allergic reactions to the grain. Psyllium is also generally palatable, though it may cause abdominal distress and bloating.

Other varieties of soluble fiber can also lower blood cholesterol levels. Guar is one example, pectin another; pectin isn't palatable as a supplement, but it's naturally present in many fruits and vegetables, particularly apples and citrus fruits. Soy fiber lowers cholesterol, too, but less dramatically. Finally, a 1993 study found that a synthetic soluble fiber, hydroxyprophylmethylcellulose, could lower LDL cholesterol by 15 percent in just 1 week; the only "side effect" was weight loss. Acacia gum is the exception that proves the rule; it's a water-soluble dietary fiber that does not lower blood cholesterol levels.

With so many options, you can fight atherosclerosis by adding soluble fiber to your diet even if you never touch an oat. You'll get help in setting your goals for dietary fiber later in this chapter; for now, you can think of 30 grams a day as a reasonable target, with about one-third coming in the form of soluble fiber. Table 8−2 lists the soluble fiber content of representative foods.

Dietary Fiber and Heart Disease Risk Factors

Winning the fight against atherosclerosis depends on more than just lowering LDL cholesterol levels. Dietary fiber lowers cholesterol; al-

Table 8-2
SOLUBLE FIBER CONTENT OF SELECTED FOODS

Food	Portion Size	Soluble Fiber (grams)	Total Fiber (grams)
Oat Products			
Oat bran cereal	¹/₃ cup (dry)	2.0	4.4
Oat bran muffin	1 large	1.6	3.3
Oatmeal	¹/₃ cup (dry)	1.3	2.8
Other Grain Products			
Brown rice	¹/₂ cup	0.4	5.3
Whole wheat bread	1 slice	0.4	2.1
Rye bread	1 slice	0.3	1.7
White bread	1 slice	0.2	0.4
Cornflakes	1 oz.	0.1	0.3
Legumes (cooked)			
Kidney beans	¹/₂ cup	2.0	6.7
Pinto beans	¹/₂ cup	2.0	6.7
Lima beans	¹/₂ cup	1.3	5.4
Vegetables (cooked)			
Brussels sprouts	¹/₂ cup	2.0	3.8
Broccoli	¹/₂ cup	1.1	2.6
Cabbage	¹/₂ cup	0.6	1.5
Spinach	¹/₂ cup	0.5	2.1
Zucchini	¹/₂ cup	0.2	1.6
Nuts			
Peanuts (roasted)	¹/₂ cup	2.4	6.3
Almonds (roasted)	¹/₂ cup	0.8	7.9
Fruits			
Prunes	6	3.0	8.0
Grapefruit	1 medium	2.2	3.6
Orange	1 medium	1.8	2.9
Apricots	1 cup	1.3	3.1
Apple	1 medium	1.2	3.6
Cantaloupe	1 slice	0.6	1.1
Grapes	1 cup	0.3	1.1
Supplements			
Psyllium	1 teaspoon	2.9	3.9

though the evidence is less extensive, it can also help improve other important cardiac risk factors.

Diabetes. Soluble fiber is the asset here, as it is for lowering cholesterol. Soluble fiber in the diet slows the passage of food from the stomach into the intestinal tract. Sugar is absorbed into the bloodstream more slowly and evenly; as a result, the pancreas releases insulin gradually instead of delivering a jolt to the bloodstream. People who eat lots of soluble fiber have lower blood sugar levels, and they use less insulin to maintain good sugar levels. These metabolic effects of soluble fiber should reduce heart attack risk. One caution: patients with diabetes often experience a drop in blood sugar when they begin high-fiber diets; as a result, they need to monitor themselves carefully with an eye toward reducing their medication dosages.

Hypertension. Both soluble and insoluble fiber appear beneficial for blood pressure control. People eating high-fiber diets have lower blood pressures than people on "normal" diets. But since vegetarian and other high-fiber diets are also lower in sodium, fat, and calories and higher in potassium, it's been hard to prove that the fiber itself is responsible for lower blood pressure readings.

Two 1992 studies illustrate the interaction between fiber and blood pressure. In India, 120 people with hypertension were divided into two groups; one continued their usual diets, while the other added guava, a fiber-rich fruit. At the end of 12 weeks, the patients in the fiber group had lowered their blood pressure by about 10 points, a major improvement; they had also lowered their total cholesterol levels by 10 percent while raising their HDL cholesterol by 8 percent.

Although the Indian results are spectacular, it may be hard for you to eat 6 guavas a day. Closer to home, however, an American study supports the benefits of fiber. During a 4-year period, 30,681 healthy male health professionals were observed for the development of hypertension. A high intake of dietary fiber was associated with a significantly lower risk of developing high blood pressure, even after weight, dietary fat and sodium, alcohol consumption, and age were taken into account. Although all forms of fiber were beneficial, cereal and vegetable fiber was a lot less helpful than fruit, possibly because of the potassium in fruit.

Dietary fiber is far from a cure for hypertension — but it's a step in the right direction.

Obesity. Excess body fat is not the most dangerous cardiac risk factor, but it's surely the most visible. Because of its many effects on human health and happiness, it's important to combat obesity. An abundant intake of fiber can help in part by slowing the passage of food from the stomach, thus reducing hunger. Chapter 15 explains how increasing the fiber in your menu can help reduce the size of your waistline.

Dietary Fiber in the Treatment of Atherosclerosis

The ultimate test of any technique used to conquer heart disease is its ability to treat patients who already have the condition. How does dietary fiber meet the test?

The data are scant but encouraging. In a 1992 study from India, 505 patients with new heart attacks were randomly divided into two groups. Both received the best conventional medical care, and both were instructed to consume low-fat diets; one group was also instructed to consume more fruit, vegetables, nuts, and grain products, all of which are high in fiber. At the end of 1 year, the patients who ate more fiber weighed less and had lower cholesterol levels. More important, the fiber-rich diet was associated with a significantly lower risk of recurrent heart attacks and of death from all causes.

More studies will be needed to confirm these results and to establish their applications to patients in America. Even so, all the available evidence confirms that dietary fiber fights atherosclerosis — both before and after the disease has made its way into the coronary arteries.

Fiber and Health

Psalm 104 tells us, "Here is bread, which strengthens man's heart and is therefore called the staff of life." The Bible doesn't specify fiber as the active ingredient, but modern science has known for 30 years that dietary fiber can fight atherosclerosis.

We've known for 2,400 years that fiber can fight intestinal diseases; in 400 B.C., Hippocrates prescribed whole grain bread for its "salutary effect on the bowel." Ancient wisdom notwithstanding, the modern study of fiber and health began in the 1960s with the work of two medical missionaries in Kampala, Uganda. Drs. Denis Burkitt and H. C. Trowell noticed that their African patients were remarkably free of high blood pressure, heart disease, diabetes, and obesity — and of other "Western" disorders, including constipation, appendicitis, diverticulosis, hemorrhoids, hernias, and gallstones. The good doctors also noticed that their African patients had much more rapid and bulky bowel movements than their British counterparts. These simple observations led to the fiber hypothesis, the theory that dietary fiber protects against many of the intestinal, metabolic, and cardiovascular disorders that plague industrialized societies.

It seems too good to be true. Over the years, many studies have set out to challenge the fiber hypothesis; the great majority have eventually confirmed its validity. And these studies have added a very important disease to the roster of fiber's benefits: colon cancer is much less common in people who eat high-fiber diets. Nigerians, for example, have less than 10 percent as many colon cancers as African-Americans.

Soluble fiber lowers cholesterol and blood sugar levels, protecting against atherosclerosis and diabetes. Both soluble and insoluble fiber are associated with a lower risk of hypertension and obesity. Insoluble fiber is the major type that protects against intestinal diseases, including cancers.

Dr. Burkitt himself explained how fiber works in the intestinal tract. His African patients digested and eliminated their high-fiber meals in less than 12 hours, while his English patients took 3 to 5 times longer to eliminate their refined foods. Because insoluble fiber increases fecal bulk, the colon can empty without forceful contractions; this lack of straining protects against hernias, hemorrhoids, and diverticulosis. Because stool is eliminated rapidly, its toxins are expelled before they can injure cells lining the colon; it's this rapid transit that protects against colon cancer.

Most people think of fiber as a remedy for constipation. They're right, but they may not realize that fiber can also help control the diarrhea and cramps associated with irritable bowel syndrome.

All in all, it's soluble fiber for your heart and insoluble fiber for your gut. Your mother got it right (again!): roughage *is* good for you.

Setting Your Goals for Dietary Fiber

There is no Recommended Daily Allowance for dietary fiber, but most authorities recommend an average intake of 20–35 grams per day. Even 20 grams would represent a big improvement for the average American diet, but you can do better. Take 20 grams as your minimum goal, then gradually increase your consumption of fiber to at least 30 grams per day.

What type of fiber is best? Both. Aim for a mixture of dietary fibers from a variety of sources. As a rough guide, about two-thirds of the total should be insoluble fiber, the remainder soluble fiber that protects against atherosclerosis.

Are fiber supplements right for you? It depends on your blood cholesterol levels (Table 2–2), and your overall cardiac risk profile (Table 2–11). It's best to get your fiber from foods that also supply much-needed vitamins and minerals. But if you can't make it to your fiber quota with foods, supplements make sense. And if you have a high cholesterol level and/or a high cardiac risk score, you may want to enrich your high-fiber diet with supplements.

Because constipation is so common in America, many fiber supplements are available. Because your goal is to reduce your cholesterol and fight atherosclerosis, select a supplement that contains soluble fiber. Psyllium is ideal; it contains both forms of fiber, but it's about 75 percent soluble. It has been carefully studied, and its ability to reduce blood LDL cholesterol levels is well documented. Psyllium is a natural grain; except for the rare person who is allergic to it, psyllium is well tolerated.

The trick to using psyllium successfully is to increase your dose slowly. Start with 1 teaspoonful before breakfast, than build up to one dose before each meal. If you are troubled by bloating and diarrhea, reduce your dose temporarily, then gradually work your way back up. And always take plenty of water with your psyllium.

Psyllium is available in many preparations. The most widely used is Metamucil, a powder. Many of my patients prefer Perdiem Fiber, a granular preparation. If you choose to supplement your diet with psyllium, experiment with various preparations until you find the one that suits you best.

Can you get too much fiber? Probably not, as long as you build up your dose slowly and you're careful to include plenty of iron, calcium, zinc, and other nutrients in your diet. Count the grams of fiber in your diet until you reach your goal. After you've reached your target, you can increase your intake without additional counting; your gut's instinct will let you know if you're getting too much! One exception: people with diverticulosis should probably avoid seeds — but apart from that, they should get all the fiber they can; most doctors, in fact, recommend psyllium supplements for diverticulosis.

A Word About Legumes

Chapter 4 provided some practical tips about whole grains, vegetables, and fruits. But legumes are the neglected nutrients — more the shame because they provide soluble fiber. Legumes are inexpensive and delicious, but they do take some planning, both to cook them right and to eat them without getting intestinal gas. Still, it's not inconvenience, or even gas, that has banished beans from the typical American diet. Instead, I suspect that cultural prejudices play a role, since legumes are a dietary staple in much of the developing world.

Legumes come in almost endless varieties: black beans, kidney beans, navy beans, pinto beans, black-eyed peas, green or yellow split peas, red or green lentils, lima beans, soybeans, and garbanzo beans (chickpeas) are but a few of the legumes you can add to your menu. All are versatile and healthful. Soybeans are particularly excellent as a source of protein, iron, and calcium; tofu is useful in many vegetarian recipes. Garbanzos contain more fat and calories than other beans, but they're still very healthful. Remember, though, that commercial processing can add undesirable amounts of salt and fat to legumes; canned baked beans and split pea soups are examples.

Legumes will give you an opportunity to enjoy recipes from around the world, such as black beans or kidney beans in chili (which can be meatless or made with ground turkey), refried black beans, lentils in Indian dal or Hungarian Magyar stew, or navy beans in minestrone. Beans are wonderful with grains, and the combination provides a fine mix of amino acids as well as great taste. Legumes can be used as meat substitutes in many dishes. Leftover beans freeze well, so you can always have a supply handy for salads, soups, or casseroles.

Cooking with legumes takes some advanced planning because of the need to soak them overnight and the 60–80 minutes needed to boil beans and peas. But when you learn to cook with legumes, you'll find them easy to use. They're also very easy on your budget.

Smoothing Out the Roughage in Your Diet

As good as it is, dietary fiber has its flaws: abdominal bloating, intestinal distress, diarrhea, and gas can be the price you pay if you eat too much too soon.

Many people avoid legumes because they are concerned with intestinal gas. You can minimize this problem by increasing your portions slowly and by soaking legumes overnight prior to cooking, remembering to discard any excess water. For extra flavor, add spices to the water in which your legumes are soaking; try thyme for lentils, cumin for kidney beans, and garlic for black beans. If soaking doesn't solve your gas problem, try using Beano, a nonprescription enzyme preparation, with your first bite of legumes.

Even though fiber is good for you, you can actually enjoy it. Increase the fiber in your diet slowly. Experiment with a variety of fiber-rich foods until you find the ones that you like best and that like you best. If gas is a problem, try Beano even if the culprit is broccoli or cabbage rather than beans. Eat slowly, chewing your food carefully to avoid swallowing air. And always be sure that your high-fiber diet is accompanied by a generous intake of fluids; it's especially important if you're using fiber supplements.

With a little trial and error you can avoid both the errors of a fiber-deficient diet and the trials of injudicious fiber consumption.

Finding the Fiber

When it comes to finding dietary fiber, you can simply forget all animal products; they contain no fiber. In contrast, fruits, vegetables, beans and legumes, seeds and nuts, and whole grains are excellent sources of fiber. Fresh produce is especially desirable, all the more if the skins of vegetables and potatoes are left in place.

Because they contain soluble fiber, oats, barley, prunes, beans and other legumes, and various fruits are particularly valuable. Choose whole grain breads, whole grain pastas, and brown rice, all of which contain much more insoluble fiber than their refined counterparts. Among snack foods, popcorn is a good source of fiber (hold the salt, butter, and margarine, please); rye crackers and dried fruits are also fine.

The rule, then, is to favor fresh foods over preserved foods. Even so, it can be very hard to reach your goal of 30 or more grams per day without eating a high-fiber breakfast cereal. Pick your cereal carefully; many boxes boast of bran and fiber in large print on the front, only to give disappointing details in the fine print on the side panel. Choose oat

Table 8-3
SOURCES OF DIETARY FIBER

Food	Serving	Fiber content (to nearest gram)	Calories
Grains and Flours			
Buckwheat	1 cup (cooked)	11	340
Whole rye	1 cup (cooked)	11	314
Whole wheat	1 cup (cooked)	10	400
Barley	1 cup (cooked)	8	700
Brown rice	1 cup (cooked)	5	230
Oats	1 cup (cooked)	3	132
White rice	1 cup (cooked)	trace	225
Refined wheat	1 cup (cooked)	trace	420
Baked Goods			
Ry-Krisp	1 square	5	55
Graham cracker	4 squares	2	120
Bran muffin	1	2	100
Whole wheat bread	1 slice	2	61
Pumpernickel bread	1 slice	1	66
Bagel	1	1	145
Pasta			
Spaghetti	1/2 cup (cooked)	1	155
Legumes			
Baked beans	1/2 cup (cooked)	9	155
Kidney beans	1/2 cup (cooked)	7	110
Navy beans	1/2 cup (cooked)	6	112
Dried peas	1/2 cup (cooked)	5	115
Lima beans	1/2 cup (cooked)	5	64
Lentils	1/2 cup (cooked)	4	97
Greens			
Kale	3 1/2 oz.	6	50
Turnip greens	3 1/2 oz.	4	27
Spinach	3 1/2 oz.	3	22
Endive	3 1/2 oz.	2	23
Romaine lettuce	3 1/2 oz.	2	23
Iceberg lettuce	3 1/2 oz.	1	13
Vegetables, raw			
Carrot	1 medium	4	30
Tomato	1 medium	2	20
Mushrooms	1/2 cup	2	10
Bean sprouts	1/2 cup	2	15
Celery	1/2 cup	1	10
Green pepper	1/2 cup	1	10
Cucumber	1/2 cup	trace	8
Vegetables, cooked			
Potato (with skin)	1 medium	3	106
Sweet potato	1 medium	3	160
Parsnips	1/2 cup	3	51
Brussels sprouts	1/2 cup	3	28
Broccoli	1/2 cup	3	20
Zucchini	1/2 cup	2	11
Turnip	1/2 cup	2	17
String beans	1/2 cup	2	16

continued

Table 8–3 *continued*

Food	Serving	Fiber content (to nearest gram)	Calories
Asparagus	¹/₂ cup	1	15
Cauliflower	¹/₂ cup	1	5
Fresh Fruits			
Apple (with skin)	1 medium	4	81
Pear (with skin)	1 medium	4	90
Orange	1 medium	3	62
Banana	1 medium	3	115
Raspberries	¹/₂ cup	3	35
Strawberries	¹/₂ cup	2	23
Peach (with skin)	1 medium	2	37
Cantaloupe	¹/₄ melon	1	30
Cherries	10	1	49
Grapes	¹/₄ cup	1	50
Plum	1 medium	1	20
Fruits, Dried			
Figs	6	19	255
Prunes	6	8	120
Dates	6	4	140
Apricots	6	4	120
Raisins	¹/₄ cup	3	106
Nuts and Seeds			
Peanuts	10 nuts	1	105
Almonds	10 nuts	1	79
Filberts	10 nuts	1	54
Popcorn (air popped)	1 cup	1	54
Breakfast Cereals			
All-Bran Extra Fiber	1 oz.	15	50
Fiber One	1 oz.	13	60
All-Bran	1 oz.	10	70
Bran Buds	1 oz.	10	70
100% Bran	1 oz.	9	70
Oat Bran (hot)	1 oz.	6	110
Bran Flakes	1 oz.	5	90
Corn Bran	1 oz.	5	98
Raisin Bran	1 oz.	5	110
Cracklin' Oat Bran	1 oz.	4	110
Shredded Wheat	1 oz.	3	90
Wheaties	1 oz.	3	110
Cheerios	1 oz.	2	110
Oatmeal	1 cup	2	108
Corn flakes	1 oz.	trace	110
Dietary Supplements			
Wheat bran	1 oz.	12	
Wheat germ	1 oz.	3	62
Psyllium (Metamucil, Perdiem, Fiberall, and others)	1 tsp. or 1 wafer	4	varies
Methylcellulose (Citrucel and others)	1 tsp.	2	varies

Principal source: "Diet, Nutrition, and Cancer Prevention: The Good News." U.S. Department of Health and Human Services.

bran or a wheat cereal that provides at least 10 grams of fiber per serving. Use low-fat or skim milk and add some fruit to enhance flavor and provide additional nutrients (and fiber!).

Read all food labels to determine how much fiber you're getting. Be sure to consider dietary fiber, not crude fiber, and to evaluate portion size. Remember, too, that although the new food labels provide a "% daily value" for fiber, it's calculated on a moderate target of 25 to 30 grams, which may be a bit below your goal.

Use food labels and Table 8–3 to find out how much fiber is in your diet. Count the grams of fiber you eat on each of 3 typical days, then add fiber-rich foods or supplements until you achieve your goals. After that, you'll find yourself choosing fiber-rich natural foods as a matter of second nature.

Dietary fiber is crucial to good health, but it's not a cure-all. Soluble fiber is an important tool in the fight against atherosclerosis, but oat bran is not a panacea. Don't settle for a token pinch of oat bran. Instead, get enough fiber of both types — and don't neglect a balanced diet or the other elements of your comprehensive program to conquer heart disease.

Chapter 9

Alcohol: Fighting Atherosclerosis with a Smile

THE FRENCH say, "*À votre santé*," the Italians, "*Salud*," and the Germans, "*Prost*." In Russian it's "*Na zdorovya*," in Yiddish, "*L'chaim*." All around the world, it seems, people offer the same salute that we do in English. Will these wishes come true? Can a drink or two actually be beneficial "to your health?"

It's a simple question, but the answer is a bit complex. First the bad news: alcohol is a major cause of death and disability. In fact, it's the second leading preventable cause of death in the United States, ranking behind smoking but ahead of passive smoking. Alcohol can be a killer. Cirrhosis of the liver is a major complication of alcoholism, but it's not the leading cause of death in alcoholics. Trauma and cancer are major killers of alcoholics, but neither is in first place. In fact, the leading cause of death in alcoholics is the same as in nondrinkers: heart disease.

Alcohol is a major health hazard, and damage to the heart is one of its many toxicities. Even so, I've included alcohol as one of your 15 ways to conquer heart disease. Am I turning my back on all the bad news just to recommend something you'll actually like to hear? Not at all — in fact, there is also important good news about alcohol: it can substantially reduce your risk of heart attack.

The news about alcohol can be good or bad depending on its dose: low-dose alcohol can protect your heart, while larger amounts can damage your heart and many other organs. Although alcohol *abuse* is a killer, proper alcohol *use* can help fight atherosclerosis. But the line between help and harm must be drawn with care; you'll need more information to decide if alcohol is right for you.

Alcohol in America

Alcohol has occupied an important place in human society since the dawn of history. People learned to cultivate plants about 10,000 years ago. Barley may not have been the first crop, but it wasn't far behind; humans learned to brew beer from barley almost as soon as they learned to cultivate grains. It took another 5,000 years or so to learn how to ferment fruits, but wine has been with us ever since. And if the pleasures of wine date to antiquity, so too, does the realization that alcohol can be hazardous; in 850 B.C. Homer decried "Inflaming wine, pernicious to mankind / [that] unnerves the limbs / and dulls the noble mind."

Like many other health hazards, alcohol abuse didn't do too much damage until the industrial revolution, when new technology made distilled spirits widely available at low prices. Public health authorities in England rapidly recognized the perils of the new "gin epidemic," but alcohol use — for good and ill — has resisted every attempt to control it. Alcoholic beverages are widely consumed all around the world today.

America is no exception. Two-thirds of all adults consume alcohol, making it the most widely used drug in the United States. As a nation, we consume 5.8 billion gallons of beer, 585 million gallons of wine, and 395 million gallons of distilled spirits each year. As individuals, we imbibe an average of 318 beers, 179 shots of whiskey, and 77 glasses of wine each year. That means that the average American adult ingests more than two and a half gallons of pure alcohol every year.

People drink for personal pleasure and to socialize with others. Because alcohol is big business, people also drink because they're persuaded to do so; each year the American alcohol industry spends more than 1.5 billion dollars to promote its products. And because alcohol is an addicting drug, as many as 19 million Americans drink because they've become alcohol-dependent.

People drink for many reasons — but few drink to protect their hearts. You should consider your heart when you decide if you should use alcohol. Drinking is a personal decision, but the health effects of alcohol — both good and bad — should play a prominent role in the decision-making process.

Alcohol and Atherosclerosis

Dr. William Heberden first recommended alcohol for patients with angina in 1789. Ever since, many physicians have advocated an evening drink to relax their cardiac patients. Despite this long history of alcohol's use for heart disease, scientific data about alcohol and atherosclerosis did not begin to accumulate until the 1980s.

The Honolulu Heart Study uncorked the modern interest in alcohol and the heart. In 1980 this distinguished project reported on how alcohol consumption influenced the health of 8,006 men of Japanese ancestry. Low-dose alcohol use was associated with a reduced death rate; the protection was substantial, and most of it was attributed to a 54 percent decrease in heart attack deaths among drinkers. But larger amounts of alcohol — above 2 ounces per day — produced a very different effect, as mortality rose in moderate-to-heavy drinkers. The excess mortality in heavier drinkers was not due to heart disease, but to cancer, strokes, and liver disease.

The results of the Honolulu Heart Study can be described as a J-shaped mortality curve. Nondrinkers are at the upper left of the curve; as alcohol use increases, the death rate falls to correspond to the midpoint of the J. But as the average daily dose of alcohol increases, the death rate rises again, eventually exceeding the mortality rate in nondrinkers.

During the past 15 years, at least 12 studies have evaluated the relationship between alcohol consumption and the risk of heart attack. All confirm the original observations from Honolulu, but because they've looked at different population groups, each study has added important information. Because they are new and controversial, it's worth a look at a few representative studies.

Whereas the Honolulu Study included only men, the equally distinguished Framingham Heart Study has been evaluating both men and women since the 1940s. Drinkers of both sexes suffered fewer heart attacks than nondrinkers; in Framingham, though, the protective dose was lower than in Honolulu: women appeared to benefit from as little as a half ounce of alcohol per day, while men required about an ounce.

The risk of heart attacks continued to decrease as alcohol consumption increased to 5 ounces per day; in all, light-to-moderate drinkers enjoyed a 30 to 40 percent reduction in heart attack risk as compared with nondrinkers.

Doctors may be slow to recommend alcohol, but health care professionals have benefited from light-to-moderate drinking. The Nurses' Health Study observed a 40 percent reduction in heart attack risk with less than 1 ounce of alcohol per day. The Health Professionals Follow-up Study collected similar information from 51,529 men, with similar findings; 1 to 4 ounces of alcohol per day was associated with a 40 to 50 percent reduction in heart attacks. In both studies, as in Honolulu and Framingham, the protection associated with alcohol was independent of other cardiac risk factors such as smoking, blood pressure, obesity, cholesterol, and exercise.

Now that the alcohol question has been opened to scientific study, the data continue to pour in. A few more examples: in 1992, the Multiple Risk Factor Intervention Trial (MR. FIT) reported a 40 to 50 percent reduction in heart attacks associated with 1 to 3 drinks per day; all 11,688 men in this study were at high risk for heart attacks because they had multiple atherosclerosis risk factors. In the same year, the Kaiser Permanente Study of 128,934 men and women in California found that 1 to 2 drinks a day was associated with a 30 percent reduction in heart attacks. In this study, as in a Danish study from 1994, heavy drinkers had an excess mortality from noncardiac causes, confirming the J-shaped curve relating alcohol intake to overall death rates. And two studies from 1993 provide additional data. In one, low-dose alcohol was protective even for men who were at an extraordinarily high risk for heart attacks because of genetic abnormalities. In the other, alcohol consumption was associated with a reduced risk of fatal and nonfatal heart attacks within 24 hours of drinking.

Studies of alcohol and heart attacks have investigated both men and women. They have accounted for all known cardiac risk factors and have included people at high and low risk. They have included foreign populations from Auckland, New Zealand, to Copenhagen, Denmark, and domestic groups from Honolulu, Hawaii, to Framingham, Massachusetts. It's a lot of information for just 15 years of study, and for all its diversity, its message is remarkably consistent: low-dose alcohol is associated with a reduced risk of heart attacks and cardiac deaths.

Can we *prove* that alcohol is protective? Absolute proof would depend on a randomized clinical trial, in which a large number of healthy people volunteer to consume varying amounts of alcohol each day while investigators track their rate of heart attacks over the years. Randomized controlled clinical trials are difficult, time consuming, and expensive, but they have produced critically important information about atherosclerosis; the protective effect of low-dose aspirin (Chapter 7) is just one example. But for obvious reasons, I doubt that a similar trial of low-dose alcohol is logistically feasible or ethically permissible. In the absence of a clinical trial, we'll just have to make do with the evidence at hand. I'm convinced; the evidence may not be 100 proof, but it's a solid 86 proof. Think it over for yourself before you decide if you should drink to the proposition that low-dose alcohol can reduce your risk of heart attacks.

The alcohol hypothesis has earned my vote because it's based on many independent studies involving thousands of subjects in diverse population groups. The studies have been conducted by epidemiologists with long years of experience studying heart disease. The studies are of excellent quality, and their conclusions are remarkably similar.

I am convinced, too, by the sheer magnitude of the protective effect that has been reported. Low-dose alcohol is associated with a 30 to 50 percent reduction in heart attacks, a result that compares favorably to the protection conferred by low-dose aspirin, smoking cessation, regular aerobic exercise, maintenance of ideal body weight, cholesterol reduction, fish consumption, and postmenopausal estrogen replacement. Low-dose alcohol is certainly no substitute for those less-controversial interventions, but under the right circumstances it can be a valuable part of your comprehensive fight against atherosclerosis.

I am convinced that alcohol retards atherosclerosis for one additional reason: there is a biologically sound explanation for the protection that has been observed in all these studies.

How Alcohol Fights Atherosclerosis

Heart attacks result from problems at three levels: the blood cholesterol, the arterial wall, and the blood clotting mechanism. Alcohol appears to help by acting on the first stage of atherosclerosis.

Alcohol consumption increases HDL, the "good" lipoprotein that carries cholesterol away from the fatty plaques of atherosclerosis so it can be eliminated from the blood by the liver. This effect of alcohol has been known for years, but doctors didn't give it much credence until recently. The reason is that HDL cholesterol comes in two subclasses, HDL_2 and HDL_3. For years alcohol was dismissed because it was thought to raise only the "wrong" subclass, HDL_3. Now we know better: alcohol consumption increases both HDL_2 and HDL_3; moreover, both subclasses of HDL are linked to a reduced risk of heart attacks.

It doesn't take much alcohol to boost the level of HDL cholesterol in the blood. In just 6 weeks, 1 to 2 drinks per day increases HDL by 5 to 10 points. A 10-point rise in HDL — whether achieved by exercise, weight loss, smoking cessation, or alcohol — is associated with a 40 percent reduction in cardiac risk. Can it be a coincidence that low-dose alcohol has been consistently associated with exactly this magnitude of protection?

New research suggests that alcohol may act in other ways as well. It may reduce blood clotting by acting on platelets or fibrinogen, both major contributors to blood clotting. It may improve glucose metabolism; a 1993 study associated low-dose alcohol use with reduced blood insulin levels. And substances in red wine may provide additional benefit by lowering LDL cholesterol in the blood or by inhibiting the oxidation of LDL in the arterial wall (see the discussion of red wine, below). But this information is still tentative, and elevated levels of HDL cholesterol remain the best explanation for alcohol's protective action.

How Much Alcohol Is Enough?

It can be very hard for doctors to determine the optimal dose of a prescription drug; it's harder still to be sure about the best way to use nonprescription drugs such as aspirin. Alcohol, too, is a drug. Like aspirin, you can buy it on your own in a wide variety of places. Although aspirin comes in a range of strengths and preparations that can be confusing, it's no match for the enormous variety of alcohol "formulations." And unlike aspirin, alcohol doesn't come with a package insert to instruct you on its safe usage. Still, the advice for alcohol is very similar to the bottom line for aspirin: if you choose to use it to conquer heart disease, use it in small doses.

The studies of alcohol and heart attacks have found protection with average alcohol doses as low as 10 grams per day; perhaps because they have higher HDL cholesterol levels to begin with, women show a better response to these very small amounts of alcohol. In general, protection increases as the average daily dose rises, up to about 60 grams per day. But noncardiac complications begin to appear at doses as low as 30 grams. All in all, an average daily intake of 15–30 grams of alcohol seems about right to provide maximal cardiac protection with a minimal risk of alcohol-related complications.

You won't get very far if you drop in at your neighborhood wineshop and request 15 grams of alcohol. Fortunately, it's easy to translate medicinal measurements to more common denominators. Fifteen grams is the amount of alcohol present in an ounce of pure ethanol. It's also the amount present in 6 ounces of wine, 12 ounces of beer, or one standard measure of distilled liquor.

How much alcohol is enough to fight atherosclerosis? When Herman Johannsen, the cross-country skier who lived to age 111, was asked the secret of his longevity, he advised, "Stay busy, get plenty of exercise, and don't drink too much. Then again, don't drink too little." I agree. The short answer is an average of 1 to 2 drinks a day, considering a glass of wine, a bottle of beer, or a mixed drink as equivalent. Women who choose to use alcohol to prevent heart disease can probably get benefit from half the amount that men require. But even low-dose alcohol can have deleterious effects — especially for women (see below).

What Kind of Alcohol Is Kindest to the Heart?

Can millions of Frenchmen be wrong? Is red wine the best way to fight atherosclerosis with a smile?

Red wine has been touted as the explanation for the "French paradox." For all their differences, the French and Americans are quite similar in their saturated-fat intakes, average blood pressures, cigarette smoking, and body mass indexes — yet heart attacks are substantially less common in France than in the United States. The explanation for this disparity is not known, but theories abound. Advocates of the Mediterranean diet suggest that olive oil is the answer, while family history experts say it's all in the genes. Both have a point, as do alcohol's partisans, who say the answer is red wine.

Red wine does have some properties that distinguish it from other types of alcohol. Theoretically, at least, one of these properties could be beneficial at each of the three stages of atherosclerosis.

Atherosclerosis begins with unfavorable blood cholesterol levels. Any form of alcohol can help by boosting HDL levels, but red wine may have the additional benefit of lowering LDL cholesterol levels. The ingredient that's responsible is resveratrol; it's not part of the alcohol itself, but it's present in the skins of grapes. Since red wine is made from grapes with the skins left in place, they contain much more resveratrol than white wine. The chemical has been shown to reduce the cholesterol in rats' livers, but its effect on humans has not been studied in detail.

The second way that red wine may fight atherosclerosis is also speculative: a 1993 study found that red wine may have antioxidant properties. Again, the active ingredient is not alcohol, but another group of chemicals called phenols. Test-tube experiments showed that phenols from red wine could protect human LDL cholesterol from oxidation. Since oxidized LDL initiates the second stage of atherosclerosis in the arterial wall, red wine may be more helpful than other alcoholic beverages — but we'll need much more data to confirm this possibility.

The third step leading up to a heart attack is activation of the blood's clotting system. Preliminary experiments suggest that red wine may have a special role here, too, since it inhibits platelet activation.

Is red wine the explanation for the French paradox? It's too early to say. But red wine — along with other forms of alcohol — is surely a factor in another difference between health in France and America: the French have twice as many deaths from cirrhosis of the liver.

Should you buy Beaujolais and chuck chardonnay? Not so fast. For one thing, red wine is more likely to trigger migraine headaches because its phenolic compounds cause platelets to release a chemical called 5-HT. More important, a 1992 study by Drs. Arthur Klatsky and Mary Anne Armstrong found that red wine was no more effective than white wine in reducing the risk of heart attacks. In this study of 81,825 men and women, white wine was actually a little more effective than red wine, and both appeared better than beer or liquor.

When in France, do as the French (except when it comes to foie gras!). When in America, choose the alcoholic drink you like best, if you choose to drink at all. As things stand now, the amount of alcohol seems much more important than the type of alcoholic beverage. And the amount is very important indeed.

Low-Dose Alcohol's Potential Health Hazards

If heart attacks were the only consideration, we could all wash down our low-dose aspirin with low-dose alcohol. Unfortunately, it's not that simple: even low doses of alcohol can have adverse consequences. Take them into account before you decide if alcohol is right for your health as well as your heart.

Alcohol and Breast Cancer: A Dilemma for Women

Heart attack is the leading cause of death in American women, but breast cancer is their second leading cause of cancer death, ranking behind only lung cancer. American women could greatly reduce their risk of death from lung cancer (and heart attacks!) by stopping smoking; preventing breast cancer is more problematic.

One in every nine American women will develop breast cancer; in this year alone, 175,000 cases will be diagnosed, and about 45,000 women will die of the disease. Early detection by clinical breast examinations and mammograms can help a great deal. But women should also take every possible step to lower the risk of developing breast cancer in the first place.

Some of the things that fight atherosclerosis will also protect against breast cancer. Although the data is better for cardiac protection, it appears that regular aerobic exercise, maintenance of ideal body weight, low dietary fat consumption, and high-fiber, vitamin-rich diets may help prevent both problems. But one thing that can protect womens' hearts may possibly increase their risk of breast cancer; Chapter 16 discusses the pros and cons of estrogen replacement therapy.

Alcohol consumption reduces the risk of heart attacks in both men and women, but it increases the risk of breast cancer in women. Although it's woefully underpublicized, the association between drinking and breast cancer has been firmly documented by more than three dozen medical studies from around the world. All types of alcoholic beverages appear equally culpable. And if that were not bad enough, there's even worse news: even the very low doses of alcohol that reduce the risk of heart disease can increase the risk of breast cancer. For example, doctors at Harvard Medical School found that as little as 3 to 5 drinks per week increases risk by 30 percent, while larger amounts may increase a women's risk of breast cancer by up to 60 percent.

There is still a lot to learn about the link between drinking and breast cancer. We don't know how alcohol increases risk; increased estrogen levels are a possibility. Nor do we know if all women who drink are equally vulnerable; most studies link alcohol to breast cancer in women of all ages, but the 1993 Canadian National Breast Screening Study found a link only in premenopausal women, while the 1992 Iowa Women's Health Study reported that alcohol increased the risk of breast cancer only in postmenopausal women who also used estrogen replacement therapy.

Even if low-dose alcohol increases the risk of breast cancer by 30 percent, it could save many lives. That's because American women are 6 times more likely to die of heart disease than breast cancer. Alcohol can reduce the risk of heart attack by about 40 percent, so the net result for American women is a substantial gain of life expectancy. Faced with a choice between the risk of heart disease and breast cancer, however, few women will be comforted by national statistics. Fortunately, there is a better way to decide if low-dose alcohol is likely to help or harm.

What's a woman to do? I advise individual decisions based on competing risks and benefits. Women who are at high risk for heart attacks (Table 2–11) might choose to use low-dose alcohol to reduce their risk, particularly if they have low HDL cholesterol levels or if they don't choose to take estrogens after menopause (see Chapter 16). On the other hand, women with a high risk of breast cancer might be best advised to avoid alcohol; to help with that decision, Table 9–1 lists the major breast cancer risk factors.

A decision about alcohol can be difficult for men, but it's substantially harder for women. People of both sexes should think it over and discuss their questions with their doctors. And in addition to considering the medical data, they should take account of their personal feelings about the potential pleasures and hazards of low-dose alcohol.

Trauma
Accidental injuries are a major hazard of alcohol abuse. Even low-dose alcohol can slow reflexes and impair judgment. The remedy, though, is simple: don't drive or operate dangerous machinery after you drink, even if you've limited yourself to just one or two.

Table 9-1
BREAST CANCER RISK FACTORS

Factors That Increase Risk	Previous cancer in the other breast
	Family history (especially a mother or sister with breast cancer at an early age)
	Advanced age
	Early onset of menstruation
	Late menopause
	No pregnancies
	Obesity
	Dietary fat (?)
	Prolonged estrogen use (?)
Factors That Decrease Risk	Early pregnancy
	Exercise
	High-fiber, vitamin-rich diet (?)

Addiction

Alcoholics consume large doses of alcohol — but they had to start somewhere. People who limit themselves to a maximum of 2 drinks per day will not become dependent on alcohol. Still, people who are at increased risk of alcohol dependence might choose to avoid exposure to even small amounts of alcohol. People with alcoholic parents or siblings are at increased risk, as are individuals who've had problems with substance abuse of any kind.

If you think you may be a problem drinker, ask yourself four questions:

1. Have you ever tried to cut down on your drinking?
2. Have you ever been annoyed by criticism of your drinking?
3. Have you ever felt guilty about your drinking?
4. Have you ever had a morning "eye opener?"

Answering yes to one or more of these questions doesn't mean that you are a problem drinker, much less an alcoholic. But it does mean that low-dose alcohol may not be right for you, even if it's good for your heart.

Pregnancy

Alcohol increases the risk of fetal damage. Women should not consume even small amounts of alcohol while they're pregnant.

Medication

Alcohol is a drug, and it can interact with other drugs. Sedatives and tranquilizers head the list. If you require daily medication, check with your doctor, nurse, or pharmacist before you use alcohol in any dose.

Calories

Alcohol is calorie-dense; at 7 calories per gram, it has nearly twice the calories of carbohydrates and proteins (4 per gram) and almost as many as fats (9 per gram). Two drinks a day will add 210 calories to your diet — even without the mixers. It's not a major consideration for most people, but if you're fighting the battle of the bulge, calories should be a factor in your decision about using alcohol to fight heart disease.

High-Dose Alcohol: A Major Health Hazard

Low-dose alcohol has its good points. Alcohol abuse is a major health hazard, lacking any redeeming features.

Although low-dose alcohol protects against atherosclerosis, high doses can cause cardiovascular diseases. Even moderate amounts of alcohol can contribute to hypertension, strokes, and brain hemorrhages. Alcohol can precipitate arrhythmias, disorders of the heart's pumping rhythm; some people are vulnerable to this "holiday heart syndrome" even if they imbibe only modestly. Heavy drinking has been linked to sudden cardiac death, especially in the presence of alcoholic liver disease. Finally, heavy drinking can damage the heart muscle itself; called alcoholic cardiomyopathy, this condition leads to congestive heart failure.

Alcohol abuse can lead to many problems beyond the cardiovascular system. Table 9–2 summarizes the hazards of heavy drinking.

If all this illness and suffering were not bad enough, alcohol abuse also imposes a substantial burden on the American economy. In all, the medical expense, lost productivity, and property damage caused by alcohol amounts to about $117 billion annually — nearly the same amount as cardiovascular disease. It's a hidden tax of $300 annually on each of us.

All these problems, both medical and fiscal, result from alcohol abuse rather than responsible low-dose alcohol use. But they are undoubtedly the reason that so few doctors recommend low-dose alcohol

Table 9-2
HEALTH HAZARDS OF ALCOHOL ABUSE

Body System or Function	Alcohol-Related Disorders
Heart	Rapid or irregular heart action Weakened heart-muscle function Heart failure Increasing angina
Circulation	High blood pressure
Nervous system	Stroke due to brain hemorrhage Confusion and dementia Seizures Acute intoxication Withdrawal symptoms, including hallucinations and DTs Brain degeneration Peripheral nerve damage
Intestinal and digestive	Inflammation of the esophagus and stomach Ulcers Bleeding Inflammation of the pancreas Hemorrhoids Cancer of the esophagus Cancer of the stomach Cancer of the colon
Liver	Fatty liver Alcoholic hepatitis Cirrhosis
Musculoskeletal	Osteoporosis Muscle weakness Fractures due to trauma
Breast and reproductive	Fetal damage, including mental retardation and growth retardation Fetal alcohol syndrome Breast cancer in women Breast enlargement in men Male impotence
Kidney	Excessive urination
Blood and immune system	Anemia Low white blood cell counts Low platelet counts Abnormal bleeding Impaired immune function

continued

Table 9–2 *continued*

Body System or Function	Alcohol-Related Disorders
Metabolic	High blood triglycerides
	Low blood sugar levels
	Low blood protein levels
	Low blood magnesium and phosphorus levels
	Malnutrition
	Acidosis
	Altered metabolism from various medications
Head and neck	Cancer of the mouth
	Cancer of the larynx
Skin	Itching
	Rosacea and other abnormalities
Infections	Increased susceptibility to many infections
Trauma	Motor vehicle accidents
	Many other accidents
	Falls
	Fires
	Drownings
	Violence
Psychological	Addiction
	Depression
	Anxiety
	Antisocial behavior
	Impaired work performance
	Impaired family interactions

to fight atherosclerosis, and they should be part of your database when you consider using alcohol to protect your heart.

Is Alcohol Right for You?

If you're like most of my patients, you want a yes-or-no answer. But, like them, you'll have to settle for my usual reply: maybe.

I'm convinced that low-dose alcohol can fight atherosclerosis, and I recommend it to selected people. The key factor is an individual's risk of heart attack. Review your risk score from Table 2–11; if you're in a high-risk group, you should seriously consider low-dose alcohol, particularly if your HDL cholesterol is low.

An equally important factor is the potential of low-dose alcohol to cause harm. For women, the major worry is breast cancer, and it's a major drawback indeed. In general, I recommend low-dose alcohol to women only if they are at high risk for heart disease (especially because of low HDLs) but have a low risk for breast cancer. Women shouldn't drink at all if they are pregnant. No one should drink before driving. People at risk for alcohol dependency should exercise great caution before they choose to drink.

The third factor is often overlooked, but it's important, too. It's the issue of personal preferences. If you enjoy a drink or two, take pleasure into account even when you're planning a medical program to conquer heart disease. If you find drinking unpleasant, don't force alcohol into your stomach just to protect your arteries. Since it's a personal choice, let me share some personal decisions. I know alcohol would reduce my heart attack risk, but even a glass of wine makes me sleepy, so I don't drink. My decision is easier because I've brought my overall risk score way down and my HDL way up with diet, exercise, and smoking cessation. On the other hand, my wife enjoys wine with dinner, so she has a glass or two nearly every evening — even though her HDL is high and, like every woman, she is concerned about breast cancer.

If you decide to make alcohol part of your fight against atherosclerosis, be sure to keep the dose low. One to 2 drinks per day is about right; just 1 a day is probably better for women. Although red wine is in fashion and its use is supported by preliminary experiments, the best current evidence suggests that any form of alcohol will do.

Most physicians are reluctant to recommend alcohol to their patients. Having seen the ravages of alcohol abuse all too often, I can see why recommending alcohol runs against the medical grain. But all physicians prescribe drugs with potential side effects; some can be addictive, and many are far more hazardous than low-dose alcohol. We explain the benefits and risks of drugs and keep an eye on our patients to be sure things are going well. In my view, physicians should approach low-dose alcohol for atherosclerosis in just the same way — including follow-up visits to check HDL levels, obtaining mammograms as indicated, and keeping an eye out for alcohol's toxicities.

If you choose to use low-dose alcohol to help conquer heart disease, keep your doctor informed and be sure to drink responsibly. Above all, don't rely on alcohol alone to keep your heart healthy — it's neither a panacea nor a substitute for other measures. Atherosclerosis is a multifactorial disease — be sure you fight it on *all* fronts.

Chapter 10

Fish: Tipping
the Scales
to Health

ATHEROSCLEROSIS is a complex disease, and fighting it is no easy task. The basic rule is simple enough; indeed it's "back to basics," back to the patterns of diet and exercise that kept human blood vessels healthy before the bodily abuse and disuse of the industrialized lifestyle put fatty plaques into our coronary arteries. But the fight against atherosclerosis also requires details; deciphering them can be hard for you, but fishing out the facts is also difficult for medical investigators.

Science uses many techniques to discover the facts you need to plan your program to conquer heart disease. Computer models provide useful predictions, laboratory experiments investigate fundamental mechanisms, and animal studies permit preliminary treatment trials. Human studies range from investigations of individual patients and families to large epidemiological observations that may encompass thousands and thousands of subjects. The gold standard of human studies, though, is the controlled clinical trial, in which subjects volunteer to be randomly assigned to try a new intervention or to serve as controls, carrying on with their usual treatments.

To provide the best care for their patients, clinicians should respond to the results of controlled trials, incorporating new discoveries into their practice patterns. Do they? To find out, let's compare the results of two clinical trials.

In a 1982 study, 3,837 patients who had survived heart attacks were randomly assigned to receive a new treatment or to continue with standard medical care. Both groups were observed for 2 years. When the code was broken, the patients who had received the new treatment were the clear winners, having enjoyed a 26 percent reduction in overall mortality.

In a 1989 study, 2,033 patients who had survived heart attacks were randomly assigned to receive a new treatment or to continue with standard medical care. Both groups were observed for 2 years. When the code was broken, the patients who had received the new treatment were the clear winners, having enjoyed a 29 percent reduction in overall mortality.

The two trials are remarkably similar in their designs and results. But doctors have responded to them very differently. Within a matter of months the treatment used in the 1982 trial had found its way into standard medical practice — but the treatment used in the 1989 trial has been overlooked. The treatment studied in 1982 was a prescription drug, propranolol (a beta-blocker); most heart attack survivors are given a prescription for a beta-blocker when they leave the hospital. In contrast, the treatment studied in 1989 is rarely incorporated into the directions given to heart patients; the neglected treatment is eating fish.

Fish Consumption and the Risk of Heart Attacks

When you were growing up, your mother may have told you that fish was "brain food"; perhaps because it was supposed to be good for you, you may have learned to dislike fish. I don't know if fish is good for your brain, but eating it is a smart thing to do for your heart — and you can learn to enjoy fish.

Credit for the first observations of fish and atherosclerosis goes to a group of Danish doctors. In 1971, they noticed that the Eskimos of Greenland had a very low rate of heart attacks. To find out why, they compared Eskimos with Danes. Despite eating high-fat diets, the Eskimos had lower LDL and higher HDL cholesterol levels. Carrying their studies one step further, Drs. Bang, Dyernerg, and Nielson determined that this difference depended on the fact that the Eskimos' dietary fat came from marine animals, while most of the fat in the Danish diet came from land animals.

Not surprisingly, Eskimos eat enormous amounts of seafood, often consuming more than a pound of fish or whale meat daily. But you don't have to aspire to the Eskimo diet or emulate the Eskimo lifestyle to get the benefits of fish; recent studies suggest that much smaller amounts of fish are beneficial.

The best study was published in the *New England Journal of Medicine* in 1985, but its observations began in 1960, when investigators carefully recorded the dietary habits of 852 healthy middle-aged men in the Netherlands. These men, from the town of Zutphen, were observed for the next 20 years. When the data were analyzed, it became clear that the men who ate the most fish had the lowest rate of death from heart attacks. The protective effect of eating fish held up even after other dietary factors, lifestyle patterns, and cardiac risk factors were taken into account. The protection was substantial, amounting to a 50 percent reduction in heart attack deaths. And it didn't take much fish to reduce the risk of heart attack; as little as 1 ounce per day was associated with significant protection. After studying all the results, Dr. Daan Kromhout and his colleagues concluded that eating fish just once or twice a week might protect against coronary artery disease.

Greenland and the Netherlands are not the only places where fish consumption appears to reduce the risk of heart attacks. In Norway, heart attacks declined during World War II, when fish consumption increased, but rose again after the war, when fish consumption fell. In Japan, fish consumption is high, averaging three and a half ounces daily, and heart attacks are uncommon; the Japanese who eat the most fish have the least atherosclerosis. In Sweden, a 14-year study of 10,966 subjects reported that people who ate fish regularly had 30 percent fewer heart attacks than non–fish eaters. In Chicago, male employees of the Western Electric Company were tracked for 25 years; the men eating the most fish had the fewest deaths from coronary artery disease. Similar results were obtained by another American study, the Multiple Risk Factor Intervention Trial (MR. FIT), in which a high intake of fatty acids from fish was associated with a 40 percent reduction in the heart disease death rate, as well as a reduction in deaths from other causes. And a 1994 study tells us that eating fish provides protection against another devastating manifestation of atherosclerosis, strokes.

Although these results are impressive, they are not uncontested, since a study from Norway and another from the United States fail to document a protective effect of fish. More studies will be required to reconcile these apparent contradictions; at present, the weight of the epidemiological evidence favors fish. Adding this evidence to the trial of fish in heart attack survivors and to laboratory studies of fish oil, it seems clear that eating fish can help fight atherosclerosis.

Fish in the Treatment of Atherosclerosis

The ultimate test of any technique used to conquer heart disease is its ability to treat patients who already have the condition. How does fish consumption meet this test?

Very well. The 1989 Diet and Reinfarction Trial (DART) study from England tells the story best. As discussed at the start of this chapter, heart attack patients who were assigned to eat fish had 29 percent fewer deaths than similar patients who received medical care that was identical in all respects except for the fish. Patients in the treatment group were advised to eat oily fish at least twice a week. It didn't take a whole lot of fish to have a protective effect; on average just 10 ounces per week significantly reduced the risk of dying during the first 2 years after a heart attack.

How Fish Consumption Fights Atherosclerosis

Land animals and marine animals differ in many respects. Hunters and fishermen explain the differences in one way, zoologists and marine biologists in another. But for cardiologists and nutritionists, the critical difference between the creatures that live on land and those that dwell in water is their fat content.

Land animals contain saturated fats, fatty acids in which all the carbon atoms are surrounded by their maximum complement of hydrogen atoms (see Figure 4–1). Vegetables contain unsaturated fats, fatty acids in which some of the slots for hydrogen remain unfilled. In most vegetable oils, the final empty slot is located on the sixth carbon from the end of the carbon chain; for this reason, vegetable oils are called omega-6 fatty acids. Fish oils are unique. They are composed of long-chain fatty acids with 20 or more carbons linked together; as many as 6 carbons have empty slots for hydrogen, making them highly unsaturated. And in fish oils, the final empty hydrogen slot is located on the third carbon from the end of the chain; that's why fish oils are called omega-3 fatty acids.

The two most abundant omega-3 fatty acids in fish are eicosapenta-enoic acid (EPA) and docasahexaenoic acid (DHA). EPA has 20 carbons, 5 of which are unsaturated; DHA has 22 carbons, 6 of which are unsaturated.

Omega-3s are crucial for marine life. Among other things, these oils remain liquid at cold temperatures. As a result, fish and marine mammals that live in cold, deep waters have the highest omega-3 contents. You'll recognize them by their dark, oily flesh.

Omega-3s do a lot for marine animals — and they can also do a lot for people who eat them. EPA and DHA are absorbed by the intestinal tract and are carried by the blood to all the body's tissues. Omega-3s are incorporated into the membranes that surround human cells, including the cells involved in atherosclerosis: endothelial cells that line the inner layer of arteries, white blood cells that migrate into arterial walls, and platelets that initiate the blood clotting process. Once they're part of the cell membrane, omega-3s exert many effects on cell metabolism and functions; one important effect is to change the balance of prostaglandins, the same chemicals affected by low-dose aspirin (Chapter 7).

Although the effects of omega-3s are not entirely understood, they may fight atherosclerosis at all three stages of the disease.

The most obvious possibility was noted in the early Eskimo studies; omega-3s lower LDL and raise HDL cholesterol levels. They also reduce the concentration of triglycerides in the blood. Obvious or not, changes in blood cholesterol levels may not actually explain the protective action of fish. It takes very large amounts of fish oil to improve blood cholesterol levels; Eskimos eat enough fish to do it, but the Dutch, British, and Americans who are protected by much smaller amounts of fish don't display similar changes in their blood cholesterol profiles. And even if purified fish oils are administered in amounts large enough to improve blood cholesterol levels, the improvements tend to dissipate within just a few months.

Omega-3s might act on the second stage of atherosclerosis, in the arterial walls. It's a possibility that has not been fully investigated, but I think it merits more study. Remember from Chapter 1 that plaque formation involves inflammation in the arterial wall. Macrophages and other white blood cells gobble up oxidized LDL; in the process, some white blood cells are damaged and die, releasing toxic substances, while others secrete small proteins that stimulate further inflammation. Omega-3s from the diet are incorporated into the membranes of white blood cells, and they inhibit the release of inflammatory proteins. In fact, omega-3s are being used experimentally to treat rheumatoid arthritis and other inflammatory diseases. It's tempting to think that EPA may fight atherosclerosis in arterial walls by reducing inflammation; it's only speculation, but it's an interesting possibility.

The most important way that omega-3s protect against heart attacks is by their effect on the third stage of the process, blood clotting. Omega-3s are incorporated into platelet membranes, where they decrease stickiness, inhibit platelet function, and reduce clotting.

Fish Versus Fish Oil

Why go to all the trouble of buying, cooking, and eating fish to fight atherosclerosis? Why not swallow down a few fish oil capsules and get on with business?

Ever eager for a quick fix, Americans began to consume fish oil capsules in record numbers during the 1980s. It took scientists a few years to catch up with the trend; the early studies of fish oil capsules have been completed, however, and their net results should serve to reel in the omega-3 capsule industry. Fish oil is not snake oil — but it's not the answer to atherosclerosis, either.

Doctors have tried fish oil capsules for high cholesterol and triglyceride levels — they help, but only temporarily. Fish oil capsules have been used to treat hypertension — they help, but only minimally and inconsistently. Fish oil capsules have been administered to patients following angioplasties in the hopes of preventing their coronary arteries from narrowing again — they work, but only in a minority of patients.

Heavily promoted as nonprescription remedies, omega-3 capsules have proved to be fishful thinking. One reason for the disappointing results may be that they contain only modest amounts of omega-3s; the fat content of a typical fish oil capsule is 12 percent EPA and 18 percent DHA, while the remaining 70 percent is a mix of saturated, monounsaturated, and polyunsaturated fatty acids. Three and a half ounces of mackerel provide 2,500 milligrams of EPA and DHA; a typical omega-3 capsule contains only 300 milligrams.

Table 10–1
OMEGA-3 FATTY ACIDS (DHA & EPA)
IN REPRESENTATIVE MARINE SPECIES

Species	Omega-3 Contents in Milligrams per 3½ oz.
Mackerel	2,500
Salmon (Pacific)	2,000
Tuna (Albacore)	2,500
Tuna (canned in water)	1,500
Herring	1,600
Trout (rainbow)	1,000
Cod	300
Snapper	300
Flounder	200
Swordfish	200
Crab (king)	500
Shrimp	300
Lobster	200

There's plenty of evidence to recommend eating fish to fight atherosclerosis, little to support fish oil capsules. It's a continuing tale with an important moral: the natural food works, but the shortcut extract does not.

We have a long way to go to understand fully omega-3 fatty acids. But until we land new insights, you'll be much more likely to shore up your health by getting your omega-3s from fish rather than from capsules. Table 10–1 lists the omega-3 contents of various fish and shellfish.

Seafood Safety

Fish oil capsules have two major side effects: expense and disappointment. Although they don't have much to offer in the fight against atherosclerosis, they are at least safe. Blood sugar levels may rise in a few diabetics who take the capsules; other people may be bothered by a fishy taste or by a tendency toward easy bruising.

Conquer heart disease the old-fashioned way: eat fish instead of taking fish oil capsules. Eating fish is more beneficial — but it also involves more worry about side effects. Apart from swallowed bones and stressed budgets, fish themselves (excluding certain shellfish) have no toxicities for humans. But the things that humans do to fish can come around to catch up with people who eat fish. Because people pollute the earth's waters, we must choose our fish with care.

For all its benefits, industrialization has its drawbacks as well. Abuse of the human body is one; atherosclerosis, hypertension, diabetes, and obesity are among its consequences. Abuse of the environment is another; water pollution is among its many consequences.

Industrial pollutants, agricultural byproducts, and human wastes all contribute to the contamination of our waters. Industry discharges gasses and particles into the air; what goes up must come down, and air pollutants often end up in water. Heavy metals, synthetic chemicals, and petroleum products are among the many industrial materials that may enter water from accidental spills, faulty storage tanks, or just plain dumping. Agriculture contributes pesticides and fertilizers, and organic wastes from humans and animals can pollute our waters with bacteria and viruses.

The Environmental Protection Agency estimates that 10 percent of America's lakes, rivers, estuaries, and coastal waters contain potentially dangerous levels of toxic chemicals and heavy metals. Your drinking water is protected by the high standards and tough testing of the EPA and local authorities. But what protects fish?

Not much.

Enormous volumes of water pass through the gills of all fish. Chemicals and metals can be absorbed from the water, then stored in the fish's intestinal organs and fat. If the process continues, pollutants can build up to higher levels in the fish than in the water. And the chemicals can pass up the food chain, first to larger predatory fish, and eventually to humans who consume fish with the best intentions of pleasant eating, healthful protein, and omega-3 fatty acids that fight atherosclerosis.

The most worrisome pollutants than can pass from industry to water, then fish, and finally humans are polychlorinated biphenyls (PCBs) and methyl mercury, which are reproductive toxins, and PCBs, dioxins, and chlorinated hydrocarbon pesticides, which can cause cancer. Worrisome, too, are viruses that can cause hepatitis and bacteria that can cause diarrhea.

It's enough to make you sick — but not enough to deter you from eating fish. In the long run, of course, the problem can best be solved by correcting water pollution. In 1994, the FDA introduced a series of new regulations that shore up seafood inspections and safety standards. It's only a first step, but we can expect it to initiate a stream of improvements that will make a whale of a difference to consumers who are at sea over fish safety. But even before the new standards take effect, you can protect yourself and your family by selecting and preparing your fish properly; you can eat fish to protect your heart without jeopardizing the rest of your body.

Even now, most seafood is perfectly safe for human consumption. Still, you should take steps to avoid the most hazardous species.

Raw clams, oysters, and mussels present the greatest risk, not because of contaminants, but because of natural toxins. One in 1,000 people who eat raw mollusks become ill; fortunately most cases are mild. Raw fish of other types are next on the hazard list, principally because they may contain bacteria and viruses that would have been killed by cooking. Doctors don't share restaurateurs' enthusiasm for sushi: you can pay your money and make your choice, but children, pregnant women, and people with serious medical problems should always cook their fish.

Proper cooking and handling will rid seafood of biological contaminants but won't provide protection against chemical contaminants. Freshwater fish are the most likely to contain chemicals. Commercial fishing is banned in polluted rivers and lakes, but sport fishing may still go on. Bottom-dwelling fish are the most likely to ingest chemicals, and fatty species are the most likely to accumulate toxins. Catfish, lake trout, and lake whitefish are the most worrisome freshwater fish; brook trout, perch, and freshwater bass the safest.

Among ocean fish, fatty coastal species are of greatest concern; examples include herring, sardines, chum salmon, and pink salmon. Deep water, off-shore species are safest; because they have less fat, cod, haddock, and pollock are even less likely to contain chemicals than tuna, flounder, and halibut. Swordfish are a special case, since they may be contaminated with mercury; migratory species such as bluefish and striped bass may contain PCBs.

The safest fish are those raised down on the farm; aquaculture has revived the ancient oriental art of growing fish in controlled environments. Because they are processed at high temperatures and are inspected more vigorously, canned fish are also safe (though they may contain undesirable amounts of salt).

Don't let this rising tide of concern about seafood safety stop you from eating fish; weighing the benefits to your heart against the potential risks of chemicals, fish will net you important health benefits. Here are five tips to ensure that your fish is safe:

1. Buy your fish from reputable markets, and look it over yourself. Fresh fish should have smooth skins, moist flesh, a translucent sheen, and clear bulging eyes. Avoid fish with a strong fishy odor.
2. Handle your fish properly; store it below 35°C in the coolest part of your refrigerator, and serve it within a few days.
3. Cook your fish thoroughly, maintaining the recommended temperature for at least 5 minutes. Oysters, clams, and mussels should be steamed for at least 6 minutes.
4. Eat a variety of species, favoring deep-water off-shore fish over coastal species. Favor small young fish that have had less time to accumulate chemicals.
5. Don't eat the internal organs or gills, including the green tomalley of lobsters and the "mustard" of crabs.

Setting Your Goals for Fish Consumption

It's an easier decision than alcohol or aspirin. It doesn't involve tallying up grams of fat or fiber. You don't have to review your cardiac risk score or recheck your cholesterol. Just make a few simple safety precautions part of your routine, then don't flounder around: eat fish.

How much fish should you eat? Two or three meals each week would be excellent; aim for 4 to 6 ounces of fish per portion.

What type of fish is best? All species can help fight atherosclerosis, but those with the most omega-3s are best. Experiment with a variety of fish. Let personal pleasure and preference guide your choice, but if all things are equal, try to get your share of dark-fleshed fish from cold, deep waters. Table 10–2 provides some vital statistics for various fish species. As usual, the less cholesterol the better. When it comes to fish, though, a *high* fat content is desirable; fatty fish contain more omega-3s; tuna, salmon, bluefish, and mackerel are examples. Two reminders: first, contaminants tend to concentrate in fatty tissues, so you should avoid fatty fish from contaminated waters. Second, oily fish tend to *taste* fishy, so if you prefer cod, flounder, or sole, enjoy them with the assurance that they also contain valuable omega-3s.

Table 10-2
FACTS ABOUT FISH

Species	Fat (to the nearest gram per 3½ oz.)	Cholesterol (milligrams per 3½ oz.)	Calories (per 3½ oz.)
Catfish	3	55	130
Clams (hard-shell)	1	55	80
Cod	1	40	105
Haddock	1	74	112
Halibut	3	41	140
Lobster	1	72	98
Mackerel	18	75	262
Mahimahi	1	85	102
Ocean perch	2	54	121
Pike	1	50	113
Pollock	1	96	113
Rockfish	2	44	121
Salmon (coho)	8	49	185
Sea bass	4	53	124
Scallops	trace	50	82
Shrimp	1	195	99
Sole	1	45	70
Snapper	2	47	128
Swordfish	5	50	155
Trout	4	73	151
Tuna (fresh)	6	49	184

Shellfish have been a dietary dilemma, moving back and forth between the good column and the bad without much rhyme or reason. Part of the confusion exists because there are actually two nutritionally distinct types of shellfish. Oysters, clams, mussels, and scallops live quietly on the ocean floor eating phytoplankton; they are the vegetarians of the sea, and like other vegetarians, they have low cholesterol levels. In contrast, lobsters and crabs do have high cholesterol contents. Shrimp have the most cholesterol of all; perhaps it's just a coincidence, but Americans eat more shrimp than any other fresh or frozen seafood, consuming 640 million pounds annually. But even these shellfish have very little saturated fat, which is why they belong back in the acceptable column, in moderation, of course.

Even people who love fish have legitimate concerns about safety. Weighing the benefits of a 30 to 50 percent reduction in heart disease against a tiny risk of toxicity from pollutants, the scales still balance in favor of fish; careful shopping and cooking are your best defense.

The greatest threat to the healthfulness of fish, however, doesn't come from water, but from people. It's not what's in the fish, but what we do to the fish after they are out of the water. Fried fish are high in fat; hardly a health food, a fast-food fish fillet sandwich provides 53 percent of its calories from fat, even without tartar sauce, which is also loaded with fat. Smoked fish is very high in salt. Canned fish is also high in salt, but low-sodium alternatives are now available. To save on fat and calories, choose canned tuna packed in water instead of oil; you'll also get more omega-3s, since the soy oil used in oil canning can leach out the omega-3s.

Instead of frying your fish, try broiling, baking, poaching, steaming, and grilling — or use your microwave to save time and flavor as well as to reduce fat. For a garnish, try vegetables, lemon slices, or spices instead of cream sauces. Experiment with new recipes and new varieties of fish — liking fish is an acquired taste, and cooking fish is an acquired art. Help is just a cookbook away.

All too often, the American idea of nutrition is a "see-food" diet — Americans see food and they eat it. A seafood diet would be far better. Fortunately, America is catching on to fish; per capita fish consumption rose by 33 percent between 1980 and 1990. But we still average only 16 pounds per year — far below the 63 pounds eaten by the average Japanese citizen each year. Let's try to catch up on fish; we'll close the health gap, if not the trade gap.

Why don't more doctors recommend fish? I wish I knew. The reason, I suspect, is that my profession is hooked on prescription medications and high technology. We should cast aside preconceptions and encourage you to include fish in your nonprescription fight against atherosclerosis.

Chapter 11

Antioxidants: New Help on the Horizon

IT'S HARD to live in the America of the 1990s without despising cholesterol. It takes only a little more medical sophistication to realize that not all forms of cholesterol are equally despicable — LDL cholesterol is the legitimate foe, while HDL cholesterol actually helps protect against atherosclerosis. But now I'm asking you to carry revisionism one step farther: I'm asking you to take good care of your LDL cholesterol.

It's still indisputably true that LDL is a major cause of coronary artery disease and that the lower your LDL the better for your heart. But not all LDL is equally culpable. In fact, normal or "native" LDL appears innocent, even though it is able to penetrate into arterial walls. But in the arterial wall LDL can be oxidized, and it's this modified LDL which is so toxic, initiating the chain of events that leads to atherosclerosis. So while you should do everything you can to lower your LDL, you should also do everything you can to take care of the LDL that's left, protecting it from oxidation.

Because oxygen is essential for life, we're used to thinking of it as a good thing. It is — but too much of a good thing can be harmful. In the case of atherosclerosis, the problem is not too much oxygen, but the wrong kind of oxygen. To be exact, the problem is oxygen free radicals — not human rebels from the '60s, but oxygen molecules with excess electrons.

What Are Free Radicals?

You don't have to be a physicist to understand free radicals, but it helps. Physicists tell us that all matter is composed of atoms. At the center of each atom is its nucleus, a dense region containing particles called protons and neutrons. The nucleus is surrounded by electrons, tiny particles that spin around the nucleus much as planets orbit the sun.

Electrons follow very precise rules in their endless travels around atoms. Electrons are neatly confined to regions of space called orbitals. Each orbital can hold only two electrons. In normal circumstances, the two members of each electron pair spin through their orbital in opposite directions, effectively counterbalancing each other. Most of the billions of molecules in the human body are constructed in just this way, containing only paired electrons. Free radicals are different; they are missing an electron, so the lone electron remaining in its orbital is not counterbalanced. As a result, the molecule is literally charged up — it has extra energy and is unstable.

Nature abhors instability. Free radicals try to rid themselves of extra energy by reacting with other molecules. If two radicals meet up, they can combine their unpaired electrons to form a stable molecule. But if a free radical reacts with a normal molecule, it will dump its unpaired electron or snatch an electron away, creating another free radical in the process. It's a true chain reaction, in which one free radical produces another.

Free radicals have a central role in many of nature's chain reactions. Combustion is one example, so you can thank free radicals for transforming your bread into toast each morning. Chemists have harnessed free radical chain reactions to produce polythene and the other plastics we find so useful. Free radical reactions allow paint to dry, but they also contribute to deterioration that affects painted surfaces as they age; it's a useful example that may help you picture the good and bad aspects of free radicals in nature.

Free Radicals in the Human Body

Like the free radicals in nature, the free radicals in the human body can be helpful or harmful.

Free radicals are generated by the body's metabolic processes. In particular, free radicals are produced as a byproduct of oxidative metabolism, in which oxygen is used to burn carbohydrate molecules for energy. Oxidation is the most efficient way to release the energy from fuel; it's what puts the "air" in aerobics.

Oxygen free radicals — charged, high-energy, unstable oxygen molecules with extra electrons — are more than just incidental byproducts of the body's metabolism. In fact, these so-called superoxide radicals are essential to killing bacteria; children born with a rare genetic defect called chronic granulomatous disease cannot generate superoxide radicals, and they are plagued by recurrent bacterial infections. But while oxygen free radicals are a boon when they attack bacteria, they can be a bane when they attack the body's own tissues.

The body has an elaborate series of mechanisms designed to keep free radicals in check. Oxidative metabolism takes place only in mitochondria, tiny furnace-like sacks within cells that contain the oxygen free radicals, protecting other cell structures from damage. In addition, cells contain a series of enzymes that can sop up or inactivate free radicals that may leak out of mitochondria.

It's a complex system. On one side are free radicals: oxygen free radicals from normal metabolism, and other reactive molecules such as hydroxyl radicals and peroxyl radicals. While not free radicals themselves, hydrogen peroxide, iron, and copper in the body promote the activity of free radicals. On the other side are the control mechanisms that fight free radicals: mitochondrial membranes, enzymes, and proteins that bind excess iron and copper. On the control side, too, are the antioxidant vitamins that are now generating so much interest and hope.

The body is a battleground between free radicals and the control systems that hold them in check. The food we eat also participates in the struggle. Although free radicals are not present in natural foods, they can be produced when foods are processed or cooked; in particular, heating and frying can generate toxic oxidation products from polyunsaturated fatty acids. On the other side are the natural antioxidants in foods; in particular, vitamin C, vitamin E, and vitamin A and its precursors work to counteract oxidized free radicals.

In health, the body's checks and balances control free radicals so they work for you, not against you. But if free radicals gain the upper hand, they can attack the body's own tissues, causing chain reactions that may ultimately contribute to disease. Free radicals can react with any of the body's molecules. If they attack DNA, the genetic mastercode, they can cause mutations that could lead to unchecked cell growth — cancer. If they attack proteins in the eye's lens, they can alter the clarity of normal proteins — cataracts. If they attack cell membranes, they may cause damage leading to neurological disorders, inflammatory diseases such as arthritis, or even to accelerated aging.

Free radicals are everywhere, and they have the potential to damage many parts of the body. But there's no need to panic: in most cases, free radicals are effectively neutralized, and even when they injure DNA and proteins the body has ways to repair the damage. Because of these complexities, scientists are not even sure that free radicals play an important role in cancer or cataracts, much less aging. But while studies to answer these questions are getting under way, research has already established a probable role for free radicals in causing America's leading killer, atherosclerosis.

Oxygen Free Radicals and Atherosclerosis

Atherosclerosis occurs in three stages. The process starts in the blood, triggered by high levels of LDL cholesterol or low levels of HDL, the "good" cholesterol that carries LDL away from arteries.

The second stage of atherosclerosis takes place in the wall of vulnerable arteries. LDL starts the process by penetrating the arterial wall. The higher the LDL in the blood, the more will penetrate. LDL will also penetrate more readily when the artery's lining membrane is damaged by smoking, high blood pressure, diabetes or other factors. You should fight these early steps in atherosclerosis by lowering your LDL, raising your HDL, and keeping your arteries healthy.

Atherosclerosis does its greatest damage right inside the arterial wall, and it's here that free radicals play a key role. All the cells in the arterial wall — the endothelial cells that line the inner membrane, the smooth muscle cells of the middle layer, and the white blood cells that wander through the wall — generate oxygen free radicals. In turn, oxygen free radicals go on the attack. The molecule they attack most vigorously is LDL cholesterol. The result is a modified form of cholesterol, a "sick" LDL, analogous, perhaps, to fat that's turned rancid in your pantry.

Normal LDL cholesterol is quite harmless — but oxidized (rancid) LDL is another matter altogether. Free radicals initiate the process, which is known to the initiated as lipid peroxidation. By any name, the result is LDL cholesterol that's transformed into fatty acid free radicals. The modified cholesterol radicals attack other cholesterol molecules — it's the very chain reaction predicted by our physicist friends. The chain reaction proceeds until the excess electron on the free radical cholesterol is neutralized; by that time, however, a single free radical may have produced thousands of modified cholesterol molecules.

If modified LDL cholesterol confined its damage to other cholesterol molecules it would make an interesting story for scientists to study. Unfortunately, modified LDL cholesterol damages the arterial wall itself, making it the culprit in atherosclerosis.

Modified LDL cholesterol is taken up by white blood cells called macrophages, transforming them into fat-filled foam cells. The cells are damaged and many die, releasing their fatty gruel into the arterial wall — where it triggers further cell damage. Cholesterol free radicals also cause smooth muscle cells in the arterial wall to enlarge and multiply.

At first, the process is only a small yellow dot on the arterial wall, then a fatty streak. But as the chain reaction continues, the damaged area slowly enlarges, eventually forming a plaque that narrows the artery's channel. Now, at last, it's easily recognizable as the deadly disease called atherosclerosis.

Not content with causing atherosclerosis, oxidized LDL cholesterol has another nasty trick at its disposal. It inhibits arteries from producing a substance that normally relaxes the muscles in the arterial wall, causing the arterial channel to widen. Without this "endothelial-derived relaxing factor," coronary arteries are narrower and more vulnerable to the complete blockages that cause heart attacks.

Oxygen free radicals play a crucial role in the second stage of atherosclerosis. New research suggests that they may also contribute to the final stage of heart attacks, in which blood clots form on atherosclerotic plaques, completing the process of arterial blockage. Free radicals appear to accelerate blood clotting by activating platelets, the tiny blood cells that trigger the clotting mechanism.

With free radicals causing chain reaction damage to LDL cholesterol, and oxidized LDL causing self-perpetuating damage to arteries, it's a wonder that all our blood vessels aren't covered with atherosclerosis. It's easy to image this as the end result of our high-fat, high-stress modern world. But the body can fight back if we provide the weapons it needs: antioxidants.

What Are Antioxidants?

You don't need a physics lesson to understand antioxidants; quite simply, they're molecules that neutralize free radicals. Some free radicals are so unstable that they break down within microseconds; fortunately the most reactive and toxic of all free radicals, the hydroxyl radical, is in this category. But other free radicals are more persistent and will go on damaging human molecules unless they're neutralized; this group includes the oxygen radicals, superoxide radicals, and peroxyl radicals that set off the chain reaction which damages LDL cholesterol. The good news is that antioxidants are on hand to fight back.

The human body produces a large number of enzymes and proteins that function as antioxidants. One of the most effective free radical scavengers (glutathione peroxidase) requires the trace nutrient selenium as a co-factor. Another important enzyme (superoxide dismutase) attacks the superoxide radical. Hydrogen peroxide is not a radical, but in the presence of iron or copper it generates the extremely reactive hydroxyl radical; the body fights back with enzymes that break down hydrogen peroxide (catalase) and proteins that bind iron (transferrin) and copper (ceruloplasmin).

It's comforting to know that your body will go on producing all these antioxidants without any particular care or feeding. But don't let comfort turn to complacency; your LDL cholesterol — along with many other vulnerable molecules — depends on another group of antioxidants that do require careful feeding. They're the antioxidant vitamins.

It's easy to remember the antioxidant vitamins; just think of vitamins A, C, and E as your ACE in the hole. Mnemonics notwithstanding, the antioxidant vitamins are actually a bit more complex.

Vitamin A is just one member of a complex group of chemicals called carotenoids. At least 600 different carotenoids have been identified in nature; the best known is beta-carotene. Most, if not all, of the carotenoids function as very efficient antioxidants. In animals, including the human animal, the carotenoids from plants are converted into vitamin A, itself an antioxidant. Vitamin A is subsequently metabolized into important chemicals called retinoids; among other things, retinoids are crucial for vision.

Vitamin C is easy; the only other name it goes by is its chemical name, ascorbic acid.

Vitamin E, though, is a member of a complex family of substances called tocopherols; alpha-tocopherol is the major antioxidant in the vitamin E family.

Although the antioxidant vitamins are chemically unique, they team up to quench oxygen free radicals. In a sense, they produce their own chain reaction; in this case, it's a chain of protection.

Vitamin E (alpha-tocopherol) is the first line of defense. It enters the arterial wall in the very same particles that carry LDL cholesterol, so it's in an ideal position to prevent cholesterol oxidation. Vitamin E binds oxygen free radicals, neutralizing their harmful energy. In the process, however, vitamin E is consumed. Not to worry: carotenoids (beta-carotene and vitamin A) are on hand to carry on as antioxidants. But even if there are too many free radicals for vitamin A to neutralize, the antioxidant counterattack has an additional resource: vitamin C (ascorbic acid). Vitamin C has two important roles. It neutralizes free radicals, and it also regenerates the activity of vitamin E, restarting the molecular struggle against atherosclerosis in the arterial walls.

Beta-carotene and vitamin A, vitamin C, and vitamin E are far and away the most important dietary antioxidants. But preliminary research suggests that some other nutritional factors may play a role, including flavenoids in apples, tea, and onions, olive oil (Chapter 4), magnesium (Chapter 6), phenols in red wine (Chapter 9), and trace metals such as selenium (Chapter 13). Until we have more evidence, though, you'll need only to concentrate on providing enough of the antioxidant vitamins that your body needs to fight atherosclerosis.

Free Radicals and Antioxidants: The Current Evidence

The theory is compelling, but it's a new story that is still being written. Before you jump on the antioxidant bandwagon, spend a minute or two considering the current evidence.

The first chapter of the story is more complete than the second. The evidence that free radicals and oxidized LDL cholesterol cause athero-sclerosis is quite secure, but the evidence that antioxidant vitamins can prevent atherosclerosis is just starting to accumulate.

Cells derived from human arterial walls have been studied in test tubes. In these laboratory experiments, it's clear that oxidized LDL is toxic to arterial cells and that it's avidly taken up by white blood cells, turning normal macrophages into fat-filled foam cells. Many experiments have confirmed that oxidized (rancid) LDL causes the inflammation of atherosclerosis.

Test-tube experiments are great, but they don't tell the whole story. In the case of atherosclerosis, however, the lab experiments are complemented by actual human studies. A study of 35 heart attack victims found that the LDL cholesterol in their blood was unusually susceptible to oxidation. The fatty plaques from patients with atherosclerosis contain oxidized LDL cholesterol. A study of 60 men found that antibodies to oxidized LDL predicted the progression of atherosclerosis. And a study of 300 people found that patients with atherosclerosis had more free radical activity in their blood than did healthy individuals. Increased free radical activity has also been identified during actual heart attacks.

If free radicals and oxidized LDL cholesterol cause atherosclerosis, it stands to reason that antioxidants should be able to interrupt the process. The available data support this hypothesis, but more investigations will be needed to be sure it's true. In the laboratory, test-tube experiments have shown that antioxidants can neutralize free radicals, preventing LDL cholesterol from becoming rancid. In a compelling series of animal experiments, antioxidants have proved able to prevent experimental atherosclerosis. Needless to say, studies in rabbits and humans don't necessarily follow the same results. Still, a study of 78 men found that antioxidant supplements diminished blood free radical activity and reduced platelet activation.

The only way to be *sure* that antioxidants can help will be to conduct controlled clinical trials in which volunteers are randomly assigned to receive antioxidants or placebo pills. In fact, such trials are under way, but it will take years to see if the people taking antioxidants have fewer heart attacks than the placebo users. Until then, we'll have to make do with epidemiological studies that already provide intriguing clues about each of the antioxidant vitamins.

Beta-carotene and Vitamin A

First discovered in 1909, vitamin A is essential for night vision and for healthy skin, hair, bones, and teeth. Beta-carotene and other carotenoids were discovered in the 1930s; present in plants, the carotenoids are converted to vitamin A by the tissues of herbivorous animals. For years, beta-carotene was considered important only as a precursor of vitamin A; it's now clear, however, that the carotenoids have important activities of their own, including antioxidant activity. Average Americans get about two-thirds of their vitamin A from meat and dairy products; the remainder is supplied by beta-carotene from deep green and yellow-orange vegetables.

The U.S. Recommended Daily Allowance for vitamin A is 5,000 international units (IUs); that's the dose that will prevent vitamin A deficiency diseases (night blindness, skin disorders) from developing in healthy people. There is no USRDA for beta-carotene. Because vitamin A is fat soluble, it's stored away in the body's fat cells. Over time, high doses can build up to toxic levels capable of causing brain swelling, liver damage, eye disorders, and skin problems; daily doses in excess of 100,000 IUs for two years or longer may result in vitamin A toxicity. Alcohol abuse increases the risk of vitamin A toxicity.

Like vitamin A, beta-carotene is fat soluble and will accumulate in the body. Unlike vitamin A, beta-carotene is nontoxic; yellowing of the skin is the only known adverse effect in humans, even in patients taking huge doses (300 milligrams per day) to treat a rare metabolic disease (porphyria). Like other carotenoids, beta-carotene is a potent antioxidant. High-dose supplements of beta-carotene reduced the oxidation of LDL cholesterol in the blood of normal volunteers. An interesting experiment in humans proved that beta-carotene gets to where it's needed, actually entering atherosclerotic plaques; patients who were given beta-carotene supplements before undergoing surgery had a 50-fold increase in the beta-carotene contained in the walls of their diseased arteries. Another preliminary human trial found that beta-carotene supplements may increase HDL cholesterol levels; if this is confirmed, beta-carotene would be the only antioxidant vitamin that can boost the HDL cholesterol while also preventing oxidative damage to LDL cholesterol.

The best current evidence linking carotenoids to a reduced risk of atherosclerosis comes from a cross-cultural comparison of people living in 8 different countries. In this study, people with the highest blood levels of vitamin A had the lowest risk of heart attacks, even after taking cholesterol levels and other risk factors into account. Similar results were obtained in a 1991 study of 504 Scotsmen, which found that high levels of beta-carotene reduced the likelihood of nonfatal angina attacks. Closer to home, a 5-year study of 1,299 elderly residents of Massachusetts found that people who consumed the most beta-carotene had 73 percent fewer heart attack deaths than did people eating the fewest beta-carotene-rich vegetables and fruits. And a 1993 European study that actually measured beta-carotene concentrations in the body's fat cells found that people with the highest beta-carotene levels had the lowest risk of heart attacks.

Despite these hopeful results, the beta-carotene story is not uniformly favorable. The 1993 U.S. Nurses' Health Study did not find a protective effect of beta-carotene consumption. The 1993 U.S. Male Health Professionals Study reported protection only in current and former smokers, but a 1994 study of 29,133 men in Finland did not find any cardiovascular protection from beta-carotene in smokers — in fact, in the Finnish study, smokers taking beta-carotene had an increased death rate due to more cases of lung cancer (see antioxidants and health, page 264; Chapters 13 and 16 also discuss the proper way to interpret new studies).

The ultimate test of any technique used to conquer heart disease is its ability to treat patients who already have the disease. How does beta-carotene meet this test?

Because antioxidants are such a new approach to atherosclerosis, we don't yet have enough data to answer fully this important question. But the early clues are encouraging. Beta-carotene or placebos were randomly administered to 333 men with angina as part of the U.S. Physicians' Health Study; the men receiving 50 milligrams of beta-carotene every other day experienced a 49 percent reduction in their chances of having a heart attack, stroke, bypass operation, or cardiac death. It took 2 years for the protection to be evident; it will take many more years of observing the other subjects in the study to define fully beta-carotene's role in preventing atherosclerosis.

What should you do about beta-carotene while awaiting the results of controlled trials? The question of vitamin supplements is complex and will be discussed at the end of this chapter. But there is no debate about the great value of eating lots of foods rich in antioxidant vitamins.

Table 11-1
THE BETA-CAROTENE CONTENT OF SELECTED FOODS

Food	Portion Size	Beta-carotene (milligrams)
Apricots	3	1.7
Cantaloupe	1/2	5.2
Carrots	1/2 cup	11.5
Collard greens	1/2 cup	1.3
Mango	1	4.9
Papaya	1	3.7
Pumpkin (canned)	1/2 cup	16.1
Spinach (cooked)	1/2 cup	4.5
Squash (butternut, cooked)	1/2 cup	4.3
Sweet potatoes	1/2 cup (mashed)	13.0

Get your carotenoids from the beta-carotene in vegetables and fruits, not the vitamin A in meat and dairy products; deep-green and yellow-orange vegetables are the best sources.

Table 11-1 lists the beta-carotene content of selected foods. Table 11-2 is a more extensive list of the vitamin A equivalence of representative foods; as a rule of thumb, about 1,666 IUs of vitamin A activity equals one milligram of beta-carotene.

Vitamin C
Although vitamin C wasn't discovered until 1912, it was actually the subject of the first controlled clinical trial in medical history. The year was 1746, the investigator Dr. James Lind. A British navy surgeon, Lind believed that citrus fruits could treat scurvy, a common disorder affecting sailors during long sea voyages. To find out if his theory was right, he divided his sailors into 6 groups; one got a normal ship's diet, while the others received supplements of cider, vinegar, sea water, elixir of vitriol, or lemons and oranges.

After several months at sea, Lind's experiment proved his theory correct: the sailors who ate citrus fruits recovered, while the others remained ill with the abnormal bleeding and diseased skin, gums, and hair characteristic of scurvy. Despite the success of his experiment, Dr. Lind experienced the same frustration that many of today's scientists do: it took the bureaucrats of the British Admiralty 50 years to endorse citrus fruits as a standard sailor's ration.

Table 11–2
ANTIOXIDANT VITAMINS IN SELECTED FOODS

Food	Serving Size	Vitamin A (international units)	Vitamin C (milligrams)	Calories
Cruciferous vegetables				
Cabbage	1 cup	90	33	15
Cauliflower	1 cup	20	72	25
Broccoli	1 spear	2,540	113	50
Brussels sprouts	1 cup	1,110	96	60
Kohlrabi	1 cup	60	89	50
Vegetables				
Asparagus	4 spears	2	16	15
Beets	1 cup	20	9	55
Beet greens	1 cup	7,340	36	40
Carrot	1 medium	20,250	7	30
Corn	1 ear	170	5	85
Kale	1 cup	8,260	33	50
Parsley	10 sprigs	520	9	5
Green pepper	1 medium	390	95	20
Potato	1 medium	0	26	220
Pumpkin	1 cup	2,650	12	50
Spinach	1 cup	3,690	15	10
Squash, summer	1 cup	520	10	35
Squash, winter	1 cup	7,920	20	80
Sweet potato	1 medium	24,880	28	115
Tomato	1 medium	1,390	22	25
Turnips	1 cup	7,920	39	30
Turnip greens	1 cup	13,080	36	30
Fruits and juices				
Apple	1 medium	70	8	80
Apricot	3 medium	2,770	11	50
Banana	1 medium	90	10	105
Cantaloupe	1/2 melon	8,610	113	95
Cherries	10	150	5	50
Grapefruit	one half	10	41	40
Grapes	10	40	5	35
Lemon juice	1 cup	50	112	60
Lime juice	1 cup	20	72	65
Orange	1 medium	270	70	60
Orange juice	1 cup	190	97	110
Peach	1 medium	470	6	35
Pear	1 medium	30	7	100
Strawberries	1 cup	40	84	45

Principal source: "Nutritive Value of Foods." U.S. Department of Agriculture.

Lind's sailors may not have been true volunteers; it's most unlikely that they gave informed consent to the study, and we don't know if their assignment into treatment groups was really random. His experiment surely lacked a true placebo and, of course, modern statistics were not available. Today, some 250 years after Dr. Lind's experiment, we still need clinical trials to find out if vitamin C — and other antioxidants — really can prevent atherosclerosis. Even without these trials, though, we do know a lot about vitamin C, and we surely won't want to wait 50 years before deciding how much to consume.

Vitamin C, ascorbic acid, is essential for healthy blood vessels, normal connective tissues and bones, and proper wound healing; it also promotes the absorption of dietary iron. The U.S. Recommended Daily Allowance for vitamin C is 60 milligrams per day. Because vitamin C is present in many fruits and vegetables (Table 11–2) deficiency diseases are rare in the industrialized world. As a water-soluble vitamin, ascorbic acid is not stored in the body to any appreciable extent. Still, very large "megadoses" can have side effects, including diarrhea and kidney stones.

Vitamin C is an efficient antioxidant, but optimal antioxidant activity may require substantially more vitamin C than the USRDA, which is based on the dosage needed to prevent scurvy. Vitamin C traps free radicals and reactive oxygen molecules; it also regenerates vitamin E, enabling it to continue functioning as an antioxidant.

The best evidence that vitamin C can fight human atherosclerosis comes from a 1992 study of 11,348 adult Americans; over the course of 10 years, men with the highest vitamin C intake, either from food or supplements, experienced a 42 percent reduction in heart disease deaths, while women who consumed the most vitamin C enjoyed a 25 percent reduction in cardiovascular deaths. The same study also linked a high intake of vitamin C to a reduced rate of cancer deaths. A 1993 study from Europe looked at the role of vitamin C from another angle, checking actual blood levels and comparing them with heart attack deaths in 16 population groups; low blood levels of vitamin C were associated with an increased risk of heart attacks in both men and women.

Although these careful studies from the United States and Europe support a protective role for vitamin C, other data are less encouraging. In America, neither the Nurses' Health Study nor the Male Health

Professionals Study found an association between vitamin C consumption and cardiac risk. Similarly, the 1991 study of 504 Scotsmen found that low blood levels of vitamin C were linked to angina only in smokers. Various studies attempting to relate vitamin C to cardiac risk factors such as cholesterol and blood pressure have also yielded conflicting results.

It's clear that we have a lot more to learn about vitamin C and atherosclerosis. A controlled clinical trial will be needed to sort out the contradictions. It's Dr. Lind redux.

Vitamin E

Vitamin E is the most potent of the antioxidant vitamins. The evidence that vitamin E protects humans against heart disease is even better than the evidence that beta-carotene and vitamin C are protective. But if vitamin E scores first among the antioxidants in these respects, it lags in another category, since it's much harder to get abundant amounts of vitamin E from foods.

First discovered in 1922, vitamin E (alpha-tocopherol) is essential to the body for its antioxidant properties. Although a distinct vitamin E deficiency disease (analogous to scurvy from vitamin C deficiency) has not been identified, lack of vitamin E may be related to various neurological diseases and cancers — and to atherosclerosis. The U.S. Recommended Daily Allowance for vitamin E is 30 international units, but much higher amounts may be required for optimal antioxidant activity. Because it's fat soluble, vitamin E can be stored in the body's tissues. Although there is concern that very high doses of vitamin E may interfere with normal blood clotting or with the body's ability to fight infection, toxic effects from vitamin E have not been documented. In one small, brief study, huge doses of 8,000 units per day appeared to be well tolerated, but much more information will be needed before we're sure that large doses of vitamin E are indeed safe.

Vitamin E is present in many foods including vegetable oils, wheat germ, leafy green vegetables, margarine, butter, and liver. In addition, most cereals are fortified with vitamin E. It's easy to meet the USRDA for vitamin E from dietary sources — but very hard to get the 10-times-higher doses that seem to fight atherosclerosis from foods alone. Table 11–3 lists some dietary sources of vitamin E.

Vitamin E is a potent antioxidant; current evidence suggests that it's

Table 11-3
VITAMIN E CONTENT OF SELECTED FOODS

Food	Portion Size	Vitamin E (international units)
Abalone	3¹/₂ oz.	12
Apricots (dried	1 cup	11
Avocado	1	5
Cereals (fortified)	1 cup	40
Corn oil	1 tbsp.	5
Escargots	6	5
Filbert nuts	¹/₄ cup	12
Kale	3¹/₂ oz.	12
Mango	1	3
Margarine	1 tbsp.	5
Mayonnaise	1 tbsp.	6
Nuts (mixed)	¹/₄ cup	5
Olive oil	¹/₄ cup	20
Peanuts	¹/₄ cup	5
Pumpkin seeds	¹/₂ cup	5
Safflower oil	1 tbsp.	8
Sunflower oil	1 tbsp.	11
Sunflower seeds	3¹/₂ oz.	66
Sweet potato	1	9
Wheat germ	3¹/₂ oz.	21
Wheat germ oil	1 tbsp.	39

the first line of defense against free radicals. Moreover, about half of the blood's vitamin E is transported in the very same lipoprotein package that carries LDL cholesterol; if you feed your body enough vitamin E, your body will automatically put it where it's needed most. Vitamin E also improves the action of insulin, an extra benefit for the heart.

Many test-tube experiments demonstrate that vitamin E can protect LDL cholesterol from being oxidized by free radicals. Studies in rabbits show that vitamin E supplements can protect against experimental atherosclerosis. Most impressive of all are the epidemiological observations that vitamin E is protective in humans. A 1991 cross-cultural comparison of men from 12 European populations found that high blood levels of vitamin E were associated with a low risk of death from heart attacks, even after accounting for other risk factors, such as cholesterol and blood pressure. Similarly, the study of 504 Scotsmen found that men with the lowest vitamin E levels had the highest risk of developing angina.

Chauvinism notwithstanding, the best evidence that vitamin E protects the heart comes from two American studies, both published in 1993 in the *New England Journal of Medicine*. Both evaluated vitamin E consumption and heart disease, making them nice complements to the European studies that measured vitamin E in the blood but not in the diet.

The U.S. Nurses' Health Study has been tracking 87,245 women since 1980. Detailed questionnaires permit investigators to evaluate vitamin intake along with diet, cholesterol, body weight, blood pressure, smoking, exercise, and other risk factors. After comparing all these factors, the study found that vitamin E consumption protected against heart attacks. All in all, the women with the highest vitamin E intake suffered about 40 percent fewer heart attacks than the women who took in the least vitamin E. Protection was confined to women who took vitamin E supplements; an average daily dose of about 200 international units appeared optimal. It took at least 2 years of supplement use for vitamin E to produce protection against heart attacks.

The Male Health Professionals Study has been evaluating 39,910 American dentists, veterinarians, and pharmacists since 1986. It uses techniques similar to the Nurses' Study, and its conclusions about vitamin E are also similar: vitamin E protected against heart attacks, but optimal protection required about 100 units a day, doses that are achieved with vitamin E supplements rather than from dietary sources. As in the Nurses' Study, men who took vitamin E supplements for 2 years or more demonstrated the best results; they experienced nearly 40 percent fewer heart attacks than did the men who consumed the least vitamin E.

These large studies of vitamin E are encouraging but not conclusive. In fact, the 1994 study of 29,133 Finnish men found no cardiac protection from vitamin E supplements; even more discouragingly, the men taking vitamin E had a slight increase in brain hemorrhages. But despite its size, this study has important limitations. For one thing, the vitamin E dose was quite modest (50 milligrams of alpha-tocopheral per day, or about 75 International Units of vitamin E). In addition, all the subjects were smokers, averaging more than one pack per day for over 35 years. Smoking lowers vitamin C levels, but the study neither measured vitamin C levels nor administered supplements. If antioxidant protection requires a chain reaction involving vitamin E, carotenoids, and vitamin C (see page 254), vitamin C may be the missing link in the Finnish smokers study.

Many Americans get less than 10 units of vitamin E a day from their diets. Typical multiple vitamin supplements contain 30 units of vitamin E per pill. The Male Health Professionals Study found the best protection from 100 units a day; the Nurses' Study suggests that 200 units is an optimal daily dose of vitamin E. All in all, the fight against atherosclerosis may require an entirely new way of thinking about vitamin E. But before you place your order for vitamin pills, consider antioxidants in their proper perspective; the Roman poet Cicero reminds us that "Nothing new is quite perfect."

Antioxidants and Health

Although the evidence is just coming in, it seems likely that antioxidant vitamins may help conquer heart disease; at present, the evidence is strong for vitamin E, hopeful for beta-carotene, and suggestive for vitamin C. Antioxidants may also prove important for other areas of human health, but the scientific data supporting these hopes is less complete than the heart disease data.

Stroke. Like heart attacks, most strokes result from atherosclerosis. A 1993 study found that women eating antioxidant-rich fruits and vegetables had a 71 percent reduction in the risk of strokes — and a 33 percent reduction in heart attack risk.

Cancer. Free radicals can damage cell membranes and DNA, which carries the genetic code governing cell division. Scientists estimate that the DNA in each cell of the human body sustains 10,000 oxidative hits every day. Most of the damage to DNA is repaired, but if it's not, it may lead to uncontrolled cell growth, resulting eventually in malignant tumors. Can antioxidants help fight cancer as they do heart disease?

More than 130 studies have evaluated this question in all parts of the world; at least 120 agree that diets high in vitamin-rich vegetables and fruits are associated with a significantly reduced risk of cancer. The protection is much stronger for some cancers than others; diet seems particularly important in cancers of the lung, mouth, stomach, colon and rectum, bladder, and cervix. Most studies cannot determine exactly which components of vegetables and fruits are protective; the leading candidates are dietary fiber (Chapter 8) and antioxidant vitamins.

The data is best for beta-carotene and vitamin A. At least 17 studies have demonstrated that diets high in carotenoids reduce the risk of lung cancer by about 50 percent; substantial protection against cancers of the mouth, intestinal tract, and female reproductive tract has also been documented. A synthetic vitamin A derivative, isotretinoin is now being prescribed for patients with head and neck cancer; it's the first (and so far, only) vitamin to have a scientifically valid role in cancer therapy. High intakes of vitamin C also appear to reduce cancer risk; at least 75 studies have evaluated this question, with 54 reporting significant protection associated with high consumption of vitamin C–rich foods. The evidence supporting a protective role for vitamin E is less persuasive, but a 1993 study of 35,215 women in Iowa found a link between vitamin E intake and protection from colon cancer.

The most exciting evidence that antioxidant vitamins may reduce cancer risk comes from a controlled clinical trial conducted in Linxian, China by a team of Chinese and American scientists. Nearly 30,000 volunteers were randomly assigned to receive 1 of 4 different dietary supplements every day for 5 years. The people who took a combination of beta-carotene, vitamin E, and selenium experienced a 13 percent reduction in their cancer death rate and a 9 percent reduction in their overall death rate. The doses used were modest, amounting to only 2 to 3 times the USRDA for each supplement.

Although these results are very encouraging, they don't necessarily apply to Americans. Linxian is in the Asian "cancer belt," a zone with an extraordinarily high rate of stomach cancer. In addition, the typical diet in the region is deficient in many nutrients. Remember, too, that the 1994 study of vitamin E and beta-carotene supplements in Finland found an *increase* in lung cancer in men taking beta-carotene; vitamin E had no effect on lung cancer, but it was linked to a slight reduction in prostate and colon cancer.

More studies will be needed to evaluate the effects of antioxidant supplements on cancer. Until the results are in, prudence dictates that smokers should *not* take beta-carotene *supplements*. But they *should* eat lots of vitamin-rich *foods* — even in the Finnish study, consumption of fruits and vegetables was linked to protection from lung cancer. It's a good lesson for nonsmokers, too: vitamin-rich foods, yes; supplements, maybe.

Cataracts. Cancer is second only to heart disease on the list of America's leading killers; it's reassuring that antioxidants may help with both. Cataracts are much less serious — but even though they're no threat to life, they impair vision in 45 percent of Americans older than 75. Cataract surgery also drains the Medicare budget of more than \$3.2 billion annually. Although not all studies agree, many report that diets containing lots of vitamin-rich fruits and vegetables substantially reduce the risk of cataracts. The data are best for beta-carotene and vitamin C. In the U.S. Nurses' Health Study, for example, women who took vitamin C for 10 years or more enjoyed a 45 percent reduction in cataracts; a 1991 study of 1,380 Bostonians reported that vitamin supplements were associated with a 37 percent reduction in cataracts.

Aging. There is good scientific evidence that antioxidants may confer protection against heart disease, cancer, and cataracts. When it comes to aging, there is much more speculation than evidence. Many gerontologists speculate that free radicals accelerate the aging process. A 1994 study, in fact, found that antioxidants increased life span by an astounding 30 percent. But before you fly down to the vitamin store, you should know that the subjects of this study were fruit flies. If the theory proves valid in humans, antioxidants might slow the aging process; despite all the vegetables and fruits in my diet, I'll be an old man before there's evidence to validate or refute this possibility. The same is true of another theory I almost forgot to mention; some neurologists believe that free radicals may contribute to Alzheimer's disease and other forms of memory loss in the elderly.

A Word About Vitamin Supplements

It will be hard for you to decide rationally about using antioxidants to fight atherosclerosis without considering the broader question of vitamin supplementation. Few issues generate more controversy — or more passion. On one side are consumers; more than 50 percent of American adults take vitamin pills during the course of a year, and 25 percent take vitamins daily. On the other side are doctors; most physicians dismiss vitamin pills as unnecessary and wasteful. Far from abating, the controversy is actually escalating as the Food and Drug Administration proposes restrictions on the claims made for nutritional supplements, and the $2.7 billion a year vitamin industry fights back.

Although there is still a lot to be learned about antioxidants and other vitamins, many facts are clear.

Thirteen different vitamins are essential for health. All are organic molecules that are vital for the body's metabolism; since none can be manufactured by the body, all must be consumed.

Only tiny amounts of vitamins are required to prevent deficiency diseases. These amounts are the basis for the Recommended Daily Allowances for vitamins.

The average American diet provides more than enough vitamins to meet the recommended allowances. The only people who need vitamin supplements to meet their RDAs are people who are very malnourished; examples include some cancer and liver disease patients, some alcoholics, and some people with intestinal diseases. In addition, the elderly and poor may have vitamin-deficient diets. Ironically, perhaps, heart-healthy vegetarian diets are deficient in one vitamin, B_{12}; women who eschew red meat often need supplementary iron as well. Finally, pregnant women may need extra vitamins to meet their extra requirements.

Except for these special groups, ordinary vitamin supplements are wasteful. Promotional claims notwithstanding, they do not provide energy, fight infections, enhance sexual prowess, improve athletic performance, cure insomnia, relieve stress, or treat arthritis.

"Megadoses" of vitamins can be toxic. Because they are stored in the body's fat deposits, this is a greater concern for fat-soluble vitamins (A, D, E, and K) than water-soluble vitamins (B_1, B_2, B_3, B_6, B_{12}, folic acid, pantothenic acid, biotin, and vitamin C).

Natural vitamins are no better than synthetic vitamins. If you choose to take vitamins, use the least expensive preparation available from a reputable supplier. Select products that are fully labeled as to content, dosage, and expiration date, and that conform to the standards of the United States Pharmacopoeia.

Food is the best source of vitamins. In particular, vegetables, fruits, and whole grain products supply dietary fiber and many other important nutrients along with vitamins. Excessive cooking and processing can remove vitamins from fresh and whole foods.

Vitamin pills should never be used as substitutes for good nutrition. Even if vitamins are taken as supplements, it's important to maintain a healthful diet. Foods are smarter than chemists; vitamins, minerals, and food extracts may not retain the beneficial properties of whole foods. Remember the cautionary example of fish (Chapter 10): eating fish fights atherosclerosis, but taking fish oil capsules does not.

All these facts argue against the routine use of vitamin supplements, which is why most scientific organizations and doctors discourage them. But these well-established facts also may explain why so few doctors recommend antioxidants even though they are a very special case.

Antioxidant Supplements

Antioxidants are special because the dosages that may help fight athero-sclerosis are about 10 times higher than the dosages needed to prevent deficiency diseases. The Recommended Daily Allowances are based on the lower doses — it's easy to get them from foods, but it may be hard to get the larger amounts from dietary sources alone.

The sad fact is that most Americans do not get enough antioxidants. The official recommendation is to get these vitamins from fruits and vegetables. A 1991 government survey, however, found that only 9 per-cent of Americans consume the recommended 5 or more portions a day, and 11 percent don't average even 1 portion a day. The average Ameri-can consumes less than 1.9 milligrams of beta-carotene per day; even among people with incomes above 300 percent of the poverty level, 25 percent are below the RDAs for vitamin E.

Fruits and vegetables? By all means! You'll find tips for increasing your intake of these wonderful and essential foods in Chapter 4, along with ways to boost your consumption of whole grains. But when it comes to antioxidants, consider supplementing your high intake of fruits, vegetables, and grains with extra doses in pill form.

Are Antioxidants Right for You?

As a scientist, I readily admit that I don't know the answer to this ques-tion. Laboratory data, animal experiments, and observations of human population groups all suggest that antioxidants can help fight atherosclerosis. But final *proof* will depend on the result of randomized trials similar to the trials that have demonstrated aspirin's protective function (Chapter 7).

Clinical trials of antioxidants are already under way; examples include the U.S. Physicians' Health Study (beta-carotene), the newer Women's Health Study (beta-carotene, vitamin E), the CARET trial (beta-carotene, retinoic acid) and the French SU.V1. Max study (multiple antioxidants). It will take years, however, for the results of these trials to tell you if you should take antioxidants — and more trials will be needed to determine what dosage is best. What to do in the meanwhile?

The expert committees agree: fruits and vegetables, yes, antioxidant pills, not yet. It's scientifically unassailable advice; I can't assail it, but I don't agree with it. Fruits and vegetables, yes. Antioxidants, perhaps.

From my viewpoint, patients who already have atherosclerosis may not want to wait for clinical trials. The same is true even for healthy people with moderate to high cardiac risk scores (Table 2–11). Antioxidants take at least a year to begin demonstrating protection. Because the stakes are so high, I recommend antioxidant supplements to people with an urgent need for all possible tools to fight atherosclerosis. Pick an inexpensive preparation containing reasonable, nontoxic doses, so you'll have little to lose. Stay alert for the results of ongoing trials; if they surprise us with negative findings, stop the antioxidants, but if the trials confirm benefit you'll have the benefit of a head start.

Since the benefits of antioxidant supplements are unproved, the optimal dosages are unknown. At present, vitamin E seems the most beneficial; it's also the hardest to get from foods. Supplementary vitamin E doses between 100 and 400 units per day seem reasonable. Fruits and vegetables can provide enough beta-carotene and vitamin C, but daily supplements supplying 15 to 25 milligrams of beta-carotene and 250–500 milligrams of vitamin C are also reasonable, except for smokers, who should omit beta-carotene supplements. For convenience, consider a single tablet containing all three antioxidants; reputable mail order suppliers can provide them at a cost of less than 10 cents per day. Beta-carotene and vitamin E require fat for their absorption. Take them with meals; if you are on a low-fat diet, you probably eat little or no fat until dinner, which would be the best time to take antioxidant supplements.

I believe that antioxidants are an important new tool in the fight against atherosclerosis. Further studies will be needed to find out if I'm right. But even if antioxidants prove beneficial, they won't end the American epidemic of atherosclerosis. Consider antioxidants now, but don't neglect the comprehensive tried-and-true program of diet, exercise, smoking cessation, and stress reduction that will conquer heart disease.

Chapter 12

Niacin: Natural Vitamin or Powerful Drug?

IMAGINE a single pill that would lower your LDL and raise your HDL cholesterol levels. Suppose you could get the pill without going to your doctor for a prescription. Think of a pill that's much less expensive than the prescription drugs usually given for high cholesterol levels. While you're at it, suppose that this pill has been in use for nearly 40 years, so there's much more experience with it than with the high-priced prescription medications. Imagine a pill that's entirely natural. And consider that clinical trials have demonstrated that this inexpensive, natural, nonprescription pill protects against heart attacks and reduces death rates.

Too good to be true? Not at all; in fact, you've conjured up vitamin B_3, niacin.

Niacin really does have all these properties. You can get it on your own in any pharmacy and start taking it tonight. You can — but should you?

No.

For all its wonderful attributes, niacin also has deleterious properties. It's effective and inexpensive, but it can be unpleasant and even toxic. Think of it not as an innocent vitamin supplement, but as a powerful medication. Think it over before deciding to take niacin — and if you choose to take it, do so with the same care you would use with other medications.

You don't need a prescription to get niacin, but perhaps you should. Like postmenopausal estrogen therapy (Chapter 16), but unlike the other items in your 15-point program to conquer heart disease, niacin requires your doctor's help to use it safely and appropriately.

Niacin As a Vitamin

Niacin may be more familiar to you as vitamin B_3; if not, perhaps you'll recognize it by one of its other names, nicotinic acid and nicotinamide. By any name, niacin is essential to health.

Like the other B vitamins, niacin is water soluble. As a result, it's not stored up in the body's fat cells but is required in the daily diet. As with other vitamins, only tiny amounts of niacin are needed to prevent illness; unlike other vitamins, though, niacin can actually can be manufactured by the human body as long as the diet provides sufficient amounts of its precursor, an amino acid called tryptophan.

The human body needs niacin to permit it to release energy from foods; niacin is important for the metabolism of carbohydrates, fats, and proteins. People who don't get enough niacin develop pellagra, a deficiency disease characterized by diarrhea, fatigue, mental confusion, a skin rash, and irritation of the mouth and tongue. Although pellagra is still a problem in some Third World countries, it's rarely seen in the United States; one of the few good things about the typical Western diet is that it provides plenty of vitamins.

It doesn't take much niacin to prevent pellagra; the U.S. Food and Drug Administration recommends a daily allowance of 20 milligrams for adults. Niacin is provided by many foods, including legumes, peanuts, fish, poultry, meat, and eggs. Although niacin is quite stable, some is lost when foods are cooked in liquids that are discarded. Still, foods that are baked, broiled, steamed, and roasted retain nearly all their niacin. Niacin is also present in whole grains, but, like many other nutrients, it's lost in the refining process; because niacin is added back to fortified flour, however, it's available in pasta, breads, and cereals.

You don't need to take supplements to prevent pellagra or maintain your metabolism; a normal diet will give you more than enough niacin. But no matter how much you eat, your foods can never provide enough niacin to improve your cholesterol and fight atherosclerosis. Niacin the vitamin is one thing, niacin the medication, quite another.

Niacin As a Medication

Niacin fights atherosclerosis by acting on the first stage in the process, the blood cholesterol. Even though it has no effect on subsequent events in the arterial wall and the blood clotting mechanisms, niacin can have a major effect on atherosclerosis and heart attacks. But to fight atherosclerosis, niacin must be consumed in an amount 25 to 150 times greater than its recommended daily allowance as a vitamin. Unfortunately, in these very high doses niacin can do harm as well as good.

Niacin and Cholesterol

Niacin was first used to correct high cholesterol levels in 1955, making it by far the oldest cholesterol-lowering drug still in use today. Many potent cholesterol-lowering prescription drugs have been introduced in the 1980s and 1990s; it will take years for doctors to learn as much about these new medications as they already know about niacin. But one thing about the new drugs is already clear: all can lower LDL cholesterol, but none is able to substantially elevate HDL levels. Niacin can do both; seniority notwithstanding, its ability to lower LDL compares favorably to the prescription medications, and its ability to boost HDL levels is unrivaled.

As if to illustrate how long it can take to understand medications, doctors have not yet determined exactly how niacin alters blood cholesterol levels. Two major mechanisms appear to be involved. First, niacin reduces the production of LDL cholesterol by the liver; it may also reduce the liver's synthesis of triglycerides. Second, niacin slows the rate at which HDL cholesterol is removed from the blood. These two chemical activities explain the two clinical benefits of niacin: lower LDLs and higher HDLs. Preliminary research also suggests that niacin may reduce the rate at which adipose cells break down fat, thus reducing the discharge of fatty acids into the blood. True or not, this possibility shouldn't worry you, since obesity is *not* a side effect of niacin.

Niacin's effect on LDL cholesterol is substantial; most studies agree that it reduces LDL levels by 20 to 40 percent, and that these reductions can be sustained for as long as the drug is administered. The higher the dose of niacin, the greater its effect on LDL cholesterol; in most studies, daily doses of 1,500 to 3,000 milligrams produced maximal benefits. These doses also produce major reductions in blood triglyceride levels of 40 to 60 percent; it's nice to see these changes, but the reductions on LDL are much more significant in the fight against atherosclerosis.

Niacin's effect on LDL cholesterol and triglyceride levels is impressive — but its effect on HDL levels is even more important. True, the magnitude of the effect is smaller, since niacin typically boosts HDL levels by 10 to 30 percent. These HDL elevations, however, are extremely important because they're so hard to achieve with other medications. And they can often be achieved with somewhat lower doses of niacin, generally in the range of 500 to 1,500 milligrams per day.

Niacin and Atherosclerosis

It's one thing to improve blood cholesterol levels, another to prevent heart attacks and cardiac deaths. There is, of course, every reason to believe that treatments that achieve the former will produce the latter. It doesn't take long for studies to demonstrate that a drug can improve blood cholesterol levels, but it takes years to be sure it's also effective where it counts, in reducing heart attacks. Studies of the new prescription drugs are still in progress — but niacin has passed both tests.

The ultimate test of any technique used to conquer heart disease is its ability to help patients who already have the disease. How does niacin meet this test? The best evidence comes from the Coronary Drug Project, a major collaborative study involving 53 research centers throughout the United States. Beginning in 1966, 8,341 patients were recruited for the study; all were men between the ages of 30 and 64, all had suffered at least one prior heart attack, and most had high cholesterol levels (which were not subdivided into HDL and LDL fractions because the project was started before these tests were available). The volunteers were randomly assigned to receive 1 of 5 treatments or to serve as controls who took only placebos. Four of the 5 treatments were ineffective — or harmful — and were abandoned. Only niacin was able to reduce the rate of recurrent heart attacks in these patients with atherosclerosis. Most important, a final analysis performed after 15 years found that the benefits of niacin held up over the years; in all, the niacin-treated patients enjoyed an 11 percent reduction in total mortality compared with untreated patients. And, remarkably enough, a 1986 study reported that the protection was sustained even in men who had stopped taking niacin up to 9 years earlier.

Low cost and easy availability, dramatic improvements in both HDL and LDL cholesterols, protection against heart attacks and cardiac deaths — niacin sounds great. But before you rush out to get some, consider the disadvantages of this powerful drug.

The Toxicities of Niacin

Niacin is the least expensive cholesterol-lowering drug. It's as good as any for lowering LDL cholesterol and better than others for raising HDL levels. But it also has more side effects than the other cholesterol-lowering drugs.

Like most medications, the toxicities of niacin are dose-related, occurring most often in patients taking the most medication. Most of niacin's side effects don't do any lasting harm — but they are unpleasant enough to force many people to give up the drug. For example, a 1993 study in the *American Journal of Cardiology* reported that 27 percent of patients were unable to tolerate even moderate niacin doses of 1,500 milligrams per day, and a 1994 study in the *Journal of the American Medical Association* found that 59 percent of patients could not tolerate full doses of 3,000 milligrams per day. Most patients who abandon niacin do so because of flushing, itching, or headaches, by far the most common niacin side effects. Others have heartburn, nausea, or abdominal distress; these intestinal symptoms rank second among niacin's problems.

The obvious side effects of niacin disappear promptly when the drug is discontinued, leaving no residual damage. Patients can recognize these ill effects by themselves and can often learn to minimize them by adjusting the way they take niacin. More worrisome, though, are niacin's internal toxicities. They can be hard to recognize; although they are much less common, they can be much more serious than flushing, itching, and gastric distress.

Niacin can cause hepatitis. In most cases it's mild, showing up only in abnormal blood test results. But niacin-induced hepatitis can cause nausea, loss of appetite, and upper abdominal pain. If the drug is continued despite these warning symptoms, it can cause jaundice (yellow skin and eyes). And in a few cases, niacin-induced hepatitis can be very severe or even fatal.

Niacin can elevate blood sugar levels. In most cases, this will show up only in abnormal blood tests, but some patients develop symptoms of diabetes; most often, symptoms occur in patients who are known to have diabetes before starting niacin.

Niacin can cause peptic ulcers and even intestinal bleeding, particularly in patients who have preexisting gastritis or ulcers. The drug can also increase blood uric acid levels, sometimes resulting in attacks of gout. In other cases, niacin can lead to abnormal heart rhythm; fortunately, this is uncommon and is usually quite mild in any case. Finally, a skin condition called acanthosis nigricans has been reported as a complication of niacin.

Flushing, itching, hepatitis, diabetes, and ulcers — niacin sounds dreadful. But before you cross it off your list, consider ways the drug can be used safely.

Niacin Preparations

It's much easier to buy nonprescription drugs than to obtain prescriptions. Nonprescription drugs are often less expensive than prescription medicines. That's the good news about over-the-counter medications. The bad news is they're not subject to the same strict government standards that apply to prescription drugs. Niacin reflects both the good news and the bad news about nonprescription drugs.

Niacin is available in drug stores and health food stores and by mail and telephone. It's sold under a bewildering variety of names in a tremendous range of strengths. Niacin preparations vary enormously in price. Worst of all, niacin preparations are poorly standardized, so that two tablets of the same size may actually deliver different doses of the drug to a patient's body.

A few guidelines may help you through this quagmire.

Nicotinic acid is the form of niacin that improves blood cholesterol levels. If you choose to use niacin, get a preparation labeled as niacin or nicotinic acid, not nicotinamide, which is less effective.

Nicotinic acid comes in two major forms, regular (crystalline, rapid-release) and sustained release (SR, slow-release). Rapid-release forms of nicotinic acid are much more likely to cause immediate side effects such as flushing, itching, and headaches. Sustained-release preparations are much more pleasant to take; unfortunately, however, they are also much more likely to produce internal side effects, particularly hepatitis.

An exception may be a new wax-matrix sustained-release preparation (Endur-acin, and other brands); a 1991 study of 201 patients found that it was well tolerated and safe, but more data will be needed to confirm these hopeful results.

Niacin is sold under many generic and brand names. Generic preparations generally cost $5 to $10 a month, but some brand names cost well over $100 for a month's treatment, as much as prescription cholesterol-lowering medications. If you choose to use niacin, pick a generic brand sold by a reputable firm — and stick with that same preparation so you'll always be getting the same amount of drug.

Is Niacin Right for You?

Like so many other questions, this one can't be answered without exploring three other questions:

First, are you at risk for a heart attack? Review your blood cholesterol profile (Table 2–3): and your overall cardiac risk score (Table 2–11). If your cholesterol ratio is high — above 5.5 or 6 — *and* you have other major cardiac risk factors, you may be a candidate for niacin.

Second, can you correct your cholesterol profile and lower your risk score without medications? Although it doesn't require a prescription, niacin *is* a medication, and medications should be a last resort. Use diet, exercise, and all the other ways to fight atherosclerosis to their maximum. In most cases, they'll do the trick — but if you are the exception, consider niacin before prescription medications. And even if you decide to take niacin, remember you must also continue the other parts of your program.

Third, is niacin safe for you? If you have liver disease, diabetes, gout, or peptic ulcers, you shouldn't use niacin. Even without these problems, you'll have to use niacin carefully to use it safely. The key is appropriate monitoring for niacin's toxicities.

Despite my concern about its side effects, I believe in niacin as a medication to improve undesirable blood cholesterol levels, and I think it should be considered before more expensive prescription drugs. In fact, I've recommended niacin to hundreds of patients, more than I've placed on prescription drugs. Some of my patients have been unable to tolerate niacin in the doses they need because of headaches, flushing, or itching.

A much larger number have done very well and are enjoying improved LDL and HDL cholesterol results. But a few of my patients have had serious side effects, including intestinal bleeding severe enough to require transfusions, hepatitis serious enough to produce jaundice, and elevations of blood sugar high enough to produce symptomatic diabetes. Fortunately, all have recovered fully after stopping the drug, as have my patients with less-serious side effects such as gout, fluid accumulation, and sexual dysfunction.

Many of my patients have had better results with niacin than with prescription drugs, particularly with regard to their HDL levels. But they've also had more side effects. As a result, I monitor patients taking niacin every bit as carefully as I monitor patients taking prescription drugs.

First, monitor yourself. Itching, flushing, and headaches won't escape your attention. Because these side effects don't reflect any damage to your body, you can continue taking niacin even with these symptoms, if they're not too unpleasant. But you'll also have to monitor yourself for more subtle and serious side effects. Be alert for nausea, loss of appetite, upper abdominal distress, unexplained weight loss, and jaundice; they could indicate niacin-induced hepatitis. Watch for excessive thirst and urination, blurred vision, fatigue, and weight loss; they could reflect diabetes exacerbated by niacin. Check for dark, tarry stools and abdominal distress; they might be a sign of internal bleeding. And if you develop a painful, swollen joint, remember that it may be a symptom of niacin-induced gout.

If you note any worrisome symptoms, stop niacin immediately and report promptly to your doctor. Even without symptoms, though, you should consult your doctor for regular monitoring.

The second step you need to be sure niacin is safe is to ask for your doctor's help. Although niacin is a nonprescription drug, it should be taken every bit as seriously as prescription medication. That includes blood tests for hepatitis, gout, diabetes, and anemia. I generally obtain these tests 6 to 8 weeks after patients start taking niacin; I repeat them every 12 to 16 weeks during the first year of treatment, and every 16 to 24 weeks thereafter. I also recheck blood cholesterol levels with each test — it's the only way to be sure that niacin is both effective and safe.

Using Niacin

Niacin is a powerful medication. Use it only after you've exhausted non-medicinal remedies for your cholesterol problems, and then as a supplement to your diet and exercise program. Although you can obtain it on your own, treat niacin as a powerful medication. Always discuss it with your doctor before you take it, and ask for medical supervision of niacin treatment.

If you and your doctor agree niacin is right for you, use it the way that's most likely to work. Most doctors are far better at spotting niacin's side effects than they are in educating patients about its proper use. It's unfortunate, particularly since it reflects the profession's bias toward expensive prescription drugs, which require fewer instructions. Here are some tips for using niacin; if they work for you, share them with your doctor!

Start with an inexpensive generic form of regular (rapid-release, crystalline) nicotinic acid from a reliable source. Begin with 100 milligrams 3 times a day; take your niacin with meals, but never with hot beverages. Even if you have mild to moderate flushing or itching, try to stick it out for a while, since these side effects often diminish with time. You can also reduce these side effects by taking an aspirin tablet 30 minutes before the niacin; consider, though, how that will affect your low-dose aspirin program (Chapter 7).

Once you're comfortable at the starting level, begin to increase your niacin dose to therapeutic levels. Go slowly and gradually, nudging up your dose once a week by adding 100 milligrams to each of your 3 daily doses. If all goes well, you'll be taking 500 milligrams three times a day after 5 weeks; for greater convenience, you can switch to tablets of 250 or 500 milligrams at any time — as long as the niacin preparation remains unchanged. At a total dose of 1,500 milligrams a day you should start seeing some results — and you should start seeing your doctor to be sure niacin is safe and effective for you. Some people require 1,000 milligrams, 3 times a day; needless to say, you shouldn't attempt these doses without medical consultation and supervision.

If flushing, itching, headaches, or heartburn prevent you from adjusting to regular niacin, you can switch to SR (sustained-release) niacin. Try a wax-matrix preparation first. Use sustained-release niacin just as regular niacin, beginning with low doses and gradually building up to therapeutic levels. Always remember to listen to your body for symptoms of niacin toxicity, and be sure to have monitoring tests by your doctor.

It sounds complex — and it is. But niacin can be worth the trouble. It can be uniquely beneficial for your blood cholesterol profile without busting your budget, and it should be safe if it's used properly.

Is niacin a natural vitamin or a powerful drug? It's both. In the doses needed to improve cholesterol and fight atherosclerosis, niacin is a powerful drug. Use it as such: only if you need it, only as a supplement to a good lifestyle program, only with care, and only with medical supervision.

If you understand niacin and use it with respect, you'll respect its ability to help you conquer heart disease.

Chapter 13

Chromium and Other Metals: Can You Steel Yourself Against Heart Disease?

NUTRITION is a major determinant of human health. When it comes to diet and atherosclerosis, cholesterol has gotten all the blame, but fat is finally getting the attention it deserves. Your 15-point plan to fight atherosclerosis goes beyond cholesterol and fat, enlisting fiber, fish, vitamins, and minerals in its nutritional program. Now it's time to consider dietary metals; although they're generally lumped together as trace nutrients, they can have a major impact on health.

To keep you healthy, your diet should contain at least 15 mineral compounds. Most are required in only tiny amounts; because a balanced diet provides more than enough of them, you don't have to think about most trace nutrients. But some minerals can affect your cardiovascular system. Chapter 6 discusses four well-known minerals that affect your blood pressure. In addition, four little-known metals may have a role in atherosclerosis; they merit your attention, even though the data about them ranges from scant to very scant.

Chromium

It's not your car bumper that makes chromium important — it's your heart. Instead of bashing chromium as a shiny emblem of the industrialization that has created atherosclerosis, I'd like you to think about this trace nutrient as a way to help conquer heart disease.

Unfortunately, doctors haven't given chromium much more thought than you have. But the data are intriguing, if preliminary. They suggest that chromium supplements may help raise HDL cholesterol levels. Doctors are not very successful at improving HDL levels with prescription medications. You can do much better with exercise, weight loss, and smoking cessation; in the right circumstances supplementary alcohol (Chapter 9) and niacin (Chapter 12) can help — as can chromium.

What Is Chromium?

Nutritionists agree that chromium is a trace metal that is vital to human health; they're not sure, however, exactly what chromium does in the body or how much is needed to maintain health.

It is clear that chromium is important for normal metabolic functions, particularly for carbohydrate metabolism. In experimental animals, chromium deficiencies can provoke diabetes. In humans, too, chromium plays a significant role in regulating blood sugar; that's why an important organic form of chromium is called "glucose tolerance factor" (GTF). Small trials of supplementary chromium, however, have not proved beneficial in the treatment of human diabetes.

A Recommended Daily Allowance has not been established for chromium. Still, the Food and Nutrition Board of the National Academy of Sciences suggests a daily intake of 50 to 200 micrograms. By this standard, 50 to 90 percent of Americans are not getting enough chromium in their diets.

Although trace amounts of chromium are present in many foods, the best dietary source is brewers yeast, which contains chromium in the form of GTF (glucose tolerance factor). Other good sources of chromium include peanuts, legumes, and whole grains; various meats and cheeses can also provide chromium, but their high fat content outweighs their value as a source of trace nutrients.

Chromium and Atherosclerosis

Chromium's role in glucose metabolism and diabetes wasn't suspected until 1959; its role in cholesterol metabolism and atherosclerosis is just now being explored.

Appropriately enough, the first studies of chromium and atherosclerosis utilized animal models. Chromium deficiency increases the blood cholesterol levels of rats, and chromium supplements bring the cholesterol values back down. More impressively, some rats actually develop fatty plaques of atherosclerosis in their arteries as a result of chromium deficiency.

Impressive or not, studies in rodents don't necessarily apply to humans. In the case of chromium, though, the animal data may pertain to human cholesterol and atherosclerosis even better than to blood sugar and diabetes.

Between 1968 and 1982 at least 6 independent trials investigated the effects of chromium supplements on blood cholesterol levels in healthy volunteers. Some of the human subjects had normal cholesterol levels, while others had abnormally high levels. Some of the studies administered yeast, others used GTF, still others prescribed supplements of inorganic chromium salts. Despite these differences in study design, chromium supplements appeared to produce small reductions in serum cholesterol levels; much more important, though, HDL levels rose by an average of 10 percent.

A 1978 study looked at the chromium question from another viewpoint. It checked blood chromium levels in patients undergoing coronary angiograms and found that low chromium levels could account for 17 percent of their atherosclerotic lesions, even after considering cholesterol and other cardiac risk factors.

Despite these clues, chromium received little medical attention for the next 10 years. Only a handful of nutritionists and physicians recommended chromium supplements during the 1980s. I was not among them; because most of the early trials were small and incompletely controlled, I elected to wait for further studies.

The study that has begun to change my mind was published in 1991 in the *Annals of Internal Medicine.* Dr. John Roeback and his colleagues studied 63 men in North Carolina. All had hypertension and were taking beta-blockers, prescription drugs that have the unfortunate side effects of lowering HDL and raising LDL cholesterol levels. Half the volunteers were randomly assigned to receive chromium, while the others took a placebo. The chromium and dummy pills were identical in appearance and taste; in this beautifully designed experiment, neither the patients nor the doctors knew which group got the real chromium until the study was completed.

Complete cholesterol profiles were obtained at the start of the trial and after 2 months of treatment. The results were significant: chromium supplements boosted HDL cholesterol levels by an average of nearly 6 points, a 16 percent increase. No changes occurred in total cholesterol, triglycerides, or body weight. All the subjects were carefully monitored for side effects; none were observed.

A 16 percent increase in HDL may not seem like much — until you've tried to raise your own HDL levels. It can be hard to do, but it's very important. A 6-point increase in HDL, which was achieved in the chromium trial, should reduce the risk of heart attack by about 20 percent.

More studies will be needed to extend these observations to people who are not taking beta-blockers and to women. It will be important to study chromium in larger groups and to continue treatment for longer periods. It will also be important to test various chromium preparations and dosages.

It's clear that more information will be needed before chromium can be recommended to everyone. But it will take years to accumulate these data. Atherosclerosis won't wait. In this relentless disease, HDL plays an important protective role, but it can be very hard to boost HDL levels in some people. Chromium is a natural product, a vital nutrient that is lacking in the majority of Americans' diets. At about $5 a month, it's inexpensive, and it appears to be very safe. All in all, chromium merits serious consideration as a nonprescription supplement to fight atherosclerosis; it's not for everyone, but it may help the very people who need help the most.

Is Chromium Right for You?

To decide if chromium supplements are right for you, simply test your mettle. Return to your overall cardiac risk score (Table 2–11); if it's moderate to high, consider an additional factor: your HDL cholesterol. If your HDL is below 35 or even 40, you should try to raise it. Exercise, maintenance of ideal body weight, and smoking cessation should be part of everyone's plan. But if these critical changes don't bring your HDL up to protective levels, consider the three supplements that raise HDL — alcohol (Chapter 9), niacin (Chapter 12), and chromium. Of the three, we know the least about chromium — but we do know it's the least toxic and least expensive of the three.

Chromium is available without prescription in pharmacies; you can also find it in health food stores and mail order catalogues. Many preparations are available. I generally recommend glucose tolerance factor because it's been studied best. The usual dose is 200 micrograms 3 times a day; this dose will provide about three times more chromium than is contained in an ideal diet, but it appears to be extremely safe.

If you decide to try chromium, remember that it's a supplement to your diet, not a substitute for the other ways to fight atherosclerosis. Continue your full program, then recheck your HDL after several months of chromium; I hope you'll find it's helping to keep your arteries shiny and smooth.

Iron

The iron story began with a bang in September 1992, when the respected journal *Circulation* reported that a high level of iron in the blood was an important heart attack risk factor. The study raised great concern because it was entirely new. Until then, iron was not considered a cause of atherosclerosis; many physicians, in fact, recommended iron supplements to their patients.

Iron is a vital nutrient; it's an essential component of hemoglobin, the oxygen-carrying pigment in red blood cells. Although Americans have a lot of heart disease, they're often low in iron; iron deficiency, in fact, is the most common cause of anemia in the United States.

Iron deficiency is particularly common in women, who lose red blood cells with each menstrual period; smaller amounts of iron are also lost through the skin and intestinal tract in both men and women. To replace these losses, women should consume 15 milligrams of iron daily; for men, 10 milligrams is enough to prevent anemia.

The best dietary source of iron is red meat — hardly the best food for the heart. Iron is also present in deep green vegetables, legumes, and certain fish. Even so, American women get only two-thirds of the iron they need from their diet. To correct this, the food industry has been adding iron to grain products for more than 50 years; iron is the supplement that gives baked goods the designation "fortified." In addition, physicians often recommend iron tablets to women who are menstruating, pregnant, or lactating. Beans and greens notwithstanding, vegetarians are also candidates for iron supplements.

We've been adding iron to our food and promoting nonprescription iron supplements for years. Suddenly in 1992 it appeared that iron may increase the risk of heart attacks. Have we been inadvertently contributing to the atherosclerosis epidemic? Let's take a closer look.

The study that raised the alarm was performed in Finland, where 1,931 middle-aged men were observed for an average of 3 years. Serum iron levels were measured in each man, and each was asked to provide a detailed dietary history. In this careful study, all the conventional cardiac risk factors were also evaluated. When the results were tallied, iron was strongly associated with the risk of heart attack. The men with the highest blood iron levels were 2.2 times more likely to suffer heart attacks than men with low blood iron. Dietary iron was also a risk factor; each milligram of iron in the daily diet increased heart attack risk by 5 percent. The association between iron and heart attack persisted even after other risk factors were considered; in fact, iron was second only to smoking as a risk factor.

Although the Finnish study was the first to implicate iron, it caused great concern because it was biologically plausible: iron promotes the formation of free radicals, which can oxidize LDL cholesterol, thus promoting atherosclerosis. And so the speculation began. Women, long-distance runners, and vegetarians all tend to have low iron levels and less heart disease — is low iron the protective factor? Should we stop administering iron supplements, accepting anemia as a lesser evil than atherosclerosis? The *New York Times* even wondered if the leeches used by medieval physicians to remove blood from patients might have been therapeutically useful after all.

Despite all this speculation, experts called for more studies before abandoning the use of iron supplements. Although the Finnish study was conducted carefully, it studied a unique population: men in eastern Finland have the highest incidence of heart disease in the world.

The results of four American studies became available in 1993. One study evaluated the body iron stores of 22,071 men in the U.S. Physicians' Health Study. Another evaluated dietary iron intake in 45,720 male health professionals. The third study checked blood iron levels in 14,916 men, and the fourth monitored iron levels in 171 men and 406 women older than 62. A 1994 study evaluated body iron stores in 4,518 Americans who had been tracked for over 20 years. All five American studies exonerated iron; no link was found between heart attacks and dietary iron intake, blood iron levels, or body iron stores. And, returning to the other side of the Atlantic, a 1994 study from Iceland found no link between iron levels and heart attacks in 2,036 people who were observed for more than 8 years.

What's a person to do in the face of these contradictory results? The easy answer is that if you're in Finland, stop taking iron supplements, but if you're an American, it's okay to keep pumping up your blood iron. Facile or not, it's the best answer we have at present. Until more studies iron out the uncertainties, it seems reasonable to go on taking iron, but only if it's really needed to prevent anemia.

There is another lesson to be learned from the debate about iron: don't panic every time you hear about a new risk factor. Ever hungry for headlines, the media tend to dramatize medical data, dividing complex issues into black-and-white categories of "new hope" or "no hope." Look behind the sound bites; for example, keep the short-lived concern generated by the 1992 Finnish iron study in mind when you evaluate the 1994 Finnish study of beta-carotene and lung cancer in smokers (Chapter 11). Before you change your lifestyle, get more facts. Here's how to proceed:

Find out if you are similar to the population in the study. There are differences between men and women, youngsters and older adults, Finns and Americans. Pay greatest attention to the studies that are most relevant to you and your family.

Find out if the study was large or small, brief or long-term. In general, large, long-term studies warrant more attention.

Find out the magnitude of the purported risk. You shouldn't dismiss anything that increases your risk of atherosclerosis, but weak associations are clearly less worrisome than potent ones.

Find out if the association makes sense and if it fits with previous observations of humans and animals. The iron story was unprecedented when it surfaced in 1992, which should have encouraged skepticism — but it was biologically reasonable, which helped justify concern.

Find out if the risk factor is correctable, but don't make drastic changes in your lifestyle until you're sure they're warranted. Even then, consider the effort, cost, sacrifice, and potential hazards of any change before you take the plunge.

It can be hard to get all these facts from your daily newspaper, much less a TV sound bite. Take your time and collect all the information you need. The Appendix lists excellent sources for additional information — and your doctor should also be willing and able to offer balanced advice about new developments in atherosclerosis research.

Copper

Another trace metal, another trace of data.

Copper plays an important role in human metabolism and in the formation of red blood cells. It only takes one and a half to 3 milligrams of copper per day to fulfill these needs. Most Americans get more than enough copper from cereals, barley, legumes, nuts, shellfish, and meats.

Might we be getting too much of a good thing? Studies from 1991 and 1992 reported an association between high blood copper levels and heart attacks. The association was strong; the highest copper levels were linked to a 4-fold increase in heart attacks. The link is reasonable; copper can promote oxidation of LDL cholesterol. But the only subjects in both studies were Finnish men.

We'll need more data to determine whether copper can contribute to atherosclerosis. It's an interesting question, but since copper is not used as a dietary supplement, we can wait patiently for the answer.

Selenium

Selenium is sold without prescription in various dietary supplements. Can it help fight atherosclerosis?

Perhaps.

Selenium is intriguing because it functions as an antioxidant; it may help prevent oxygen free radicals from damaging cells and from oxidizing LDL cholesterol. For men, the Recommended Daily Allowance for selenium is 70 micrograms, for women it's 55 micrograms. Selenium is provided by many foods including tomatoes, poultry, shellfish, garlic, meat, and egg yolks.

A 1982 study of 11,000 men and women found that people with low blood selenium levels had an increased risk of developing coronary artery disease. After accounting for other risk factors, 22 percent of the heart attack deaths in this population were attributed to low selenium levels; as you might have suspected, the study population was in Finland. And a 1991 study of Finnish men linked low selenium levels to atherosclerosis of the carotid arteries.

These reports are interesting enough to warrant additional studies, possibly including a trial of selenium supplements. Until more data becomes available, though, it's far too early to recommend selenium pills. Despite its potential role as an antioxidant, selenium is still just a glimmer on the horizon.

Chapter 14

Stress Control: Winding Down for a Happy Heart

AT ONE TIME or another, all of us have experienced a pounding heart or racing pulse brought on by stress, fear, or excitement. Most of us have lived through the heartache of loss or loneliness. And we've all heard of heart attacks triggered by strong emotions and of people who were literally frightened to death. Each of these events makes it clear that there is a powerful link between the mind and the body, the heart and the soul.

Psychological stress can strain your heart, and mental depression can be heartbreaking — if you let negative emotions get the upper hand. But if you learn to control stress and counter depression, you'll enjoy the benefits of a happy heart in a healthy body.

The Stress Response

Species survive by adapting to their environments, both friendly and hostile. Over millions of years, evolution has equipped human beings with an intricate set of responses that promote survival during stress.

Stress produces a state of arousal involving the whole body. The mind becomes more alert and vigilant. The pupils dilate, improving vision in dim light. Breathing speeds up and the bronchial tubes widen to admit more oxygen. The heart beats faster and pumps more blood with each beat, and the blood pressure rises. Arteries that carry blood to the intestines narrow, slowing the digestive process. Circulation to the skin also diminishes, making the skin feel cool and clammy. At the same time, arteries carrying blood to the muscles widen, so muscles will have all the oxygen they need for maximal effort. Muscles become tense and taut, ready to spring into action on a moment's notice.

The body's metabolic machinery is also dramatically activated by stress. At the very first sign of danger, adrenaline surges. Cortisone, another stress hormone, also pours into the bloodstream. In contrast, blood insulin falls and blood sugar rises, providing instant energy for the brain, heart, and muscles. Even the blood itself is changed by stress, as the clotting system is activated, readying it to staunch any wound.

Although it's a fundamental part of human nature, the stress response wasn't understood until the early years of the twentieth century, when the pioneering studies of Dr. Walter Cannon demonstrated that the nervous system, the heart and circulation, the metabolism and endocrine glands, and the blood itself all play a part in the body's carefully orchestrated response to stress.

Dr. Cannon characterized the stress response as the "fight or flight reaction," understanding it to be a rapid call to action that would quickly revert to normal when the stress subsided. Another scientific giant, Dr. Hans Selye, took the story one step farther by studying the effects of repeated or persistent stress. Dr. Selye found that prolonged stress can actually deplete the body's coping mechanisms: arousal turns to exhaustion, vigilance to impaired concentration, metabolic mobilization to abnormal eating patterns and disordered blood chemistries, and endocrine enhancement to reproductive dysfunction. In everyday terms, the transition from Cannon's state of arousal to Selye's state of exhaustion is proof that when it comes to the body's stress response, there can indeed be too much of a good thing.

Stress control does not mean eliminating all stress; instead it involves preventing *excessive* arousal, which can lead to dysfunction and disease. And stress control also requires restricting arousal to circumstances in which it's appropriate and beneficial.

Changing circumstances, in fact, explain why the stress response is so often inappropriate and harmful. The fight or flight response evolved in the days of the saber-toothed tiger, when physical survival was a very real issue. But in the modern world, our major challenges are not physical but mental. Human physiology has not changed, but the world around us has; the stress response that served humanity so well in the forest can be a disservice in the corporate boardroom, to say nothing of rush-hour traffic or supermarket check-out lines.

In biological terms, the stress response is an intricate series of reflexes that have survived intact since primitive times. Even today, the stress response can be helpful. It's essential to achieve peak athletic perfor-mance and to survive accidents and physical threats. A state of height-ened alertness and energy can also help people rise to the mental challenge of a big exam or an important presentation. But when the stress reaction spills over into everyday life, it becomes harmful. The fight or flight response is not designed for life in the fast lane. It's all too easy for arousal to become anxiety; is it any wonder that the modern era is called the age of anxiety?

The Response to Loss

If arousal is the response to stress, withdrawal is the response to loss.

Medical science has done a better job of unraveling the puzzle of stress than of illuminating the physiology of withdrawal. But even if we don't understand the neurology and chemistry of withdrawal, we can chart its effects on human health and happiness. At times, those effects can be heartbreaking.

In arousal, the body's processes speed up; in withdrawal, they slow down. Physical energy is sapped, replaced by lethargy and fatigue. Men-tal vigor also drains away, with only apathy and torpor to fill the void. Sleep is disturbed; in some people the result is excessive somnolence, in others it's insomnia. Appetite, too, can increase or decrease in response to loss; the subsequent weight gain or loss can be unwanted but uncon-trollable. Among the many bodily activities that slow down are sexual performance and bowel function.

The heart, circulation, and metabolism are all stimulated by stress but all function normally during the withdrawal reaction. Still, just as unrelieved stress accelerates atherosclerosis, prolonged withdrawal can lead to heart disease. And even if the heart and blood vessels seem nor-mal, life is not.

People who experience loss can't concentrate normally. They lose interest in the world around them, often becoming preoccupied with the minutiae of their bodily functions. At the same time, they neglect their appearance and grooming. Relationships suffer, producing social isolation. If unchecked, social isolation can increase the risk of heart disease and premature death.

All people experience loss and disappointment, such as defeats in sports, setbacks at work, bodily illnesses, broken relationships, and the deaths of friends and relatives. Understandably, all people feel sad and "down" from time to time, and most go through periods of bereavement and mourning. But if normal sorrow dominates everyday life, if it's triggered by inner thoughts rather than real losses, or if it persists excessively, it can develop into clinical depression.

The prototype of anxiety is fear, of depression, grief. Arousal and withdrawal are physiologically and psychologically normal; they are universal, but temporary, parts of the human condition. In contrast, anxiety and depression are abnormal, exaggerated, and prolonged. They make life difficult and unhappy. Even worse, they can lead to diseases that can shorten life itself. But both the stress reaction and the response to loss can be controlled. The rewards include a healthy heart and a successful life.

Heartfelt Emotions

People often think of the mind and the body as separate and distinct. Doctors often classify ailments as either "physical" or "mental." These divisions, however, are arbitrary and misleading. In fact, the mind and the body are inseparable aspects of each human being. And the fundamental unity of mind and body is nowhere more evident than in the interactions between emotions and the heart.

How the Heart Affects the Mind
Heart disease can certainly affect mental function. At one extreme, patients suffering through angina or heart attacks often experience apprehension, intense anxiety, or even a profound sense of foreboding and doom. At the other extreme, patients with congestive heart failure are often depressed and lethargic; in advanced cases, they may be somnolent or groggy.

How the Mind Affects the Heart
The link between the heart and the mind works in both directions: emotions can also influence the cardiovascular system. Those effects in-

clude abrupt, minute-to-minute changes in cardiovascular function as well as more subtle long-term influences that can eventually lead to atherosclerosis.

The *immediate effects* are easier to measure; doctors can take subjects to a lab and hook them up to monitors that will reveal how stress affects cardiovascular function. In both healthy people and heart patients, the effects are profound indeed.

Stress raises blood pressure. It doesn't take a wailing siren or midnight telegram to pump up your blood pressure; even the gentle stress of an arithmetic problem will cause nearly everyone's pressure to rise. Add a little embarrassment and blood pressure soars; healthy, well-adjusted volunteers who are given an insolvable puzzle with the casual assurance that an average 5-year-old can solve it in two minutes will develop extreme hypertension before the test is half over. Interestingly, a 1993 study found that subjects who were accompanied by a supportive friend developed less-severe hypertension during mental stress than did people who were alone. And another 1993 study reported that mental stress makes the blood itself more concentrated, or "thicker," perhaps making it harder for the heart to pump blood through vessels narrowed by adrenaline.

Stress can alter the heart's pumping rhythm. Whenever stress raises the blood pressure, it also speeds the pulse. The reason is simple: the rising pressure and racing heart are both caused by a stress-induced surge of adrenaline. A racing heart is one thing, a heart that misfires, quite another. And stress can quite literally cause the heart to skip a beat, to experience disordered pumping rhythms called arrhythmias. Most arrhythmias are not harmful, but sometimes, particularly in patients with heart disease, they can lead to an abnormally low blood pressure, a loss of consciousness, or even sudden death. In some people even "good" stress, such as the excitement of watching a close basketball game, can provoke unpleasant or dangerous disturbances of the cardiac rhythm.

Stress causes healthy hearts to pump stronger as well as faster. But in patients with heart disease, stress can have the opposite effect, reducing the heart's pumping ability. A 1991 study from Italy, for example, found that mental arithmetic reduced pumping function in 22 patients with coronary artery disease; 2 subjects actually developed pulmonary edema (fluid in the lungs) during the experiment. And in the same year, an American study of 27 heart patients found that simply recalling an episode of anger reduced heart function by more than 5 percent. On both sides of the Atlantic, mental stress was much more likely to impair these patients' heart function than was the physical stress of hard exercise; a 1993 study explains why: intense anger can produce coronary artery spasm, narrowing arteries and reducing the flow of blood to the heart muscle.

I'm happy to report that all the patients who volunteered for these studies recovered from their experimental stress without difficulty. Patients with heart disease are not always so fortunate. Indeed, mental stress can trigger angina, heart attacks, and even sudden death. Not surprisingly, the patients with the sickest hearts are the most vulnerable to these stress-induced calamities. But even people with healthy hearts can be scared to death. It's rare, but well documented: people with very strong beliefs can actually die from mental stress in so-called voodoo deaths. The converse is also true; the will to live can actually prolong life. Death rates among observant Jews drop before important festivals such as Passover, only to rise afterward. The same phenomenon occurs in Chinese before and after the symbolically important Harvest Moon Festival.

The *long-term effects* of emotions on the heart and circulation are harder to quantify than are the short-term effects — but they're just as real and just as important. The great physician Sir William Osler observed that "in the worry and strain of modern life, arterial degeneration is not only very common but develops often at a relatively early age." Osler penned these words in 1897; in the century that's followed, life has become much more stressful — and atherosclerosis has become much, much more common.

Contrary to popular belief, stress does not appear to raise cholesterol levels. But stress certainly alters the body's metabolism; among other things, the surge of adrenaline that accompanies stress causes the liver to break down stored fat, releasing free fatty acids into the blood, where they can serve as an emergency source of energy. Studies in the 1960s suggested that cholesterol levels might also rise as a result of stress; in these early observations, people living through the stress of natural disasters, job losses, and academic examinations appeared to have higher blood cholesterol levels, as did accountants during tax season. But even in those early days, studies found that patients suffering the stress of heart attacks had falling cholesterol levels (only temporarily, alas). And recent, more exacting studies have failed to link mental stress to altered blood cholesterol levels. So if your cholesterol is high, blame your diet, your waistline, your lack of exercise, or your genes — but not your boss or your mother-in-law.

If stress does not raise cholesterol levels, how can it contribute to atherosclerosis? Remember that atherosclerosis and heart attacks occur in three stages. Although stress does not appear to alter the first stage, the blood cholesterol, it can influence the second and third stages by affecting events in the arterial wall and the blood clotting system.

High blood pressure damages arterial walls, accelerating the vascular injury leading to fatty plaques, then narrowed, and finally blocked, vessels. And stress puts the tension in hypertension. It's been clear for decades that stress raises blood pressure; even the act of having a checkup can raise pressure ("white coat hypertension"). But these well-documented stress-induced jumps in blood pressure are only temporary, and they're much less harmful than sustained hypertension. In contrast, medical studies couldn't confirm the commonsense observation that stress increases the risk of sustained hypertension — until 1993, when the Framingham Heart Study released the results of a long-term study of 1,123 people. The subjects were middle-aged people with normal blood pressure readings. At the start of the trial, all were checked for psychological factors as well as the usual hypertension risk factors (obesity, diet, exercise, alcohol use, smoking, and family history). After 18 to 20 years, all these factors were reevaluated. The result: the men with the highest levels of anxiety and anger had an increased risk of developing sustained hypertension, even after taking the other variables into account. So even if you can't blame your job for your high cholesterol, you may be able to implicate it in your high blood pressure.

The final event causing most heart attacks is the formation of a blood clot on the surface of a fatty plaque. The clot transforms a partial blockage into a complete occlusion, and stress can activate the clotting system. The culprit is adrenaline. Adrenaline activates platelets, the tiny blood cells that initiate the clotting process. The effects of stress on platelets are brief — but it doesn't take long to form the clots that cause heart attacks.

Mental factors are important for their direct impact on atherosclerosis, but they can be even more important for their indirect effects. The mediator is not adrenaline, but human behavior. It's hard to take good care of your heart when you're tensed up or bummed out. People who are tense or depressed often seek solace in smoking, drinking, or eating rich foods; they won't find solace, but they often find illness. People who are upset often stop exercising and gain weight. In turn, their guilt and falling self-esteem lead to more mental stress, then more bodily self-abuse. But the cycle can be interrupted. In fact, taking good care of your heart and your health is also the best way to care for your psyche; the unity of mind and body can promote health instead of illness.

Stress, Anxiety, and Heart Attacks

If stress can lead to heart attacks, the most high-powered people should be at greatest risk. They are.

The first major study linking personality to coronary heart disease was published in 1959. Working in California, Doctors Meyer Friedman and Ray Rosenman found that certain high-powered individuals were extraordinarily susceptible to heart attacks. Even if you've never visited a coronary care unit, you have probably encountered this personality type. In fact, because "Type A" people are often very effective and successful, you may have hired one to be your attorney or accountant but you probably wouldn't be happy working for one. Type A people work long hours and accomplish a great deal, but they are not simply workaholics. Instead, they carry goal-oriented behaviors to extremes, tending to be perfectionistic, competitive, and demanding. Type A people are rushed and impatient, often responding to frustration or delay with bursts of hostility and anger. Typical Type A individuals walk quickly with short, choppy strides. They talk quickly, often conveying their "short fuses" through taut facial expressions, rapid breathing, and staccato speech. Always rushing from task to task, Type A people don't sit down for long, but when they do take a chair, they're restless and fidgety.

Ambition, conscientiousness, responsibility, and hard work are admirable traits, essential for success. Hard work does not cause heart attacks. But Type A people are more than hard workers. They are tense and driven, victims of the "hurry sickness" that affects so many people living in the fast lane of the modern world. Like it or not, Type A people often find their busy schedules ruined by an unplanned hospital stay.

Doctors Friedman and Rosenman found that Type A personality traits increase the risk of heart attacks by 300 percent. Although their work was careful and their findings impressive, their results have been controversial. Some investigators have corroborated the importance of the Type A personality, but others have failed to confirm that these traits triple the risk of heart attacks. Part of the difficulty stems from the fact that the Type A personality was originally described in very specific ways and was diagnosed with a highly structured interview requiring experienced investigators. Recent studies have examined the question more broadly, exploring the effects of hostility, anger, and tension on coronary risk instead of concentrating on just one personality profile. Studies using these new standards have confirmed the basic observation that stress is bad for the heart. A few examples:

A 1983 study from Duke University traced the incidence of heart attacks in physicians, all of whom were initially healthy. During a span of 25 years, the most hostile men had 5 times more heart attacks that did their docile peers. Nor are doctors unique in their heartbreaking behavior; a later study reported similar findings in male lawyers.

In 1989, the Multiple Risk Factor Intervention Trial (MR. FIT) confirmed the role of hostility, associating it with a two-fold increase in the rate of heart attacks in middle-aged men. And a 1993 study from Denmark found that men who could not relax after work suffered an increased rate of heart disease.

Although most studies of hostility, tension, and heart disease focus on men, women are also vulnerable to stress. In the 1980s, studies from North Carolina and Florida compared the results of psychological tests with the findings of coronary angiograms; in both men and women, hostility was linked to the severity of atherosclerosis. After observing women for 20 years, the famed Framingham Heart Study reported in 1993 that mental tension was significantly linked to coronary heart disease even after other cardiac risk factors were taken into account. And in 1994, a study of 501 women and 1,122 men who had heart attacks found that intense anger doubles the risk of having an attack during a 2-hour span following the anger.

Not all authorities agree on the role of stress, and the details do differ from study to study. Fine print notwithstanding, the big picture is clear: stress, anger, hostility, and tension contribute to heart disease.

Isolation, Depression, and Heart Attacks
Often overlooked in the rush to understand how stress affects the heart, isolation and depression are now emerging as cardiac risk factors in

their own right. If the overstressed heart is at risk, the lonely heart is also vulnerable, perhaps even more vulnerable.

Depression has been linked to atherosclerosis. A 1993 California study administered personality tests to 1,100 men who also underwent medical exams, including ultrasounds that measured atherosclerotic thickening of their carotid arteries. Depressed men had more atherosclerosis; in addition, depression tripled the harmful impact of smoking and doubled the damage caused by high cholesterol levels.

Depression has been linked to fatal arrhythmias. A 1990 report in the *American Journal of Cardiology* evaluated personality profiles in 342 patients with coronary artery disease and abnormal heart pumping rhythms. The patients were followed for a year; the risk of cardiac arrest was higher in patients who were depressed and withdrawn at the start of the study, even after taking other variables into account.

Depression has been linked to first heart attacks. The National Health Examination Follow-up Study performed personality tests on 2,832 men and women aged 45 to 77 who were free of diagnosed heart disease. The people were followed for more than 12 years. Even after taking other risk factors into account, mild to moderate depression was associated with a 50 percent increase in fatal heart disease, and severe depression was associated with a 100 percent increase.

Most impressive of all is the link between depression, social isolation, and reduced survival in heart attack patients. During the past 10 years, at least 5 major studies have performed detailed psychosocial and medical evaluations on patients hospitalized with heart attacks. In each study, the patients were observed for 6 months or longer to see which psychological and medical factors could best predict outcome. In each study, depression and social isolation were associated with decreased survival rates. The results were striking: patients who were depressed or socially isolated were between 2 and 5 times more likely to die of heart disease during the 6 to 12 months after their first attack. In fact, depression and isolation were linked to mortality every bit as strongly as congestive heart failure.

Death is, of course, the very worst possible consequence of a heart attack. But even in heart attack survivors, depression takes a toll. A 1994 study of heart attack patients who survived 6 months found that the patients who were the most depressed at the time of their attacks were 3 times more likely to have angina after 6 months than patients without depression. Depressed survivors were also much more likely to be disabled and out of work.

Social Networks and Longevity

It's not clear why the lonely heart is so likely to become a broken heart. But even if the mechanisms are not fully understood, it's quite clear that social support networks are good for the heart. Examples of the power of relationships can be found in diverse communities from around the world. Some examples: A landmark study from the 1960s evaluated nearly 7,000 adults in Alameda County, California. This 9-year investigation by Doctors Lisa Beckman and Leonard Syme identified one factor that increased the risk of dying during the study period by 2.8 in women and 2.3 in men. This crucial risk factor is not smoking, nor is it drinking, sloth, or nutritional neglect. Instead, the risk factor is social isolation; people with the fewest social ties had the greatest risk of dying from heart disease, circulatory ailments, and even cancer.

Another long-term American study underscores the point. In 1962, Doctors Stewart Wolf and John Bruhn began observing the residents of two neighboring towns in rural Pennsylvania. The townsfolk of Bangor and Roseto were similarly inclined to smoke, eat fatty foods, and shun aerobic exercise. Despite these similarities, the people of Roseto proved to be stronghearted, suffering many fewer heart attacks. The major difference between the towns was their social structure: Roseto was a cohesive community of Italian immigrants who lived in large extended families, sharing a strong sense of community, fervent religious beliefs, and common values. For better or worse, Roseto became Americanized in the 1970s. Prosperity brought many blessings, but health was not one of them. As Rosetians gained in education and wealth, they became more materialistic, competitive, and individualistic — and their heart attack rate rose just when the rate was falling in most of America. Losing "the power of clan," the people of Roseto fell victim to the quintessential American epidemic, atherosclerosis; losing their social supports, they lost heart.

Much the same thing happened to Japanese-Americans in California. A 1976 study evaluated 3,809 members of this community in San Francisco. Japanese-Americans who retained traditional cultural, religious, and family attitudes had only 20 percent as many heart attacks as their Americanized counterparts. True, the Western diet was much higher in saturated fat and cholesterol and lower in fish and fiber — but even accounting for these factors, social support networks appeared to exert substantial protection against heart disease.

The latest study, a 1993 report in the *British Medical Journal*, reminds us that support networks are just as important in Europe as in California and Pennsylvania. Physical and psychological tests were administered to a random sample of 50-year-old men in Göteborg, Sweden. During the next 7 years, 11 percent of the socially isolated men died, but only 3 percent of the well-connected men succumbed.

The most important support system is a good marriage. A 1990 study from Princeton University found that unmarried men have twice the mortality rate of married men; for unmarried women, the death rate was one and a half times that of married women. We know, too, from earlier studies that widows and widowers are more likely to die in their first year of bereavement than are men and women of the same age who have not experienced the loss of a spouse. Divorce also substantially increases the rate of illness during the first year of separation.

People are good medicine — but animals may be, too. Among 5,741 people who were studied in Australia, pet owners had better blood pressure and lipid profiles than did nonowners; these differences could not be explained by differences in smoking or exercise habits, age, body fat distribution, or socioeconomic status. It didn't take a lionhearted pet to do the trick; even owning a bird seemed to help. More study will be needed to see if the animal fanciers' improved risk profiles translate into actual clinical benefit. Let's hope that future research finds that our four-legged friends are truly heart-saving.

Lots of new research will be required to develop a full picture of how emotions affect the cardiovascular system. Since only half the heart disease in America can be fully attributed to conventional "physical" risk factors, there is clearly a pressing need for such research.

Emotions and Health

Emotions are heartfelt — but they are felt by other parts of the body, too. In view of the unity of mind and body, it's no surprise that psychological factors influence nearly every aspect of human health.

Emotional disturbances contribute to many diseases. One example is the nervous system itself; stress can trigger migraines, tension headaches, neck pain, and tremors. In the respiratory tract, strong emotions can precipitate asthma, a common, potentially life-threatening illness. Worry and stress are well-known contributors to gastrointestinal problems ranging from gastritis to ulcers, diarrhea, and irritable bowel syndrome. The reproductive system is also vulnerable; anxiety and depression are important causes of male erectile dysfunction and female menstrual disorders.

Among the endocrine diseases, hyperthyroidism stands out as a chemical imbalance that can be triggered by emotional stimuli. Much more common is the low back pain that is often exacerbated by mental tension and muscle tension. Deep emotions are frequently to blame for surface blemishes, as stress causes itching, hives, and other skin rashes. Much less obvious but potentially more important are subtle stress-induced changes in the immune system that might alter the body's ability to ward off infections or even cancer.

Psychosomatic illnesses are common and important, but psychosomatic symptoms are even more prevalent. At least half of all visits to doctors' offices are motivated by complaints that turn out to be "functional" or "mental." It's frustrating for patients and doctors alike, but it's important to remember that the physical distress caused by emotional factors is every bit as "real" as the pain of clearly defined physical ailments. Emotional forces can make people feel and act just as sick as if they had physical illnesses.

Not to be overlooked is the enormous burden of suffering caused by emotional illness itself. A 1994 study found that 48 percent of all Americans experience mental illness at some time in their lives, and 30 percent are affected during any one year. Although many of these problems are mild, the National Institute of Mental Health estimates that 30 million Americans are currently suffering from major psychological disorders. Anxiety disorders and clinical depression head the list; alcoholism and drug abuse are also distressingly common problems that have their roots in the psyche. In addition to causing so much suffering and disability, the 30,000 suicides in the United States each year demonstrate that mental illness can be lethal. Mental illness is also expensive, consuming more than 7 percent of all health-care dollars; depression alone rivals heart disease in its negative impact on the American economy.

It's a lot to worry about. But there is also good news about the interaction of mind and body. Mental disorders can be treated. Maintaining good physical health will help ensure good mental health. And mental forces can be harnessed to promote recovery from physical illnesses ranging from heart attacks and strokes to ulcers and colitis. Even cancer patients can benefit from the power of the mind; a 1989 study in the *Lancet* reported that women with metastatic breast cancer who were randomly assigned to receive weekly group therapy lived 18 months longer than their equally ill counterparts who received conventional therapy without emotional support.

More than 2,300 years ago the great Greek physician Hippocrates recognized that a sound mind and a sound body are equally important determinants of human health and well-being. Plato, too, understood that "the right education must tune the strings of the body and mind to perfect spiritual harmony." But in our modern world, alas, mind and body are often out of tune. Restoring their harmony could help put the civilization back into Western civilization; it would also help enhance health and prevent disease.

The healthy body is a happy body; the happy heart is a healthy heart.

Stress Reduction and the Treatment of Atherosclerosis

The ultimate test of any technique used to conquer heart disease is its ability to treat patients who already have the disease. How does stress reduction meet this test?

Quite well.

The best evidence comes from the results of treating the Type A personality. Dr. Friedman and his colleagues reported their experience with more than 1,000 heart attack survivors in the 1986 *American Heart Journal*. Patients were randomly assigned to receive special counseling or conventional care. Although smoking, exercise, diet, and medications did not differ between the groups, the risk of recurrent heart attacks was reduced by more than 50 percent in the special counseling group during nearly 5 years of observation. Patients who received counseling in the Recurrent Coronary Prevention Project reduced their level of hostility, time urgency, and impatience. They learned to contain anger and counter depression. And a 1990 study from Sweden provides another possible explanation for these striking results; it found that cardiac patients who received counseling were likely to develop social support networks, whereas other patients tended to remain isolated.

Cardiac patients may need professional help to reduce stress. But like all people, they should also learn to recognize and manage stress by themselves. So should you. Caring for your mind will go a long way toward caring for your heart.

Controlling Stress for Heart and Health

Your 15-point program to conquer heart disease allows you to construct a customized program to fight atherosclerosis based on your individual needs, goals, and preferences. Some elements of the plan belong in every program, others do not. Stress control is among the points that apply to everyone — but even here, personal considerations should dictate choices among the many options available for managing stress.

Review your emotional self-assessment test from Table 2–9 as well as your overall cardiac risk profile from Table 2–11. If personality factors are contributing to your risk, plan to make the changes that will help. Even if your risk is moderate to low, spend a few minutes sizing up your general health and personal happiness. Chances are that even the most well-adjusted among us could benefit from at least a few changes. But even after you've decided that change is right for you, think over the entire range of options before you rush into a mental fitness program; in fact, it's a good opportunity to begin the process of replacing rushed or harried decisions with a more relaxed and deliberate approach. You'll get there just the same — and your heart will thank you for a slow but steady course. Follow the advice of Reinhold Niebuhr by seeking the courage to change the things you can change, the serenity to accept the things you can't change, and the wisdom to know the difference.

Stress control can — and should — take many forms:

Physical Exercise

What's good for the body is good for the mind; exercise is *very* good for both.

Exercise is a form of physical stress. Can physical stress relieve mental stress? Alexander Pope thought so: "Strength of mind is Exercise, not Rest." Plato agreed: "Exercise would cure a guilty conscience." You'll think so, too — if you learn to apply the stress of exercise in a controlled, graded fashion.

Aerobic exercise is the key for your head, just as it is for your heart.

You may not agree at first; indeed the first steps are the hardest, and at first exercise will be more work than fun. But as you get into shape, you'll begin to tolerate exercise, then enjoy it, and finally depend on it.

Regular aerobic exercise will bring remarkable changes to your body, your metabolism, your heart, and your spirits. It has a unique capacity to exhilarate and relax, to provide stimulation and calm, to counter depression and dissipate stress. It's a common experience among endurance athletes and has been verified in clinical trials that have successfully used exercise to treat anxiety disorders and clinical depression. If athletes and patients can derive psychological benefits from exercise, so can you.

How can exercise contend with problems as difficult as anxiety and depression? There are two explanations, one chemical, the other behavioral.

The psychological benefits of aerobic exercise have a neurochemical basis. Exercise stimulates the production of endorphins, chemicals in the brain that are the body's natural painkillers and mood elevators. Endorphins are responsible for the "runner's high" and for the feelings of relaxation and optimism that accompany every good workout — or at least every hot shower after your sweating is over.

Behavioral factors also contribute to the emotional benefits of exercise. As your waistline shrinks and your strength and stamina increase, your self-image will improve. You'll earn a sense of mastery and control, of pride and self-confidence. Your renewed vigor and energy will help you succeed in many tasks, and the discipline of regular exercise will help you achieve other important lifestyle goals.

Exercise and sports also provide many opportunities to make friends and build networks. "All men," wrote Aquinas, "need leisure." Exercise is play and recreation; when your body is busy, your mind will be shielded from the stress of daily life and will be free to think creatively.

If exercise seems too good to be true, just try it for yourself. Follow the guidelines in Chapter 5 to construct the exercise program that's right for you.

Behavioral Exercises

Aerobic exercise improves your heart by making it work harder. Resistance exercise can do the same for your muscles. Mental exercise can sharpen your memory. But can behavioral exercises alter high-stress Type A response patterns?

Yes. The trick is to exercise restraint.

Behavioral patterns are learned through repetition. You can learn to change them by conditioning yourself to new patterns; again, repetition is the key. Here are a few exercises you can use to practice winding down:

- Drive your car in the right-hand lane, the slow lane.
- Use your car horn only to avert accidents, not to vent frustration or anger.
- When you drive up to a toll plaza, join the longest line, even if you have exact change.
- Put your cart in the longest supermarket checkout lane, even if your basket would qualify for the express line.
- Eat slowly, trying to be the last person to finish the meal.
- Talk slowly and don't interrupt.
- Don't put in the last word in an argument, even if you're sure you're right.
- Keep your voice down; never shout.
- Don't use expletives. Find less-hostile substitutes; "darn," "rats," and even "bad word" may serve you well.
- Don't permit outbursts of anger. Instead, wait a few moments, take some deep breaths, and express yourself calmly.
- Try not to grimace or clench your teeth. Practice smiling.
- Leave early for plays and concerts so you don't have to rush. Plan to spend 10 minutes relaxing in your seat before the curtain goes up.
- Don't do two things at once. For example, hang up the phone before you start opening your mail or emptying the dishwasher.
- Don't set your alarm clock on weekends.
- Don't set your watch ahead. Even better, don't look at your watch more than once an hour. Best of all, don't wear your watch, at least on weekends.
- Don't plan up all your time. Start by leaving an evening free, then a day, then a weekend.

Like any exercise program, behavioral exercise can be tough, particularly at first. Don't fall into the Type A trap of trying to do them all at once. Instead, pick the exercises that meet your needs and practice one at a time, moving on to the next only when you're comfortable with your progress.

There is no vaccine to prevent hurry sickness. It can't be cured with pills (though tranquilizers may provide temporary relief in some cases).

No surgery can cut it out of your personality. Hurry sickness is not an infection or a tumor, but a pattern of behavior — and it can be modified through behavioral techniques.

Aerobic exercise is essential for your heart, but it's not enough to fight atherosclerosis by itself. Behavioral exercises can help modify stress-driven response patterns, but they're not enough to fully control stress. Fortunately, many other options are available.

Autoregulation Exercises

Stress comes in many forms and produces many symptoms. Mental symptoms range from worry and irritability to restlessness and insomnia, anger and hostility, or sensations of dread, foreboding, and even panic.

Mental stress can also produce physical symptoms. Muscles are tense, resulting in fidgitiness, taut facial expressions, headaches, or neck and back pain. The mouth is dry, producing unquenchable thirst or perhaps the sensation of a lump in the throat that makes swallowing difficult. Clenched jaw muscles can produce jaw pain and headaches. The skin can be pale, sweaty, and clammy. Intestinal symptoms range from "butterflies" to heartburn, cramps, or diarrhea. Frequent urination may be a necessity. A pounding pulse is common, as is chest tightness. Rapid breathing is also typical, and may be accompanied by sighing or repetitive coughing. In extreme cases, hyperventilation can lead to tingling of the face and fingers, muscle cramps, lightheadedness, and even fainting.

The physical symptoms of stress are themselves distressing. In fact, the body's response to stress can feel so bad that it produces additional mental stress. During the stress response, then, mind and body can amplify each other's distress signals, creating a vicious cycle of tension and anxiety.

Because the root cause of stress is emotional, it is best controlled by gaining insight, reducing life problems that trigger stress, and modifying behavior. But stress control can — and should — also involve the body. Aerobic exercise is one approach; physical fitness will help promote mental fitness. But there is another approach: you can learn to use your mind to relax your body. The relaxed body will, in turn, send signals of calm and control that help reduce mental tension.

Autoregulation exercises are a series of techniques designed to replace the spiral of stress with a cycle of repose. Several approaches are available.

Deep breathing. Rapid, shallow, erratic breathing is a common response to stress. Slow, deep, regular breathing is a sign of relaxation. You can learn to control your respirations so they mimic relaxation; the effect, in fact, will be relaxing.

Here's how deep breathing exercises work:

1. Breathe in slowly and deeply, pushing your stomach out so that your diaphragm is put to maximal use.
2. Hold your breath briefly.
3. Exhale slowly, thinking "relax."
4. Repeat the entire sequence 5 to 10 times over, concentrating on breathing deeply and slowly.

Deep breathing is easy to learn. You can do it at any time, in any place. You can use deep breathing to help dissipate stress as it occurs. Practice the routine in advance, then use it when you need it most. If you find it helpful, consider repeating the exercise 4 to 6 times a day — even on good days.

Progressive muscular relaxation. Stressed muscles are tight, tense muscles. By learning to relax your muscles, you will be able to use your body to dissipate stress.

Muscle relaxation takes a bit longer to learn than deep breathing. It also takes more time. But even if this form of relaxation takes a little effort, it can be a useful part of your stress control program. Here's how it works:

Progressive muscle relaxation is best performed in a quiet, secluded place. You should be comfortably seated or stretched out on a firm mattress or mat. Until you learn the routine, have a friend recite the directions or listen to them on a tape, which you can prerecord yourself.

Progressive muscle relaxation focuses sequentially on each major muscle group. Tighten each muscle and maintain the contraction 20 seconds before slowly releasing it. As the muscle relaxes, concentrate on the release of tension and the sensation of relaxation. Start with your facial muscles, then work down your body.

Forehead	Wrinkle your forehead and arch your eyebrows. Hold, then relax.
Eyes	Close your eyes tightly. Hold, then relax. Wrinkle your nose and flare your nostrils. Hold, then relax.

Tongue	Push your tongue firmly against the roof of your mouth. Hold, then relax.
Face	Grimace. Hold, then relax.
Jaws	Clench your jaws tightly. Hold, then relax.
Neck	Tense your neck by pulling your chin down to your chest. Hold, then relax.
Back	Arch your back. Hold, then relax.
Chest	Breathe in as deeply as you can. Hold, then relax.
Stomach	Tense your stomach muscles. Hold, then relax.
Buttocks and thighs	Tense your buttock muscles. Hold, then relax.
Arms	Tense your biceps. Hold, then relax.
Forearms and hands	Tense your arms and clench your fists. Hold, then relax.
Calves	Press your feet down. Hold, then relax.
Ankles and feet	Pull your toes up. Hold, then relax.

The entire routine should take 12 to 15 minutes. Practice it twice daily, expecting to master the technique and experience some relief of stress in about 2 weeks.

Another excellent way to relax muscles and mind is through yoga. Many types of yoga are available; take a class or pick up a book to explore yoga's wide variety of postures, stretching exercises, and breathing techniques. You can use yoga strictly as a method of muscle relaxation, or you can combine it with meditation, an autorelaxation technique that begins by relaxing the mind.

Meditation is a prime example of the unity of mind and body. Mental stress can speed the heart and raise the blood pressure; meditation can actually reverse the physiological signs of stress. Scientific studies of Indian yoga masters demonstrate that meditation can actually slow the heart rate, lower the blood pressure, reduce the breathing rate, diminish the body's oxygen consumption, reduce blood adrenaline levels, and change skin temperature.

Although meditation is an ancient Eastern religious technique, you don't have to become a pilgrim or convert to put it to work for you. In fact, your best guide to meditation is not an Indian spiritualist but a Harvard physician, Dr. Herbert Benson. Here's an outline of Dr. Benson's relaxation response:

1. Select a time and place that will be free of distractions and interruption. A semidarkened room is often best; it should be quiet and private. If possible, wait for 2 hours after you eat before you meditate, and empty your bladder before you get started.
2. Get comfortable. Find a body position that will allow your body to relax so that physical signals of discomfort will not intrude on your mental processes. Breathe slowly and deeply, allowing your mind to become aware of your rhythmic respirations.
3. Achieve a relaxed, passive mental attitude. Close your eyes to block out visual stimuli. Try to let your mind go blank, blocking out thoughts and worries.
4. Concentrate on a mental device. Most people use a mantra, a simple word or syllable that is repeated over and over again in a rhythmic, chant-like fashion. You can repeat your mantra silently or say it aloud. It's the act of repetition that counts, not the content of the phrase; even the word "one" will do nicely. Some meditators prefer to stare at a fixed object instead of repeating a mantra. In either case, the goal is to focus your attention on a neutral object, thus blocking out ordinary thoughts and sensations.

Meditation is the most demanding of the autoregulation techniques, but it's also the most beneficial and rewarding. Once you've mastered meditation, you'll probably look forward to devoting 20 minutes to it once or twice a day.

Biofeedback is a high-tech autoregulation. It involves physiologic monitoring of the body's responses to stress and relaxation. The subject is hooked up to electronic monitors that measure the pulse rate, blood pressure, respiratory rate, muscle tension, and skin temperature. As the subject relaxes, audiovisual devices signal physiological improvements, reinforcing the mental acts that reduce stress.

Biofeedback requires specialized facilities and trained practitioners. It's less convenient than the other techniques, and it can be expensive. Still, if bells and whistles will help you let off steam, biofeedback is worth a try.

Autoregulation is not a panacea, but it's an excellent option for stress management. Many studies demonstrate that it can lower blood pressure in the short term, but proof of sustained hypertension control is still lacking. Remember, though, that Cannon found that stress produces rapid but temporary increases in blood pressure way back in 1914 — but we had to wait 79 years for the Framingham Heart Study to prove that anxiety contributes to sustained hypertension. Future research may or may not establish the long-term ability of autoregulation to reduce blood pressure and fight atherosclerosis. But if you make autoregulation part of your stress-control program, you'll feel better and enjoy life more while awaiting the scientific verdict.

Exercising Your Options: Making Choices for a Healthy Personality

You can't live in the modern world without experiencing stress. But you can learn to structure your world to reduce stress to manageable levels; it will take some introspection, planning, and effort, but it will be good for your heart, your health, and your happiness.

Identify your source of stress. Sound bites dramatize lurid crimes and blazing fires. Headlines announce fighting and famine over the world. Falling employment and rising interest rates. The spread of AIDS. Homelessness. There certainly is a lot of stress in the world.

There's not much you can do to reduce global and national causes of stress. Surprisingly, perhaps, the world's big crises contribute relatively little to personal stress. Most stress is local.

Think about what sets you on edge. The usual suspects include *overload, ambiguity,* and *hostile relationships.* Few things are more stressful than packed schedules and tight deadlines, simply having too many things to do and too little time to do them. Ambiguity produces stress in a different way, by putting you in a social or professional situation without a clearly defined role; not knowing what to do can be just as uncomfortable as having too much to do. And few things will raise your stress level faster than a blast of hostility or a dose of disparagement; Sartre was right when he said, "Hell is — other people!" — or at least partly right, since having good relationships with people is also one of the best ways to reduce stress by providing the supports that will keep your heart healthy.

The "big three" of stress may not apply to you. Even if they do, they may be hard to correct. It's important, therefore, to look also for other things that are stressful; even small things such as loud noises, frequent interruptions, or rushed meals can send your blood pressure soaring.

Identify the things that you find stressful; you may even want to keep a diary to help determine what makes your heart pound, your head ache, or your stomach sour. Once you know where the stress is coming from, you can plan to change things.

Restructure your lifestyle. Identifying the causes of stress is one thing, correcting them another. Here are a few tips:

- Establish priorities. Since you can't do everything, do the things that count most — and don't feel guilty about the things you can't do.
- Establish realistic expectations. Don't overload yourself by taking on too much — but don't run the risk of boredom and isolation by taking on too little. Know your abilities and use them to the fullest. Know your limits and respect them. It's the only way to master both the Scylla of stress and the Charybdis of depression.
- Be flexible. Like it or not, things will go wrong. Expect the unexpected — or at least be prepared to make the best of things, to "go with the flow."
- Pace yourself. Getting through your day is more complex than riding a bicycle; you can — and should — stop pedaling from time to time without worrying about falling off. Give yourself some downtime. Alternate stressful tasks with relaxing ones. Take your phone off the hook. Take an extended lunch hour or a three-day weekend. Spend some time doing nothing at all.
- Seek variety, both at work and at play. Routines can be reassuring, but rigidity can replace comfort with staleness and stress. Variety will keep you stimulated, enthusiastic, and fresh. Consider new challenges at work, and experiment with new forms of recreation and play.

Express yourself. You can't eliminate stress by denying it, and you can't control your response to stress by simply holding your feelings in. You don't have to wear your heart on your sleeve to express yourself, and you shouldn't blow off steam with an angry outburst whenever you're thwarted. Instead, think about your feelings and express them appropriately. If you're a very private person, you can talk to yourself, keep a journal, or write a letter that you never mail. Better still, learn to talk to other people, to express your feelings honestly without dwelling on emotional minutiae, wallowing in self-pity, or blasting away at the nearest ear. To learn how to talk your problems out, you'll also have to learn to be an empathetic, supportive listener; both skills will stand you in good stead.

Think positively. It's a hardhearted fact that not all clouds have silver linings. But there is an upside to every situation; it may not be much, but if you look for it, you can help it grow. Look for the kernel of humor hidden in every scenario. Learn to think of a glass as half full, not half empty, to taste lemonade, not lemons.

Embrace good stress. Yes, stress can be good. You don't usually think of it as stress, but as stimulation. Without challenge and excitement, life becomes dull and dreary — and depressing. Depression is as bad for your heart as stress. Develop interests that will keep your tempo brisk and your heart upbeat.

Listen to music. It's not the answer for everyone, but it can be remarkably helpful. A 1993 study even found that students who listened to Mozart performed better on standard intelligence tests. Pick the music you like best, and see if it won't help pick you up when you're low or settle you down when you're tense. The chances are you'll sing its praises.

Get enough sleep. You can't cope with stress when you're exhausted. Sleep rejuvenates both body and mind. Your body will tell you how much sleep you need — listen to it. Paradoxically, perhaps, many people need more sleep when they have the least time to sleep. Don't kid yourself — sleep deprivation will make you irritable and inefficient just when you need to be at your best. Give yourself enough time to sleep, and consider trying a 15-minute afternoon nap.

Giving yourself enough time to sleep won't do much good if you are among the 30 percent of Americans who experience sleep disturbances or insomnia. Here are a few tips for a good night's sleep:

- Establish a regular schedule, going to bed and getting up at nearly the same time each day. Don't sleep during the day if you have trouble sleeping at night.
- Be sure your bed is comfortable, and reserve it for sleeping. Use your chair for reading or watching TV, restricting your bed for sleep and other horizontal activities.
- Be sure your bedroom is quiet and dark. It should also be well ventilated and kept at a constant, comfortable temperature.
- Get plenty of exercise during the day.

- Eat properly. Avoid caffeine and alcohol, especially late in the day. Try to avoid all beverages after dinner if you find yourself getting up at night to urinate. If you enjoy a bedtime snack, keep it bland and light.
- Try yoga, meditation, or deep-breathing exercises before you get into bed. Practice progressive muscle relaxation while you're waiting to fall asleep.
- Above all, don't worry about sleep. Watching the clock never helps. Try not to lie in bed reviewing your problems or plans; instead, think of something relaxing and pleasant. If you can't manage to relax in bed, don't lie there thrashing about; get up, do something different — and then try again.

Don't rely on alcohol, nicotine, or drugs. You may run, but you can't hide. Self-medication will not resolve stress, nor will it counter depression. Quite the contrary, chemical coverups are sure to compound your problems, probably sooner rather than later. Even caffeine may amplify sensations of stress by speeding up your heart and your mind. Food is not the answer, either; "comfort foods" may provide temporary solace, but in the long run they'll just weigh down your self-image, adding to stress and depression.

Improve your interpersonal skills. Few things are more stressful than conflicts with hostile or demanding people. Learn to handle them. Listen carefully, trying to understand what's behind the anger. Instead of fighting fire with fire, acknowledge hostility, and try to defuse it ("You sound angry; how can I help?"). Stay calm but don't always retreat. Instead, learn to assert yourself to protect your own rights and interests.

Build networks. People are good medicine. Cultivate relationships with friends (and even with relatives!). Invest the thought, time, and effort needed to build the social networks that will help you get through times of crisis and stress. Remember that social isolation is a major risk factor for heart disease — don't let yourself drift away from your community. Instead, join organizations, enroll in classes, or become a volunteer. If you live alone, even getting a pet can help you stay connected — especially if you also join an animal fanciers' club.

Consider getting help. You wouldn't (or shouldn't) consider managing your physical problems without a doctor or nurse. If you have emotional problems that don't respond to the self-management techniques outlined in these pages, get help. That help can come in many forms, ranging from support groups and stress-management classes to professional counseling by social workers, psychologists, or psychiatrists. Techniques vary, but the basic goal is to work through problems by talking them out, gaining insight, and learning to control emotions, make choices, and establish healthy relationships. Sometimes just a few sessions will be remarkably helpful, but in other cases more intense therapy is needed. Physicians can also prescribe medications to treat psychological problems; ideally, they are just temporary aids used to help you get started on a long-term program for mental health.

Build a balanced life. Just as moderation is the key to a healthy heart, balance is the key to a happy life. Balance work and play, exercise and rest, discipline and indulgence. Balance independence and interdependence, solitude and companionship. Balance thought and fantasy, effort and relaxation, structure and spontaneity. Balance your needs with those of your family and your community. Balance your mind and your body to keep both healthy and fit.

Stress is everywhere. A national survey recently reported that 89 percent of all Americans frequently experience stress, and 59 percent experience substantial stress at least once a week. It's no coincidence that so many Americans also experience heart disease. To take care of your heart, take care of your head.

Chapter 15

Weight Control:
Slimming Down
for a Healthy Heart

IT'S NEW YEAR'S DAY in America. With the new year, of course, comes new resolve. For most of us, two items top the pledge list, becoming better people and becoming healthier people. And despite our nation's wonderful diversity, nearly all Americans who resolve to become better and healthier plan to start out in the same way, by losing weight.

There's no time better than today for turning over a new leaf. But there are all those football games to watch and that nice soft couch to view them from. With a bit of a headache, an easy lunch is in order, perhaps a sandwich and some frozen fries. The chips go well with the games, especially with that leftover sour cream dip. For dinner, a pizza is just a phone call away; for dessert, there's cake from the party, and some candy for snacktime.

New Year's Day in America.

You can do better. Start with the same resolution, to improve your health. But don't include weight loss on your wish list; even if you're corpulent, you can return the scale you got for Christmas. Instead, resolve to follow the 15-point program to conquer atherosclerosis. The results will please you: you'll earn a healthy heart and — without even weighing yourself — you'll become lighthearted.

What Is Obesity?

Nearly every patient who comes to my office asks the same question: "How much should I weigh?" It's the wrong question. Obesity is not an excess of body weight — it's an excess of body fat.

The human body stores energy in its fat cells, also gaining insulation from the cold, protection against trauma, the ability to process sex hormones, and a storage depot for vitamins A, D, E, and K. That's the good news about the body's 40 billion fat cells. The bad news is that when the body has more energy than it needs, it converts the excess into triglycerides that are deposited in fat cells. The result is no surprise: fat cells enlarge. And when the cells are completely full, they divide in two, doubling the body's fat storage capacity.

From a medical standpoint, obesity is defined as a 20 percent excess of body fat. As you may recall from Chapter 2, this corresponds to a body mass index of about 27 in women and 28 in men (see page 57).

The medical definition of obesity is useful, but it's arbitrary. In fact, body fat follows the same general rule as blood pressure and blood cholesterol: lower levels are associated with longer life spans. Even a 5 percent gain in fat has adverse health consequences; the lowest risk of death from heart disease occurs in men with BMIs between 19.9 and 22.6 and in women with BMIs between 18.6 and 23.0.

For your heart, the leaner the better. For your life, though, it's not that simple.

What Causes Obesity?

It's a question that has occupied thousands of scientists for hundreds of years. There are nearly as many theories as there are medical journals and TV talk shows. But the scientific debates and public controversies overlook the simple, indisputable cause of obesity:

Obesity is caused by an energy excess.

When the body takes in more energy than it uses up, that energy is stored as fat. The only people who get fat are those who take in more calories than they burn up. The only people who lose weight are those who burn up more calories than they take in.

That's the short answer. But it doesn't tell the whole story; in particular, it doesn't explain why some people are fat, others thin, why some people struggle to lose weight, while others find it just as hard to gain. Let's review some of the theories of obesity — without, I hope, losing sight of the basic fact that obesity is caused by energy excess.

Genetics

Freud explained that "anatomy is destiny"; the genetic theory of obesity asserts that destiny is anatomy, that it shapes humans' middles as well as their ends.

You don't have to be a geneticist to see the truth in this theory. Obesity tends to run in families; if your family tree has a thick trunk, you have a higher than average chance of having one, too. In fact, children with one obese parent have a 50 percent chance of becoming obese, whereas the children of two obese parents have a 63 percent risk of obesity.

But does obesity run in families because family members learn the same behavioral patterns of eating and physical inactivity, or because they have a genetic predisposition to obesity? The answer is that both components are important, but in many families, big jeans truly come from fat genes. Children who are raised from infancy by adoptive parents have body fat patterns like their biological parents, not their adoptive relatives. Similarly, twins separated at birth grow up to resemble each other despite being raised in different households.

Psychology

The psychological theory of obesity holds that people become obese because they have an emotional need to overeat. The mind and body are inseparable, and there is evidence that mental factors contribute to some cases of obesity. For example, a 1994 study found that severe parental neglect in childhood is a major risk factor for obesity in adulthood; but on the other hand, neither mild neglect nor strong parental love and support influenced body fat in adulthood.

It's true that in our affluent society the signals to eat don't come from hunger, but from habit. And it is true that eating habits can be changed. But it's not true that obesity is a psychological disorder or a simple lack of willpower and discipline. In our culture, at least, nobody wants to be fat. There is no "obese personality"; obese people do tend to be depressed, but largely in reaction to the discrimination they confront in daily life. Eating behavior can be changed, but attributing obesity to emotional problems is blaming the victim.

Overeating

In a sense, all obesity is due to overeating, since all people who gain weight take in more calories than they need. But the stereotype of obese people as gluttons is wrong; in fact, thin people actually consume more calories per pound than fat people do.

Underexercise

Again, lack of exercise plays a role in all obesity, since fat would not accumulate if enough calories were burned off. But simple sloth is not responsible for obesity. Fat people do tend to be sedentary, but in many cases the excess weight comes first, slowing people down and discouraging healthful exercise. And although few marathoners are obese, many sedentary people are thin — even if they don't deserve to be.

Hormones

Is obesity "all in your glands?" Hormones such as insulin, glucagon, thyroid, adrenaline, and cortisone play essential roles in the body's energy economy. But endocrinologists tell us that it's very, very rare to detect hormonal abnormality in people who are obese. It's not in the glands.

Metabolism

It's appealing to postulate that obese people simply burn fewer calories than lean people, that they have slower metabolisms. Appealing or not, the theory can't be substantiated: average metabolic rates are the same in the rotund and the scrawny. Still, new studies hint at subtle metabolic abnormalities in people who are obese. As scientific measurements improve, the metabolic theory may gain support. At present, though, it's just one theory among many.

The Set Point

Another theory but, I think, a good one.

The set point theory begins with a simple observation: body weight resists change. That part, at least, is not theory but fact; just ask anyone who has tried to lose or gain weight.

It's true that people lose weight when they're sick — but the pounds come right back when they recover. It's also true that the typical American gains about 2 pounds a year in middle age. Two pounds a year is not much, but over 15 or 20 years it adds up to obesity. Still, the body will gain 2 pounds a year by storing just 20 extra calories a day. Consider how much your exercise and dining schedules vary from day to day, and you'll see that the body is remarkably efficient at establishing its energy balance. A 1991 study of healthy children between the ages of 2 and 5 emphasizes the point. The kids were allowed unrestricted access to whatever foods they wanted; their caloric intake varied widely from meal to meal, but their 24-hour totals were remarkably constant from day to day.

Whether you're 2 years old or 22, your body adjusts its energy balance with remarkable precision. How does the body compensate for illness and health, exertion and rest, Thanksgiving and fasting? No one knows. But the set point theory says that each individual has a unique set point; it allows temporary ups and downs, but in the long run it brings body weight back to its predetermined set point.

Obese people, the theory says, differ from the thin people only in having higher set points. It's a discouraging theory, since we have neither tests to measure the set point nor treatments to alter it. The theory explains why conventional diets fail, but it doesn't necessarily condemn people who are overweight to a lifetime of obesity. My theory is that the set point can be changed, and that the 15-point program contains the way to do it.

Cultural Factors

Each theory of obesity has some validity, and each has some flaws. That's because obesity is multifactorial. There is no one cause of obesity; instead, there are many causes that contribute more or less to each individual's weight problem. But there is another way to look at obesity, viewing it from the cultural perspective.

Obesity is a disorder of modern Western society. Rare before the industrial revolution, obesity began to appear in the upper socioeconomic classes in the eighteenth century. During the last 100 years, obesity has spread down through society on a massive scale, until today it's actually most prevalent in the lower classes of industrialized societies. Even today, however, obesity is uncommon in underdeveloped society.

The industrial revolution hasn't changed human genetics, hormones, or metabolism. But it has changed human behavior. We've learned to mass-produce high-fat, calorie-dense foods, and we've learned how to make these foods inexpensive and how to make them appealing through advertising. We've learned how to refine foods, removing fiber and adding sugar. We've learned how to substitute machines for muscles, creating the labor-saving devices that enable us to work with our minds instead of our bodies. We've learned how to enjoy sports as spectators instead of participants. We've learned how to be fat.

We can also learn to be lean.

Obesity and Heart Disease

It's no coincidence that the epidemics of obesity and atherosclerosis have occurred simultaneously. Both, after all, have the same root cause, nutritional abuse and physical disuse.

Obesity promotes atherosclerosis. Excess body fat contributes to all the major cardiac risk factors except smoking. Obesity raises LDL cholesterol and lowers HDL cholesterol. It increases blood pressure. Obesity raises blood sugar levels and promotes insulin resistance, greatly increasing the risk of diabetes. Obesity discourages exercise. And in our weight-conscious society obesity adds to psychological stress.

Quite apart from its adverse effects on other risk factors, obesity is a cardiac risk factor in its own right. Even accounting for its effect on other risk factors, a 10 percent gain in body weight increases the risk of a heart attack by about 25 percent. Moderate to severe obesity is even worse; for example, a woman with a BMI of 29 is 230 percent more likely to have a heart attack than a woman with a BMI of 21.

All types of body fat are equally harmful for the blood cholesterol, blood pressure, and blood sugar. But in terms of direct cardiac risk, upper body fat is much more harmful that lower body fat. The cardiac impact of upper body obesity can be quantified using the waist-to-hip ratio (see Chapter 2, page 57). Ratios above 1.0 in men and 0.80 in women are linked to increased risk; for example, men with ratios above 1.0 are twice as likely to die from heart disease as are men with ratios below 0.85.

Upper body fat is worse than lower body fat — and up-and-down weight is more dangerous than a constant weight. The Framingham Heart Study found that fluctuations in body weight are associated with

FIGURE 15–1: The Relationship Between Body Mass Index and Mortality

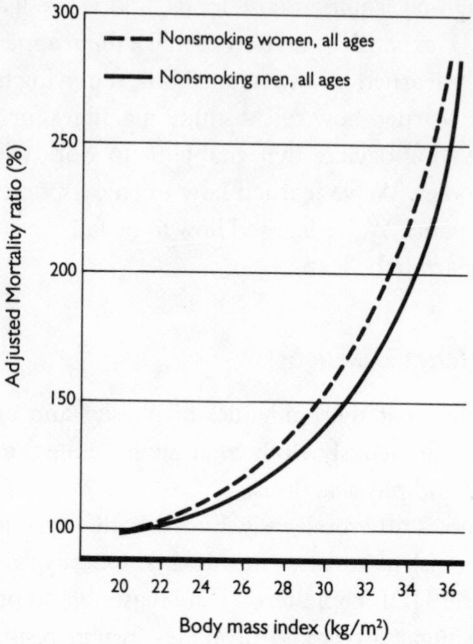

Source: Lew, E.A. and Garfinckel, L. *Journal of Chronic Diseases* 32:563,1979.

higher rates of heart attacks and deaths than sustained obesity. But these results shouldn't be interpreted as an endorsement of obesity; instead, they encourage sustained weight loss, even if it's modest, instead of temporary losses that are regained. When it comes to your weight, the yo-yo is a no-no.

Obesity and Health

In 1958, John Kenneth Galbraith observed that "more die in the United States of too much food than of too little." Professor Galbraith is an economist, but he was right: obesity is a major cause of needless disease and premature death in our "affluent society." In fact, if smokers are excluded from the analysis, body fat is directly and continuously linked to the death rate in America; Figure 15–1 displays this relationship in graphic form.

Table 15–1 lists the diseases linked to obesity. They have all increased dramatically since the industrial revolution; even today they

Table 15–1
DISEASES ASSOCIATED WITH OBESITY

Cardiovascular disease	Hypertension Angina Heart attacks Sudden death
Neurologic disease	Stroke
Metabolic disease	Diabetes (Type II) Gout
Gastrointestinal disease	Fatty liver Gallstones
Urinary tract disease	Kidney stones
Respiratory disease	Sleep apnea syndrome
Musculoskeletal disease	Osteoarthritis
Malignant disease	Breast cancer Female reproductive cancer Prostate cancer Cancer of the gallbladder
Psychological disease	Depression

are much more common in the United States and Europe than in underdeveloped countries. Like obesity itself, they are the diseases of affluence.

Obesity and its associated diseases are a steep price to pay for modernization. Obesity also has a steep monetary cost. According to conservative estimates, the aggregate cost of obesity and its associated illnesses in America is $39.3 billion a year. Only an affluent society could afford such expense; only a foolish society would allow it to continue.

Obesity in America

It's a big problem.

Even using the generous criterion of 20 percent fat excess, obesity is distressingly common in America. And it's a problem that's getting worse: Americans gained 155 million pounds in 1993 alone; the average young adult, in fact, has gained 10 pounds in the past 7 years. As a result, between 1988 and 1991 the prevalence of obesity increased from

24 to 32 percent in men and from 27 to 35 percent in women. In all, more than 25 million American adults are obese — to say nothing of the countless millions with less extreme fat excesses.

Can 25 million Americans really be wrong? Since 1 of every 3 Americans qualifies as obese, perhaps the definition itself is at fault. Should we redefine obesity, expanding our standards to fit our expanding waistlines? The Metropolitan Life Insurance Company thinks so. Over the years, their height-weight tables, which serve as the standard for much of America, have become more lenient about corpulence. For example, in 1950 the "ideal weight" for a 5-foot-10-inch-tall man was 159 pounds; in 1983, the same man was congratulated for weighing 172, and in 1990, 188 pounds. But a 1993 study from the Harvard School of Public Health reaffirmed that thin people live longer; the best weight for a 5-foot-10-inch man is actually 157 pounds. All in all, the fact that obesity is so common does not mean that it's "normal." Instead, it means that we're in the midst of an epidemic of weighty proportion.

The obesity epidemic is not unique to the United States; in fact, it affects virtually every industrialized society in the world today. Nor is obesity a secret; in fact, at any one time more than 50 million Americans are trying to practice girth control.

Americans don't want to be fat. Far from it: weight loss is a national obsession, consuming resolutions, hours, and dollars by the millions. Yet obesity is on the rise. Why does nearly every weight loss plan fail? There are three reasons: the wrong motivation, the wrong goals, and the wrong methods. You can do better.

Is Weight Loss Right for You?

It seems like a silly question; most Americans would answer it with a resounding "yes." But it's not a silly question, nor is the answer quite so simple. To answer it for yourself, first consider your own body, then evaluate the pros and cons of attempting to change your body fat.

How Do You Weigh In?

In Chapter 2 you learned how to evaluate your body fat by calculating your body mass index. You also learned how to estimate the cardiac

Table 15–2
YOUR BODY MASS INDEX

Height						Body Weight in Pounds								
4'10"	91	96	100	105	110	115	119	124	129	134	138	143	167	191
4'11"	94	99	104	109	114	119	124	128	133	138	143	148	173	198
5'	97	102	107	112	118	123	128	133	138	143	148	153	179	204
5'1"	100	106	111	116	122	127	132	137	143	148	153	158	185	211
5'2"	104	109	115	120	126	131	136	142	147	153	158	164	191	218
5'3"	107	113	118	124	130	135	141	146	152	158	163	169	197	225
5'4"	110	116	122	128	134	140	145	151	157	163	169	174	203	232
5'5"	114	120	126	132	138	144	150	156	162	168	174	180	210	240
5'6"	118	124	130	136	142	148	155	161	167	173	179	186	216	247
5'7"	121	127	134	140	146	153	159	166	172	178	185	191	223	255
5'8"	125	131	138	144	151	158	164	171	177	184	190	197	230	262
5'9"	128	135	142	149	155	162	169	176	182	189	196	203	236	270
5'10"	132	139	146	153	160	167	174	181	188	195	202	207	243	278
5'11"	136	143	150	157	165	172	179	186	193	200	208	215	250	286
6'	140	147	154	162	169	177	184	191	199	206	213	221	258	294
6'1"	144	151	159	166	174	182	189	197	204	212	219	227	265	302
6'2"	148	155	163	171	179	186	194	202	210	218	225	233	272	311
6'3"	152	160	168	176	184	192	200	208	216	224	232	240	279	319
6'4"	156	164	172	180	189	197	205	213	221	230	238	246	287	328
BMI	19	20	21	22	23	24	25	26	27	28	29	30	35	40

Source: Bray, G. A., Gray, D. S. Western Journal of Medicine 149:429–441, 1988.

impact of your body fat by calculating your waist-to-hip ratio. If you've forgotten your results, go back to page 57 and repeat the simple math. Or, if you prefer, use Table 15–2 to look up your approximate body mass index (BMI).

The BMI is the newest and best way to evaluate your body's fat, but it's not the only way. Some people still like to use the older height and weight tables; they're easier to use and understand, but because they focus on weight instead of fat, they're less accurate. If you'd like to compare the two methods, have a look at Table 15–3; when it comes to planning your personal management program, you'll also have an opportunity to choose between traditional methods that focus on calories and weight and a new method that focuses on fat in the diet and in the body.

The Advantages and Disadvantages of Weight Loss
The advantages of reducing body fat are obvious. From the viewpoint of atherosclerosis, heart disease, and the other diseases of affluence

Table 15–3
HEIGHT AND WEIGHT TABLES

Men

| Height | | | | |
Feet	Inches	Small Frame	Medium Frame	Large Frame
5	1	112–120	118–129	126–141
5	2	115–123	121–133	129–144
5	3	118–126	124–136	132–148
5	4	121–129	127–139	135–152
5	5	124–133	130–143	138–156
5	6	128–137	134–147	142–161
5	7	132–141	138–152	147–166
5	8	136–145	142–156	151–170
5	9	140–150	146–160	155–174
5	10	144–154	150–165	159–179
5	11	148–158	154–175	168–184
6	0	152–162	158–170	164–189
6	1	156–167	162–180	173–194
6	2	160–171	167–185	178–199
6	3	164–175	172–190	182–204

Women

| Height | | | | |
Feet	Inches	Small Frame	Medium Frame	Large Frame
4	8	92–98	96–107	104–119
4	9	94–101	98–110	106–122
4	10	96–104	101–113	109–125
4	11	99–107	104–116	112–128
5	0	102–110	107–119	115–131
5	1	105–113	110–122	118–134
5	2	108–116	113–126	121–138
5	3	111–119	116–130	125–142
5	4	114–123	120–135	129–146
5	5	118–127	124–139	133–150
5	6	122–131	128–143	137–154
5	7	126–135	132–147	141–158
5	8	130–140	136–151	145–163
5	9	134–144	140–155	149–168
5	10	138–148	144–159	153–173

Source: Modified from data of the Metropolitan Life Insurance Company.

(Table 15–1), the less fat you have the better. From the viewpoint of longevity, you'd benefit from reducing your BMI to 22 or even less, a lean range indeed (Figure 15–1).

For real people in the real world, however, there are disadvantages to consider. The first is disappointment and frustration. Traditional diet schemes invariably fail to achieve sustained weight loss. Frustration is bad enough, but failure can also lead to guilt, diminished self-esteem and even depression — hardly a combination that will make it easy for you to take care of your heart, much less enjoy life.

Another potential drawback is expense. Diet foods, diet pills, diet books, commercial weight loss schemes, and medically supervised treatments are all costly. They'd save money if they worked, but in the long run they don't. In contrast, the hearty option for health and weight control won't cost you any more than you've already spent on this book.

A third potential drawback to weight reduction is success, or at least partial success. Most diet plans do achieve weight loss, enabling the mother of the bride, for example, to get into her beautiful dress. But that success is short-lived at best, causing the mother-in-law, for example, to look like one. The result is a roller-coaster weight pattern, itself a heart disease risk factor. Your health — and your wardrobe — would be better off at a constant weight.

Want more drawbacks? Weight loss can make you feel tired; some people also experience itching or diarrhea as they reduce. Thin people feel cold. Very thin people, especially women, may experience sexual or reproductive dysfunction and an increased risk of osteoporosis. And even if they're very healthy, very thin people can look peaked or downright ill.

Still want to reduce? I hope so. But I hope you'll go about it in the right way. The key is to avoid the all-too-common trap of becoming preoccupied with your weight. Even better, forget about your weight. Instead, think about your heart and your health, about your fat and fiber intake and your muscular output. As you follow a balanced plan to take care of your heart, your weight will take care of itself.

Weighing Your Options

There are almost as many diet plans as there are stomachs. You couldn't possibly consider them all, nor do you have to. Instead, think over the best of the traditional approaches, and try them out if they seem to fit your needs. Understand the medical options; it's interesting to see that even in this era of advanced technology, medicine has such a limited ability to solve what is fundamentally a lifestyle problem. Finally, consider the new hearty option before you weigh in with a final choice.

Traditional Options for Weight Loss

At this very moment, about 1 of every 10 American adults is on a diet. In the course of this year, they will spend about $34 billion on diet books, diet foods, potions and pills, and weight loss clinics. Many will lose weight. But virtually all will regain the weight they lose. People who go on diets are doomed to repeat them; losing 12 pounds invariably leads to gaining a dozen.

There are hundreds and hundreds of reducing programs. For all their diversity, the overwhelming majority have three things in common: their emphasis on weight as a goal, their emphasis on caloric restriction, and their high relapse rates. The hearty option does away with the first two elements, substituting a plan designed to avoid the third. Still, you should know how to use the best aspects of the traditional approach — and what pitfalls to avoid.

Selecting a target weight. If you choose a weight-based approach, it's critical to pick a realistic, attainable goal. It's easy to look up your "ideal" weight on Table 15–3; easy or not, it's a bad idea. If your goal is unrealistically low, your reward is bound to be failure and frustration. As a rule of thumb, don't set your goal below the lowest weight you were able to sustain for a full year at age 21 or beyond. But even your "best weight" should be used as a long-term goal; for the short term, don't ask yourself to lose more than 10 percent of your current body weight.

Selecting a rate of weight loss. The message is simple: if you plan to reduce too quickly, you'll just fail quickly. Obesity is a chronic condition; to correct it, aim for slow, steady, long-term change. Losing a pound a week is a realistic goal.

Selecting a daily calorie intake. If you use caloric restriction as your method of weight loss, you'll have to plan an appropriate daily caloric intake. Here's how:

1. Calculate your resting metabolic rate (RMR). For men, RMR = 900 plus 5 x body weight in pounds. For women RMR = 700 plus 3.2 x body weight in pounds.
2. Factor in your exercise level. For sedentary people (less than 1 hour of exercise per week) multiply RMR x 1.2. For moderately active people (1 to 3 hours of exercise per week) multiply RMR x 1.4. For very active people (more than 3 hours of exercise per week), multiply RMR x 1.8. The result is the number of calories you need each day to keep your weight constant.
3. Subtract the calories you'll have to give up to lose weight. To lose one pound per week, subtract 500 calories per day; if your goal is 2 pounds, subtract 1,000.

Consider behavior modification. You now have goals for your weight and your daily caloric consumption. Setting goals is hard, but achieving them is even harder because you'll have to change your eating behavior. Still, behavior is the key to obesity; there is nothing more fattening than a fork. Here are a few tips that may help:

1. Understand your eating patterns. Few Americans eat because they are hungry. Do you eat for solace when you're tense and frustrated or as a reward when you're satisfied and happy? Do you eat when you're lonely or when you're socializing? Do you eat when you're bored or when you're busy? For many people the answer is "all of the above." Still, if you understand what triggers your eating — particularly your snacking — you may be able to substitute other responses.
2. Shop prudently. Make a shopping list and stick to it. Buy only the things you plan to eat. Never shop for food when you're hungry.
3. Store your food only in the kitchen or pantry; snacking will be much harder to resist if food is close at hand in the den or bedroom. Even in the kitchen, put "forbidden" high-calorie foods in inaccessible places.
4. Cook only what you plan to eat. If you're cooking for more than one day, put away the second portion before you sit down to eat.
5. Use small plates; small portions will seem more substantial on small dinnerware.
6. Eat regularly. Skipping meals will make you excessively hungry, backfiring in the long run. It's particularly important to eat breakfast.
7. Eat slowly. Put your utensils down between bites. Chew your food

thoroughly and deliberately; you'll enjoy the taste and texture more, and you may trick yourself into thinking you're having a large meal.

8. If you feel hungry after your meal, wait a full 15 minutes (by the clock!) before you even think about eating more food.

9. Eat only when you are sitting at the table.

10. Plan ahead for social situations and for eating out. Give yourself enough flexibility to enjoy life, but be prepared to deal with the temptation by knowing what foods you'll eat.

11. Maintain your self-esteem. Don't get down on yourself if you "cheat" ("I'm a failure and I'll always be fat"). Don't overcompensate by making unrealistic promises that are bound to fail ("I'll never look at another cookie"). Instead, think optimistically and positively, emphasizing all the things that you are doing right in your diet, and in the rest of your life.

12. Get support. Discuss your plans and progress with a friend; better yet, find a sympathetic, compatible person to start a program with you. Or consider joining a group — as long as it's nutritionally sound and reasonably priced. Aside from professional hospital-based groups, the commercial program I recommend most often is Weight Watchers.

Monitor your progress. Most weight control–based programs advise keeping food diaries and weight records at least weekly. The goal of self-monitoring is to allow your progress to reenforce your resolve; the problem is that setbacks may make your program collapse. Another problem is that even the best-intentioned food diaries are notoriously inaccurate, usually underreporting caloric intake.

Plan a maintenance phase. No plan will succeed unless it includes *permanent* maintenance. To succeed, the maintenance phase must be nutritionally sound, palatable, and realistic.

Add the missing elements. Most traditional weight loss programs stop here. Even those that go farther give little more than lip service to the two missing elements: the *quality of food* and the *importance of exercise*. In contrast, the hearty option depends very heavily on the kind of food you eat (low-fat, high-fiber; low-sugar, high-complex carbohydrate) and how much you exercise (lots). Even if you select a traditional weight-calorie program, you'd be well advised to include these elements in your plan; we'll get to them shortly.

Avoid pitfalls. Many traditional weight loss programs include additional features — usually gimmicks that promise a painless, foolproof, rapid result, often at a substantial cost. Here are some pitfalls to avoid at any and all costs:

1. The quick fix. If it's too good to be true, it's not.
2. Crash diets. Almost any diet will produce weight loss. But what goes down on a crash diet will go up again. Don't become a nutritional elevator. Avoid crash diets — at best you will lose weight temporarily, at worst your health will crash.
3. Nutritional fads. There is a reason fads don't last. A good reason.
4. Fasting for weight reduction. There may be legitimate religious, philosophical, and even political reasons to fast. A day or so without nutrition will not harm healthy people. But fasting to lose weight will not work — ever. It combines the very worse of the quick fix, the crash program, and the dietary fad.
5. Spot-reducing and "cellulite" reduction. There is no such thing as cellulite. Apart from cosmetic surgery, there is no way to "spot-reduce" body fat. Even exercise won't do it.
6. Over-the-counter diet pills. Most claim they will suppress your appetite. In the long run, in fact, they will suppress only your bank balance, sometimes adding the injury of side effects to the insult of gullibility.
7. Over-the-counter diet powders and potions. Most claim to substitute for food, providing you nutrition with few calories. Many, in fact, are nutritionally deficient, and none will produce long-term benefits. Food is better, as long as it's the right food. Food is also cheaper, especially the right foods.
8. Expensive weight-loss plans. See precautions 1 through 7.
9. Vitamins. Vitamins have many roles for health, but they have no role in managing obesity.
10. Laxatives and vomiting. There are no exceptions.
11. Weight loss wraps and devices. No exceptions.
12. Smoking. Absolutely no exceptions.
13. Radical remedies of any kind.

These precautions seem pretty obvious, and they are. Self-evident or not, they are often overlooked. They're overlooked because our culture is excessively preoccupied, almost obsessed, with weight. At every turn, we are confronted by images and slogans linking thinness to sophistication, success, and sexual allure. Common sense and scientific evidence are overlooked because people want to believe there is an easy way. And the experience of other dieters is overlooked because the diet industry wants to fatten up at the expense of the public. And, I fear, at the expense of public health.

Traditional weight- and calorie-based programs almost always fail, even if they're nutritionally sound and psychologically reasonable. Still, they have some elements you may want to bring to your consideration of other options. Quick-fix weight loss schemes always fail; leave them behind as you consider other options. Above all, don't lose heart about losing harmful fat, because there *are* other options.

Medically Supervised Options for Weight Loss

Obesity is bad for heart and health. Even so, people who are mildly to moderately obese do not need medically supervised programs. In contrast, moderately to severely obese people (40 to 100 percent excess fat) may be candidates for very low calorie diets or prescription medications, and morbidly obese people (more than 100 percent excess fat) may even be candidates for surgical treatment. Unfortunately, despite their scientific basis and medical supervision, these options are far from ideal, having more limitations than benefits for most participants. Because these medical options require professional supervision, they'll be discussed here only briefly.

Very low calorie diets. Most calorie-based weight loss programs provide 1,000–1,500 calories per day. In contrast, very low calorie diets provide only 400–800 per day.

Very low calorie diets got a bad name in the 1970s, when medically unsupervised liquid-protein diets were linked to many complications, including abnormal heart rhythms and at least 60 deaths. The current products have been reformulated to include high-quality protein, carbohydrates, and minerals. They appear safe, though some patients who lose weight rapidly on very low calorie diets develop gallstones. Still, patients with heart disease should avoid very low calorie diets, and all people using these diets should be medically supervised and monitored.

Only people who are severely obese (BMIs above 30) should consider very low calorie diets. This option requires people to give up food entirely, substituting the liquid formula for periods of 12 to 16 weeks. Up to 25 percent of enrollees drop out of these programs, but people who stick with the plan lose an average of 12 to 15 pounds. That's not much, but every little bit helps — unless it's regained. Often, despite the sacrifice and expense involved, that's just what happens.

Prescription appetite suppressants. "If only there was a pill." Now there is a pill — several, in fact.

Fenfluramine (Pondimin) is chemically related to the amphetamines ("speed"), but it's not addictive and it doesn't cause jitteriness. Drowsiness and diarrhea are the major side effects. Fluoxetine (Prozac) is widely used as an antidepressant. It's effective in that role, but some patients develop side effects that may include nausea or diarrhea, nervousness, insomnia, tremors, and sexual dysfunction.

Controlled studies have demonstrated that both fenfluramine and fluoxetine reduce appetite and produce weight loss. But the weight loss is modest, usually no better than can be achieved with behavior modification. And, as with all "easy" programs, the weight loss is temporary.

Prescription medications should be considered only by very obese people who've exhausted their other options. Careful medical evaluations and ongoing clinical supervision are required.

Surgery. "If only there was an operation." Now there is an operation — several, in fact.

Intestinal bypass operations produce weight loss, but they produce so many complications that they've been abandoned. The current operation, called a gastroplasty, limits food intake by creating a small pouch that reduces the stomach's capacity to about 2 ounces. Operations that wrap or bypass the stomach are also in use. The operations work — but they have appreciable risks and substantial limitations.

The surgical option should be considered only by really obese individuals who meet strict criteria, including medical criteria, surgical criteria, and Shakespeare's criterion: "Diseases desperate grown / by desperate appliance are relieved / or not at all" (*Hamlet*).

It's disheartening but true: the medical options are even more limited than the traditional options for weight loss. Fortunately, there is a third way.

The Hearty Option

If you've read the first 14 chapters of this book, the best solution to the problem of obesity should be clear: to take care of your weight, take good care of your heart.

What makes the hearty option different? Why should it succeed when other plans fail?

First, it provides you with the right reasons to change: freedom from heart disease, good health, and a longer life. These are long-term objectives; they're less dramatic than a goal of looking great in a bathing suit, but they are more likely to motivate long-term, durable changes. It's a lifelong plan for life.

Second, it sets the right goals. It asks you to begin by weighing and measuring yourself to calculate your body mass index and waist-to-hip ratio. After that, however, you don't have to weigh yourself at all. It takes will not to weigh; remember that your goal is not an arbitrary weight, but a steady improvement in your cardiac risk score. That's a number, too, but as your score improves you'll be rewarded by new feelings of energy and optimism, which will tell you more than any number can.

Third, it uses the right methods. Instead of asking you to restrict calories, it asks you to reduce dietary fat and simple sugar. Instead of asking you to gobble expensive supplements, it asks you to eat natural fiber and complex carbohydrates. Instead of asking you to visit a diet center, it asks you to run to a gym.

The hearty option gets the right results: less body fat in the context of a stronger heart and improved overall health. But, of course, there is a catch: it requires work, and it takes time. By changing gradually, though, you'll find this plan enjoyable. And by changing permanently, you'll achieve a healthy way of life that will become second nature to you.

Here's how it works:

Set the right goals. You've done the figures already: review your body mass index, waist-to-hip ratio, and overall cardiac risk score (Table 2–11) from Chapter 2. For longevity and health, everyone's goal is the same: to achieve a BMI of about 22 and a waist-to-hip ratio of below 1.0 for men or below 0.8 for women. But longevity curves don't tell the whole story; people come in different sizes, and the same goal won't fit everyone. Use three additional considerations to tailor your goals to fit your needs: First, your cardiac risk score; if it's low, you can set your BMI goal higher, since your prospects for cardiovascular health are so good. If, on the other hand, your risk score is high, you should set a more stringent BMI goal. But even here, consider the second factor, your personal preferences. Review your entire risk profile and decide where to make the maximum effort to improve. As you improve in one area, you'll probably be eager to take on new goals. But for starters, establish your personal priorities; a low BMI may or may not be among them. Finally, be realistic. If your BMI is 28, you're unlikely to bring it down to 22, particularly if you come from a family of 28s. Instead of setting a target you're sure to miss, aim to get your index down by 2, then re-evaluate your situation.

Set the right pace. The only way to get permanent results is to get them slowly. By the time you're 40, you'll have eaten more than 40,000 meals, to say nothing of all those snacks and all those hours spent in your easy chair. Don't try to change all at once. Instead, pick one dietary improvement and one exercise goal each week; when they're an easy, automatic part of your life, move on to the next goal. This week, for example, you might change from doughnuts to bran muffins, then next week to whole wheat toast. This week, start walking upstairs whenever you have two flights to travel, then next week make it three flights.

Reduce your dietary fat. This is one of the two key elements in the hearty option. Why is fat so crucial?

Your main goal is to have a healthy heart and body. A low fat intake is essential to meet that goal. Chapter 4 explains how dietary fat contributes to atherosclerosis and many other diseases, including cancer; review it if you need to, brushing up on the distinctions between saturated and unsaturated fats, animal fats and marine oils, hydrogenated vegetable oils and monounsaturated fats.

Your secondary goal is to reduce your body's fat content. The best way to have less fat is to eat less fat. There are two reasons for this. First, fat is the most calorie-dense food. Fats, whether saturated or unsaturated, have 9 calories per gram; alcohol has 7, but carbohydrates and proteins each have only 4 calories per gram. Second, the human body is much more efficient in converting dietary fat into body fat than it is in storing away the calories from other foods. Suppose, for example, that you eat 100 calories more than you burn up. If those 100 calories are in the form of fat, 97 will be stored as triglycerides in your body fat. But if the 100 excess calories are from carbohydrates, only 77 will be stored away, since your body will use up 23 calories turning carbohydrates into triglycerides.

Count fat instead of calories. Still, you're counting toward a target — how many grams of fat should you eat? It's a complex question, but you've already figured out the answer in Chapter 4. Review Table 4–4. For a healthy heart, a 20 percent fat intake is reasonable — unless your risk score is high, in which case you should aim closer to 10 percent. For less body fat, a 20 percent fat intake is also reasonable — unless your BMI is high, in which case you should aim closer to 10 percent.

Reduce your dietary fat for your heart and your hips. Chapter 4 tells you exactly how to achieve a fat accompli.

Increase your dietary fiber. It's not simply a question of finding something to eat instead of fat. Chapter 8 explains all the ways fiber will help your heart, your gastrointestinal tract, and your health. Reducing your body fat is among these benefits.

Fiber is present only in vegetable foods; most of these foods are very low in fat and calories. High-fiber foods take longer to eat, another advantage. Soluble fiber, in particular, reduces hunger by delaying the passage of food from the stomach. Both soluble and insoluble fiber tend to distend the stomach and intestines, making you feel full (though also, perhaps, producing gas). High-fiber foods help reduce blood levels of insulin, a hormone that stimulates appetite. Last but not least, high-fiber foods are interesting, enjoyable, and satisfying, making it easy for you to stick to the hearty option.

How much fiber should you consume? Chapter 8 sets 30 grams a day as a general target, explaining also where to find dietary fiber and how to count it. But if your goals include decreasing your body fat, consider increasing your daily fiber intake to 40 to 50 grams; for comfort's sake, go slowly, following the guidelines in Chapter 8.

Shift from simple sugars to complex carbohydrates. Even though you're not counting calories, you'll benefit from cutting down on calorie-dense foods. Fats heads the list, of course, but simple sugars can pack a lot of calories into a small morsel of candy or cake.

All carbohydrates are composed of just carbon, hydrogen, and oxygen. Simple sugars are small molecules that are rapidly absorbed into the bloodstream, boosting blood sugar levels and stimulating a surge of insulin from the pancreas. Complex carbohydrates, in contrast, are large molecules that must be digested into simple sugars before they're absorbed; as a result, they're not responsible for an appetite-stimulating jolt of insulin. Simple sugars are added to refined, processed foods, which are usually low in fiber and other nutrients; quite the reverse is true of complex carbohydrates, which are normally present in nutrient- and fiber-rich starchy foods. Sugary foods are fattening, but starchy foods are filling. A cookie and a potato, for example, may each have 100 calories; try eating eight potatoes!

America has a sweet tooth to match its fat hips. The average American consumes more than 130 pounds of sugar each year, nearly double the national average in 1900. But if our diets are high in sugars, they are low in starches. Complex carbohydrates provide only 24 percent of America's calories, compared with up to 75 percent in less industrialized countries.

The hearty option advocates reducing simple sugars. You can detect them by taste and reputation, or you can find them by reading food labels. Remember that brown sugar is as calorie-dense as white, and that the "natural" sugars in honey, corn syrup, maple syrup, and molasses are no better than the refined sugars labeled as sucrose, glucose, dextrose, maltose, fructose, and lactose.

The hearty option asks you to increase the complex carbohydrates in your diet until they provide at least 65 percent of your calories. You'll be eating pasta, potatoes, beans, cereals, and breads. Conventional dieters will envy your menu — and your results.

Eat protein in moderation. High-protein foods are the prestige items in the American diet. They are also the main fare in traditional weight loss plans; eat the steak but skip the potato is the usual creed. As usual, it's backward.

Proteins are, of course, crucial for health. They are essential for muscles, bones, tissue growth and repair, and for the enzymes that power the body's metabolism. But the entire body contains just 3 pounds of protein; as little as 2 ounces of dietary protein per day will provide all the amino acids needed to keep the body's proteins in fine repair. Excess protein will not make muscles stronger; quite the contrary, they'll be stored away just like any excess energy, as body fat. And excess protein may, over the years, contribute to kidney damage and to urinary calcium losses. As a rule of thumb, 15 percent of your daily calories should come from protein; that translates to no more than 60 grams (2 ounces) per day for most adults.

The hearty option puts protein in its place. It calls for a dramatic reduction in dietary fat and corresponding increase in dietary fiber. Simple carbohydrates, sugars, should also be reduced. What makes up the balance?

Consider again the steak and potato. A 6-ounce steak contains 53 grams of protein, just about enough for an entire day. But it also contains 15 grams of fat, 150 milligrams of cholesterol, and no fiber. The potato, in contrast, provides only 5 grams of protein but adds 3 grams of fiber, only a trace of fat, and no cholesterol. Need more convincing? The potato contains 100 calories, the steak 400.

Cut way down on fat and sugar. Boost your dietary fiber. Make up the difference with complex carbohydrates, keeping dietary protein to a modest 15 percent of calories. And remember that beans, grains, and vegetables are excellent sources of high-quality proteins that are free of cholesterol and saturated fat.

Avoid junk food. You know what it is, and that it's well named. A 1-ounce serving of potato chips has more calories than an 8-ounce baked potato. The chips have fat and salt, the real potato fiber, vitamins, potassium, and iron. The chips cost more. The chips are fast, the potato filling.

Don't be seduced by nonfat junk foods. Food manufacturers and advertising moguls are not dummies. First, they pushed NO-CHOLESTEROL foods, neglecting to tell us about the fat they contained. Now they promote NO-FAT foods. It's an improvement, but it's not good enough for the hearty option. No-fat cake, for example, has plenty of calories but no fiber and few nutrients. It's not filling, but it has the taste you've been taught to like. It's easy to eat and it's okay for a treat, but it's not the right thing to depend on. Instead, reach for nonfat natural foods, for fruits, veggies, and whole grain products.

Exert discipline early in your food chain. Planning a hearty-option menu requires no sacrifice. Shopping for low-fat foods is not taxing. Cooking right is an acquired skill, and it can be time consuming — but if you have the right ingredients and recipes, it won't require willpower. If you use discipline when you plan, shop, and cook, you won't have to struggle against temptation when you eat. Instead, you'll love your hearty meals and snacks.

Think about food. Traditional diet plans try to distract you from thinking about food. It never works. Low-fat, high-fiber eating is not a punishment. Quite the reverse: you'll find it stimulating and satisfying if you learn about it. Explore new foods and experiment with new recipes. Take it as a challenge, but give yourself time to meet the challenge slowly.

Don't try to ignore food. Instead, embrace it, learning to enjoy your new lifelong style of eating. Bruce Springsteen tells us, "Everybody has a hungry heart"; if you feed yours right, you'll have a healthy heart, and you'll meet your goals for body fat.

Exercise. It's the missing ingredient in quick-fix diet schemes but an essential element in the hearty option.

Obesity is caused by an energy surplus — not a surfeit of vim and vigor, but an excess of calories that are stored as triglycerides in the body's fatty tissues. Body fat is always determined by a simple, immutable equation: Body Fat = Energy Consumed − Energy Expended.

The only way to correct obesity is to rebalance the body's energy equation. Foods that are low in fat but high in fiber, low in sugars but high in complex carbohydrates, will reduce the caloric energy you take in. But even the best diet will not reduce unwanted body fat. Of equal importance is exercise — it's the only way to burn your excess energy.

Aerobic exercise is the best for your waist, as it is for your heart. Aerobic exercise burns calories; at rest a 150-pound person burns only

70 calories an hour, but moderate aerobic exercise can use 700 calories per hour, intense exertion even more. Exercise burns fat; during moderate aerobic exercise, muscles use free fatty acids as well as glycogen to provide the fuel they need. There is also some evidence that exercise actually increases the body's metabolic rate, so you'll go on burning away excess calories even after you've moved from gym to shower. Other studies suggest that exercise suppresses appetite, a surprise to the couch potato who thinks of a workout as a brisk trip to the fridge.

Exercise helps in two more ways. First, it dissipates stress and fights depression, both common causes of overindulgence in sweet or fatty "comfort foods"; it also provides a sense of mastery and control, making it easier to stick with the hearty option. Second, exercise seems to re-set the body's "set point." Although the set point theory hasn't been proved, it is a useful empirical explanation for the indisputable fact that body weight resists change. The only way to lower your set point and to keep it down is to exercise it down.

In theory, aerobic exercise should be able to correct and prevent obesity. In practice, it will live up to its billing, but only if it's practiced regularly. Too often, alas, exercise is just theoretical. Average Americans, its true, are eating less fat, but they are also exercising less, burning 200 *fewer* calories each day then they did 30 years ago. Is it any wonder that we're becoming ever more heavyhearted?

Exercise is the best-kept secret in weight control, but it's no secret to people who are taking care of their hearts. Chapter 5 helped you construct a safe, effective, enjoyable exercise program. It also helped you set your exercise goals; for risk reduction, optimal cardiac function, and maximum longevity, an average of 30 minutes a day is about right. But if shedding fat is an important personal objective, consider gradually building up to twice that level, or even more if you really get into it. Remember, though, that swimming is less effective for weight loss than are the other types of aerobic exercise. In any form, exercise is a big commitment, but it has big rewards — or, in the case of your profile, little rewards.

Obesity is a weighty problem. Traditional remedies are disheartening at best, and medical options are no better. The hearty option, though, can solve the problem, not quickly or easily perhaps, but permanently and enjoyably.

Instead of weighing in with more statistics, I'll reveal just one last set of figures: my own. Between ages 20 and 35 I had the all-too-common experience of a 30-pound weight gain. At 35 I changed my ways, gradually learning to take care of my heart and health. As a result, I've had the all-too-rare experience of losing 35 pounds and keeping it off. My weight has gone from 200 to 165, my waistline from 37 to 33, and my BMI from 26 to 21. They're wonderful results, but they're not what got me started or what keeps me going. I got started to lower my cholesterol, reduce my blood pressure, kick my smoking habit, and escape my family's history of heart disease and early death, and I've done them all. I keep going because the hearty option keeps me feeling fit, energetic, and happy. I have a scale, but I get on it only when my wife tells me I'm looking too thin!

Don't worry about your weight. Instead of a New Year's Day resolution to lose weight, make a Valentine's Day resolution to take care of your heart — by next New Year's Day, your weight problem will be history. If you take care of your heart, your weight will take care of itself.

Chapter 16

Estrogens: Keeping Women Young at Heart

IT'S A NATURAL PRODUCT of the human body and a powerful medication. It's a prescription drug, but the decision to take it is best made by patients, not doctors. It can cut the risk of heart attack and stroke by nearly 50 percent, but it's rarely prescribed for this purpose. It can fight atherosclerosis in half the adult population, but it increases the risk of heart disease in the other half. It's controversial, but it needn't be. It's estrogen.

Heart attacks are rare in younger women, but they become progressively more common in the postmenopausal years. Estrogen replacement therapy can keep older women young at heart, but its role in conquering heart disease is often overlooked amidst the controversies about its more obvious benefits — and its well-publicized potential risks. As scientific data accumulate, estrogen therapy can be approached rationally, not emotionally. One indisputable fact is that it's an issue for women only; men who take estrogens get more heart disease, not less. Women should learn the facts about estrogens so they can make decisions about their use jointly with their doctors.

Like the nonprescription ways to fight atherosclerosis that have been discussed in Part 2, postmenopausal estrogen replacement can be a powerful way to protect your heart. Like the prescription drugs discussed in Chapter 18, it requires your doctor's agreement and help. But more than with any other prescription drug, the final decision about estrogen therapy is each woman's responsibility.

What Is Menopause?

Atherosclerosis is not a natural condition, but menopause is entirely normal.

The female hormone estrogen is produced principally by tiny follicles in the ovaries. More than 7 million follicles are present at birth, but they don't start producing estrogens until puberty. At puberty, the brain's hypothalamus and pituitary gland begin to secrete hormones that stimulate the ovaries. At the behest of these hormones, the follicles go to work, producing large amounts of estrogen in the first half of each menstrual cycle and adding the second female hormone, progesterone, during the second half.

Cyclic production of estrogen and progesterone continue throughout the reproductive years. At menopause, however, both hormones fall to very low levels. It's a gradual process that occurs because the ovaries have used up all 7 million follicles. The brain and hypothalamus continue to pour out their stimulatory hormones, but because 99 percent of the follicles are gone, the ovaries can no longer respond.

Menopause is inevitable, but its timing is variable. The age of menopause depends on many factors, including nutrition, body fat, and heredity. In American women the average age of menopause is 50, older than in most other countries.

Few women would care about menopause if it were only a matter of low hormone levels. But menopause is much more. Heralded by the halt of menstrual cycles, menopause signifies the end of reproductive capacity and the beginning of many bodily changes. Like most changes, menopause is often greeted with apprehension and concern. But women who understand menopause can separate myth from reality, allowing them to decide whether to let nature take its course or to mimic reproductive cycles with hormone replacement therapy.

Menopause and Atherosclerosis

Most women don't even list heart disease among their concerns about menopause. Most doctors don't, either. But atherosclerosis is actually the major medical consequence of menopause, at least in industrialized societies, where the disease is so prevalent.

Heart attacks and strokes, the lethal manifestations of atherosclerosis, are rare in premenopausal women. But menopause changes things, signaling an increase in the risk of cardiovascular disease that continues to mount as women age. In the final analysis, heart attack is the leading killer of American women, just as it is for men; in fact, in each of the last 10 years, heart disease has claimed the lives of more women than men.

Heart disease increases with age in men even though their hormone levels don't change. But the age-related increase is more abrupt and dramatic in women, and menopause is the reason. More specifically, the fall in blood estrogen levels is responsible for the rise in heart disease. A 1993 Dutch study explains the link: blood cholesterol levels begin to rise 2 years before menopause, and they continue to increase for 6 years beyond menopause, after which they remain stable. In all, cholesterol levels rise by an average of 19 percent after menopause; that's enough to increase the risk of heart attack by 40 to 60 percent.

American women are beginning to fight back; between 1979 and 1989, their death rate from heart attack fell 26 percent, while their death rate from stroke declined by 31 percent. But like men, women can do better, much better. Both sexes can gain important protection from 14 points of this book's program to conquer heart disease, but women have a fifteenth strategy at their disposal: estrogen.

If heart disease and strokes were the only consideration, the decision would be simple, and doctors would prescribe estrogens for every postmenopausal women. But the decision is much more complex, involving every part of a woman's body.

Menopause and Health

Atherosclerosis is the most dangerous medical consequence of menopause. The second most dangerous is osteoporosis; declining estrogen levels are responsible for weakening bones just as they're to blame for hardening arteries.

Bones are complex, metabolically active tissues. Although growth ceases in adolescence, bone formation continues throughout life. Calcium is constantly entering and leaving bony tissue; at any one time, about 7 percent of the body's bone mass is being remodeled.

To keep bones strong, new bone formation must balance the rate of calcium removal. In women, the crucial determinant of the balance is estrogen. Bone loss accelerates in the years leading up to menopause; as estrogen levels fall further, so do bone calcium levels. The average adult has about two and a half pounds of calcium stored in bone; the average woman will lose half her bone calcium in the postmenopausal years.

Twenty million American women have osteoporosis. Osteoporosis means that bones lack calcium; as a consequence, bones are weak. Osteoporosis is responsible for the loss of height and the "dowager's hump" that affect so many women. Even worse are the 1 million osteoporosis-related fractures suffered by American women each year. The spine, hips, and wrists are most vulnerable; in all, 1 of every 3 American women will develop a fractured vertebral bone in her spine, and 1 in 7 will fracture a hip or wrist. Pain and disability are the obvious consequences. Not so obvious is the fact that hip fractures in older women carry a 1-year mortality of 20 percent and a 30 percent risk of requiring nursing home care. Another consequence is financial; osteoporosis drains the American economy of $7 billion each year.

Menopause is inevitable, but osteoporosis can be prevented. Happily some of the tools that women should use to fight atherosclerosis will also help prevent osteoporosis; exercise (Chapter 5) and a high-calcium diet (Chapter 6) are high on the list. But the best way to prevent osteoporosis is to combine exercise and diet with postmenopausal estrogen replacement therapy.

Every woman should exercise regularly and eat well. But estrogen replacement is not for every woman. Part of the decision depends on the risk of atherosclerosis, another part on the risk of osteoporosis. Table 16–1 summarizes risk factors for osteoporosis.

Atherosclerosis and osteoporosis are the major medical consequences of menopause, but other bodily changes resulting from declining estrogen levels may be of even greater personal concern.

Many women pass through menopause without any discomfort, but others experience distressing symptoms. Hot flashes are the most common. They are typically experienced as an uncomfortably warm feeling on the face, back, and chest, often accompanied by flushing of the skin. Although hot flashes last only a minute or two, they can occur up to 10 times a day, sometimes interrupting sleep. Other symptoms of menopause may include skin dryness, vaginal dryness and discomfort during

Table 16–1
FACTORS THAT INCREASE THE RISK OF
OSTEOPOROSIS IN WOMEN

Age and menopause
Family history of osteoporosis
Smoking
Alcohol abuse
Lack of exercise
Dietary deficiencies of calcium, vitamin D, or fluoride
Dietary excesses of protein, sodium, aluminum, magnesium, or caffeine
Never having been pregnant
Thin body build
Various illnesses (diabetes, thyroid and parathyroid disease, adrenal disease,
    liver disease, intestinal diseases)
Various medications (cortisone derivatives, certain antibiotics, anti-seizure
    drugs, and diuretics)

sexual intercourse, urinary burning, and diminished bladder control. Since women depend on androgen, the "male hormone," for libido, menopause itself does not diminish the sex drive. Psychological changes may occur at about the time of menopause, but it's not clear if they are actually caused by falling estrogen levels. Cognitive function may also decline with age; estrogens do not appear to affect normal age-related changes in mental function, but two 1993 studies suggest that they may significantly reduce the risk of Alzheimer's disease.

Estrogen replacement therapy will reduce or eliminate all the bona fide symptoms of menopause. Troublesome symptoms are a valid reason to favor estrogen replacement, but don't expect miracles. Hype and hope notwithstanding, estrogen will not forestall changes in the hair, skin, breasts, and body fat distribution that are part and parcel of normal aging. But even without these false hopes, estrogens can do a lot of good — as well as some harm.

Estrogen Replacement Therapy, Heart Disease, and Stroke

Postmenopausal estrogen therapy fights atherosclerosis. Its most important benefit occurs in the place where atherosclerosis starts, in the blood cholesterol. Many studies have compared the blood cholesterol levels of postmenopausal woman who choose to take estrogens with those who don't. Here at last is an area of menopause in which all the results agree: women who take estrogens after menopause are the clear winners, having lower levels of LDL cholesterol and higher levels of HDL cholesterol. And a 1994 report suggests that estrogen replacement can also reduce oxidative damage to LDL cholesterol, another plus. Importantly, the benefits of estrogen replacement occur both in normal women and in high-risk women with genetically abnormal cholesterol levels. Both the lower LDL and the higher HDL should reduce the risk of heart attacks — and they do.

Although the data are preliminary, new research suggests that estrogen may also fight atherosclerosis in its second stage, in the arterial wall. Estrogen replacement may preserve the coronary arteries' normal production of relaxing factors; without estrogen, arteries may tend to have spasms that can block the flow of blood. Since postmenopausal estrogen users have lower levels of fibrinogen and other clotting factors, it is even possible that estrogen replacement fights heart attacks in their final stage, the formation of blood clots that block blood flow. New studies have raised the possibility that estrogen replacement may improve other heart disease risk factors, including blood pressure, carbohydrate metabolism, and insulin levels, but the evidence for those benefits is still incomplete.

Doctors may debate just how estrogens fight atherosclerosis, but they agree on their net effect — and it's very favorable indeed. At least 31 studies have evaluated the risk of heart attack in postmenopausal estrogen users and nonusers. It's uncommon for all the studies of complex medical issues to agree, but here's a case in which they do: estrogen replacement decreases the risk of heart attacks in postmenopausal women. And the protection is substantial, averaging 44 percent. Since 485,000 American women die from heart attacks every year, estrogen replacement could save more than 200,000 lives annually.

Stroke is the other major manifestation of atherosclerosis, and it's the third leading cause of death in America. In study after study, postmenopausal estrogen replacement has been associated with a greatly reduced risk of stroke. For example, a 1993 study reported on 1,910 postmenopausal American women who had been observed for 12 years; estrogen users had 31 percent fewer strokes than nonusers, even after considering the impact of smoking, hypertension, diabetes, obesity, and

other risk factors. Other studies are even more optimistic, some reporting a 40 to 50 percent reduction in strokes.

Fewer heart attacks and strokes — good news about estrogen replacement. But there's more news, some good, some bad.

Estrogen Replacement and Health

In addition to fighting atherosclerosis, postmenopausal estrogen replacement has two major benefits. One applies to every woman: estrogen therapy substantially reduces the risk of osteoporosis, at least if it's
begun within 5 or 6 years of menopause. In all, postmenopausal women
can reduce their risk of fractures by 60 percent if they take estrogens.
The other benefit applies only to some women: estrogen therapy provides comfort and relief to women who have unpleasant menopausal
symptoms.

There are three major areas of benefit from estrogen replacement:
atherosclerosis, osteoporosis, and menopausal symptoms. But there are
also three potential drawbacks: symptomatic side effects, breast cancer,
and endometrial cancer.

Although most postmenopausal women feel better taking estrogens,
some complain of bloating, nausea, weight gain, breast fullness, vaginal
bleeding, or fluid retention. In most cases, these side effects can be controlled by changing the estrogen preparation or decreasing its dose.
Some women with migraines experience more headaches while taking
estrogens. Other possible side effects of estrogen include gallstones and
phlebitis (inflammation of veins).

Breast cancer is a much greater worry for women who are considering postmenopausal estrogen replacement. Despite intensive study,
the evidence here is contradictory; some studies have found an increased risk of breast cancer in estrogen users, while others have
detected no excess risk. But even when estrogen therapy seemed to increase risk, the increase was slight; often it was confined to high estrogen
doses, possibly prolonged use, or unconjugated estrogen preparations.

More studies will be needed to clarify a possible link between postmenopausal estrogen replacement and breast cancer. It's a reminder that
all postmenopausal women should have annual mammograms and regular breast exams. All women should also make the lifestyle changes that
will reduce their risk of developing breast cancer; exercise and

low-fat, high-fiber diets are the key — they should already be familiar, since they're also important ways to fight atherosclerosis (Chapters 4, 5, and 8).

Even with these precautions, worry about breast cancer is a negative in the estrogen replacement equation. Women who are at increased risk for breast cancer have more reason to be concerned; Table 9–1 reviews breast cancer risk factors (see page 231). Unfortunately, women who choose to use low-dose alcohol to fight atherosclerosis have an additional worry, since at least one study suggests the combination of alcohol and estrogen increases breast cancer risk. It's doubly unfortunate, since high cardiac risk scores and low HDL cholesterol levels would otherwise tend to favor both low-dose alcohol and estrogen replacement therapy. Until we have more information, it's probably best for women at risk to choose between these two ways to conquer heart disease instead of adopting both.

There is uncertainty about estrogen replacement and breast cancer, but no doubt about estrogens and endometrial cancer. Estrogen therapy increases the risk of developing cancer of the lining of the uterus. It's no surprise, since the conditions that predispose to endometrial cancer all involve high estrogen levels: puberty, late menopause, never having been pregnant, and a high-fat diet.

Endometrial cancer is common, affecting some 34,000 American women each year. Early detection is difficult because the Pap smears that are so useful for finding early cancers of the cervix are not effective for detecting endometrial cancers. Despite the lack of a good screening test, endometrial cancer responds well to treatment, with a cure rate of up to 70 percent.

Curable or not, endometrial cancer is a negative in the estrogen replacement equation, since estrogen users are 3 to 10 times more likely to develop cancer of the uterus. But there is a way around this problem. If postmenopausal women take progesterone as well as estrogen, their risk of endometrial cancer is no greater than if they took no hormones at all.

Progesterone is, of course, the second female sex hormone. Before menopause, estrogen is the dominant hormone in the first half of each menstrual cycle, while progesterone rises in the second half. Postmenopausal women can mimic the natural cycle by taking estrogen for the first 25 days of each month, adding progesterone for days 16 to 25. This program eliminates the increased risk of endometrial cancer without changing the possible risk of breast cancer one way or the other. But since all hormones are withdrawn at the end of each month, women on this program generally experience mild vaginal bleeding at the end of each cycle; this, too, mimics youthful nature, but the bleeding is much milder than in natural menstrual cycles. Even so, many women dislike monthly bleeding; to avoid bleeding, newer regimens prescribe low doses of progesterone, which are taken along with conventional doses of estrogen every day.

Since hysterectomies remove the uterus, women who have had this operation can take estrogen every day without adding progesterone. But other women who choose estrogen replacement should consider taking progesterone as well. We don't yet know if the combined program will be as good as estrogen alone in fighting atherosclerosis, but the evidence at hand is encouraging. Like women taking estrogen alone, women taking both hormones have lower LDL and higher HDL cholesterol levels; unlike women who take estrogen alone, they also have lower blood triglyceride levels, a possible benefit in the fight against heart disease.

Progesterone eliminates the worry about uterine cancer and estrogen replacement. For additional protection, some gynecologists recommend routine endometrial biopsies, which can be done simply in an office setting. Other authorities don't feel these tests are necessary; I'm inclined to recommend them only for women who choose to take postmenopausal estrogens without progesterone.

Is Estrogen Replacement Right for You?

It's a complex decision; in starkest terms, it comes down to the benefits for atherosclerosis and osteoporosis versus the possible risks of breast and uterine cancer.

To help you decide, consider the outlook for healthy women at average risk for atherosclerosis and cancer who do not take postmenopausal estrogens.

Imagine 2,000 women who are healthy at age 50. In each postmenopausal year:

- 20 will develop heart disease; 12 will die of it.
- 11 will develop osteoporosis; 1 will die of it.

- 6 will develop breast cancer; 2 will die of it.
- 3 will develop endometrial cancer; 1 will die of it.

As you can see, heart disease is so much more common than breast and endometrial cancer combined that estrogen therapy should produce a net gain of major proportions for postmenopausal women. And you don't have to imagine these results — direct observations have demonstrated that women who take postmenopausal estrogens do in fact live longer.

A 1991 study from the University of California reported the results of estrogen therapy in 8,881 postmenopausal women. Estrogen replacement produced a significant decrease in the death rate from heart attack and stroke. The death rate from breast cancer and all other cancers was actually lower in women who took estrogens, but this reduction was not statistically significant. Overall, estrogen replacement produced a 20 percent reduction in mortality — a highly significant benefit indeed. Importantly, the study found that the women who had been taking estrogens the longest enjoyed the greatest benefit; for example, women who had used estrogen replacement therapy for 15 years had a 40 percent lower death rate than women of the same ages who had never taken estrogen.

These favorable results for estrogen replacement therapy were confirmed by a 1992 study in the *Annals of Internal Medicine;* all things considered, it calculated that postmenopausal estrogen therapy extends overall life expectancy by 1.1 years.

Because no woman is average, each woman will have to decide if estrogen replacement is right for her. The decision involves three elements: the benefits of estrogen, the risks of hormones, and personal preferences.

The greatest benefit is, of course, substantial protection against atherosclerosis, amounting to a 44 percent reduction in the risk of heart attack and similar protection against stroke. Women who are at high risk of atherosclerosis should consider strongly taking estrogen after menopause; since estrogen exerts much of its benefit by improving blood cholesterol levels, women with high LDL and/or low HDL cholesterols are particularly good candidates for hormone replacement. To find out if you are in this category, review your risk score from Table 2–11.

Table 16–2
FACTORS INFLUENCING THE DECISION TO USE
POSTMENOPAUSAL ESTROGEN REPLACEMENT

Factors Favoring Estrogen

Major factors	Increased risk of atherosclerosis (Table 2–11)
	Increased risk of osteoporosis (Table 16–1)
	Troublesome menopausal symptoms
Minor factors	Having had a hysterectomy
	Availability of good medical follow-up, including mammograms and gynecological evaluations

Factors Discouraging Estrogen

Major factors	Increased risk of endometrial cancer (page 349)
	Increased risk for breast cancer (Table 9–1)
Minor factors	Regular alcohol consumption
	Unpleasant side effects of estrogen
	Uterine fibroids or endometriosis
	Gallbladder disease
	Recurrent phlebitis
	Frequent migraine headaches

Factors That Preclude Estrogen	Breast cancer
	Endometrial cancer
	Active liver disease

The other benefits of hormone replacement are protection against osteoporosis and control of menopausal symptoms. The major negatives are an increased risk of endometrial cancer, which can be neutralized by progesterone use, and a possible slight increase in breast cancer risk. Table 16–2 will allow you to construct your own balance sheet.

Two elements are missing from Table 16–2, and both are important. The first is personal preference. Menopause is not a disease, but an entirely natural, normal, inevitable part of life. Many women prefer to let nature takes its course, while others prefer to intervene with hormone replacement. For the average American woman, medical factors favor hormones, but it's a personal decision with no right answer. Women who choose to go natural, however, should be doubly sure to lead the natural lifestyle that will reduce their risk of atherosclerosis.

The second element in the decision process that hasn't been considered thus far is your doctor. Estrogens and progesterones are prescription drugs. Your doctor should be able to provide important advice about them as well as providing consent in prescription form. Discuss hormone replacement with your doctor to arrive at a mutual decision and a plan for medical follow-up.

Your doctor should also discuss the type of hormone to prescribe. Many forms are available. The most widely used in the United States is conjugated estrogen tablets (Premarin); other preparations include a slightly different conjugated estrogen tablet (Estratab), estrone tablets (Ogen), estradiol tablets (Estinyl), and estradiol skin patches, which are applied twice weekly (Estroderm). Estrogen pills may be preferable to patches for women with abnormal cholesterol levels, since pills deliver the hormone directly to the liver, which controls cholesterol metabolism. In contrast, patches may be preferable for women with high triglyceride levels, migraines, liver or gallbladder disease, phlebitis, or tobacco abuse. The most commonly used form of progesterone is medroxyprogesterone (Provera tablets).

Your doctor will discuss the advantages of each preparation. I generally prescribe Premarin (usually .625 milligrams) with or without Provera (usually 5 or 10 milligrams). Women who have had a hysterectomy can take the estrogen daily. For the majority who have not had surgery, there are two options. First, use an estrogen alone, taking the pills for the first 25 days of each month. Because of the risk of endometrial cancer, I recommend yearly gynecological exams for women taking estrogen alone; although proof of benefit is lacking, many gynecologists perform endometrial biopsies at the time of those exams. If vaginal bleeding at the end of each month isn't a hassle, however, I prefer to add progesterone for days 16 to 25 of each month, thus eliminating the need to consider endometrial biopsies. In either case, annual mammograms are important — just as they are for postmenopausal women who do not take estrogens.

If you decide to take estrogens, when should you start? Finally a question with an easy answer: as soon as possible after menopause, but in any case within 5 to 6 years. How long should you continue treatment? Another tough question! In fact, there is no good answer to this one. At present, most doctors recommend estrogen for about ten years, or until your mid-60s. Two 1993 studies, however, suggest that estrogens may also be helpful for older women. In the first, women who took estrogens beyond age 65 had better cholesterol levels and less atherosclerosis than their contemporaries who were not taking hormones. In the second, women with an average age of 76 lost their protection against osteoporosis when they stopped taking estrogens. Stay tuned for more data — and at any age, keep alert for changes in your body that may cause you to reevaluate treatment. You've only signed on for one day at a time, and you can change your mind at any time.

In fact, we can all anticipate changes in the guidelines for estrogen replacement as new data become available. The issue is complex, and it involves each and every woman. Careful evaluation and reevaluation are mandatory. A look back over the past three decades provides a fascinating insight into estrogen replacement. In the 1960s, estrogens were the rage — mostly for the wrong reason, the hope of remaining "feminine forever." The predictable backlash arrived in the 1970s with rising concerns about endometrial cancer. Enthusiasm returned in the '80s because of new estrogen-progesterone regimens and rising concerns about heart disease and osteoporosis. The '90s will surely be interesting, with new data about breast cancer and alternative programs to prevent osteoporosis due to arrive.

About 3 million postmenopausal American women take estrogens. In view of their susceptibility to heart attack and stroke, many more should consider hormone replacement. It's a powerful way to fight atherosclerosis, an extra option for women who choose to use it in conjunction with a comprehensive program to conquer heart disease.

Chapter 17

Facts or Fads: Other Tips That May Help

THIS CHAPTER does not present a single strategy to conquer heart disease, but a series of options for your consideration. Some are grounded in scientific fact, but their overall importance is uncertain or minor; still, they warrant consideration as you fine-tune your personal plan. Others are just possibilities, requiring much more research to determine if they have merit; they're interesting reminders that the fight against atherosclerosis will continue to evolve. Still others are but fads, based on little more than rumor and wishful thinking; even if they're harmless, they should be avoided because they add only distracting complexity and a false sense of security.

Vitamins B₆ and B₁₂ and Folic Acid

Few physicians recommend vitamin supplements; fewer still use them for cardiovascular disease. Antioxidant vitamins, though, are beginning to earn a place in the fight against atherosclerosis (Chapter 11). In the future, vitamins B_6, B_{12}, and folic acid may join them — or, on the other hand, they may not prove useful.

It's a complex story. The first chapter centers on a chemical called homocysteine. Despite its formidable name, homocysteine is just an amino acid. Like the other amino acids, homocysteine is a nitrogen-rich compound that is used by the body to build proteins; unlike most amino acids, homocysteine also contains sulfur.

Homocysteine is a normal constant of the human body. But that doesn't guarantee that it's harmless. In fact, elevated levels of homocysteine are emerging as a potentially important atherosclerosis risk factor.

Although research in this area is just now gaining the momentum it deserves, the first observations about homocysteine and cardiovascular disease date back 25 years to the discovery of a rare genetic disease called homocysteinuria. Patients with this disorder have an inborn metabolic defect that results in extremely large amounts of homocysteine in their blood and urine. Afflicted persons suffer from severe premature vascular disease, often dying in their 20s from heart attacks, strokes, or blood clots. But because of its rarity, homocysteinuria was treated as an unfortunate genetic curiosity rather than as a possible clue to the cause of atherosclerosis in people who don't have the two abnormal genes responsible for homocysteinuria.

What's bringing homocysteine into the medical mainstream? It's the observation that elevated levels of the amino acid are associated with an increased risk of atherosclerosis. And in contrast to the extreme elevations that characterize the rare genetic disease, even modest elevations are associated with atherosclerosis in genetically normal adults.

The most convincing data were reported by the U.S. Physicians' Health Study in 1992. Blood was collected from 14,916 apparently healthy men, who were then observed for a 5-year period. Men who developed heart disease during the study were compared with those who remained well; the two groups were analyzed for their blood homocysteine levels as well as for traditional atherosclerosis risk factors. The results were striking: elevated homocysteine levels were associated with a 3-fold increase in the risk of heart attack, even after other risk factors were taken into account. Nor does this study stand alone; at least 8 other studies dating back to 1984 have reported an association between high levels of homocysteine and severe atherosclerosis involving arteries of the heart, brain, or legs. In some studies, a modest elevation of homocysteine was an even stronger risk factor than smoking or elevated LDL cholesterol levels. And a 1993 study found that high homocysteine levels can activate the blood clotting system, adding the insult of clots to the injury of atherosclerosis.

Even if you're fascinated by these new observations, they won't help you fight atherosclerosis — until you consider the story's second chapter, which is about vitamins.

Biochemists are still working to understand the details of homocysteine metabolism, but they've already learned that three vitamins, B_6, B_{12}, and folic acid, play an important role in the process. A 1992 study in the *American Journal of Clinical Nutrition* tells us just how important a role: among men with abnormally high homocysteine levels, 25 percent were B_6 deficient, 57 percent were low in B_{12}, and 59 percent were deficient in folic acid.

Vitamin deficiencies appear to be associated with elevated homocysteine levels. Animal studies dating back to 1949 have shown that deficiencies of vitamin B_6 can cause accelerated atherosclerosis; unfortunately homocysteine levels were not studied in these animals, nor have B_{12} and folic acid been tested in similar experiments.

Human studies have not yet evaluated a possible role for B_6, B_{12}, or folic acid in the therapy of atherosclerosis. But the effect of vitamin supplements on homocysteine levels has been investigated. The vitamins work; daily supplements bring down homocysteine levels in just 6 weeks. And only small amounts are needed, including 2 milligrams of B_6, 0.4 milligrams of folic acid, and 6 micrograms of B_{12}.

Before you rush out to buy vitamin pills or have your blood homocysteine level checked, consider these three vitamins in perspective.

Discovered in 1934, vitamin B_6, or pyridoxine, is essential for normal nervous system function and red blood cell formation. B_6 is found in whole grains, soybeans, peanuts, bananas, poultry, and meat. The U.S. Recommended Daily Allowance is 2 milligrams; large overdoses can result in nerve cell damage.

Vitamin B_{12}, or cobalamine, was first discovered in 1926; its early investigators went on to win a Nobel Prize for their work treating pernicious anemia with B_{12}. In addition to its vital role in the formation of blood cells, B_{12} is essential for normal function of the nervous system. Because it's found only in animal products such as poultry, fish, dairy products, and meat, B_{12} is the only vitamin that may be lacking in strict vegetarian diets. The U.S. Recommended Daily Allowance of B_{12} is 6 micrograms.

Not recognized until 1941, folic acid was the last vitamin to be discovered. Like B_{12}, folic acid is essential for the formation of red blood cells; unlike B_{12}, it's provided by many vegetables, fruits, legumes, and grains as well as by poultry and meat. The U.S. Recommended Daily Allowance for folic acid is 0.2 milligrams, but women who are pregnant or are planning to become pregnant are now advised to take a daily supplement containing 0.4 milligrams to prevent neural tube defects in their babies.

Except for folic acid supplements during pregnancy and B_{12} supplements for strict vegetarians, healthy adults who eat good diets should not need supplementary B_6, B_{12}, or folic acid. Does the homocysteine story change this traditional view? To take B or not to take B? That is the question — but it's too early to answer it. We already know that elevated homocysteine levels are associated with an increased risk of atherosclerosis. We know, too, that elevated homocysteine levels are common, occurring in 30 percent of people older than 65 according to a 1993 report from the Framingham Heart Study. We know that many apparently healthy adults have suboptimal levels of one or more of the three B vitamins; in the Framingham study, vitamin deficiency accounted for two-thirds of the high homocysteine levels. We know that modest, nontoxic doses of vitamin supplements will reduce blood homocysteine levels. But we don't know if homocysteine is a cause of atherosclerosis or just an innocent bystander that reflects some other yet-to-be discovered causative factor. Nor do we know if reducing homocysteine levels with B_6, B_{12}, and folic acid supplements will reduce the risk of atherosclerosis.

Homocysteine research is at the same early stage cholesterol research was 25 years ago. Until it catches up, it's far too early to recommend routine blood tests for homocysteine, much less universal vitamin supplementation.

Join me in keeping an eye out for new discoveries about homocysteine, vitamins, and atherosclerosis. While we're waiting, I won't object if you decide to take multiple-vitamin tablets — but if you do, follow the general guidelines for vitamins in Chapter 11, and be sure to continue the basic steps that have already proved beneficial against atherosclerosis.

Nuts

It's exciting to think about new ways to fight atherosclerosis. Just a few years ago, most doctors would have said that anyone promoting nuts for heart disease was cracked. New data, however, have given nuts medical respectability; predictably, nut advocates are coming out of their shells.

Four recent studies are driving the traditionalists nuts.

In 1992, investigators from Loma Linda University evaluated nut consumption and heart disease in 31,208 men and women who were observed for at least 6 years. The results were striking: people who consumed nuts frequently had fewer heart attacks than those who ate fewer nuts. In all, eating nuts at least 4 times per week was associated with a 50 percent reduction in heart attacks. These results held up even after body weight, exercise, smoking, age, blood pressure, and cholesterol were considered. The study also evaluated other dietary factors; the only other food that seemed protective was whole wheat bread.

These results are provocative, but they should be interpreted with a bit of caution. All the subjects were Seventh Day Adventists; as a result, the population was virtually free of smoking, and meat consumption was very low. Because of their healthy lifestyle, Adventists have much less heart disease and a 7-year-longer life expectancy than other Americans. More studies will be needed to learn if the protective effect of nuts will hold up in non-Adventist populations. While we're waiting to learn more about nuts, though, we can certainly learn a lot from the diet, smoking, and exercise patterns of the Adventist lifestyle.

Preliminary results suggest the Adventist findings may apply to other groups. In 1993, the Iowa Women's Health Study reported an evaluation of 41,837 women older than 55. It found that women eating the most nuts had the fewest heart attacks, even after considering the impact of all known cardiac risk factors. A third study provided more information about nuts in 1993. It involved many fewer subjects, but its careful metabolic data provide a clue as to how nuts may work. Eighteen healthy men were randomly placed on diets containing 30 percent of calories from fat; in one group, two-thirds of the fat came from walnuts. After 4 weeks, the groups were compared; the cholesterol levels of the walnut-eaters had fallen by more than 12 percent. If sustained, this reduction might translate into a 20 to 30 percent fall in the risk of heart attack. But this study, too, has its limitations. For one thing, it's not clear if the fall in cholesterol was due to the presence of nuts or the absence of other fats that were removed from the diet. The dose of nuts was high, at least 7 times more than most Americans consume. Finally, the trial was brief and involved only a small number of subjects. Taken alone, it's not much to go on, but it adds meat to the studies of Adventists in California and older women in Iowa.

A fourth study from a very different part of the world completes the current, still incomplete, information about nuts. More than 500 heart attack victims in India were studied; all were treated with low-fat diets and standard medications, but half were randomly assigned to consume extra amounts of nuts, grains, fruits, and vegetables. The special diet group had a significant improvement in blood cholesterol levels, many fewer heart attacks, and a lower death rate than the standard care group. The study emphasizes the great value of diet in conquering heart disease, but it doesn't single out nuts as the protective element, since the special-diet group also consumed fruits, vegetables, and grains providing antioxidant vitamins, fiber, and minerals. Still, the study argues for including nuts in a comprehensive dietary attack on heart attacks.

Nuts are high in calories and fat — hardly what you consider a heart-healthy combination. Why might nuts confound expectations? It's true that 70 to 90 percent of the calories in nuts come from fat, but the fatty acids in nuts are very different from those in animal fat. Nuts contain only tiny amounts of saturated fat; instead they have lots of polyunsaturated and monounsaturated fat. The monounsaturates may be particularly helpful; they constitute 78 percent of the fat in hazelnuts, 65 percent in almonds, 49 percent in peanuts, and 23 percent in walnuts. Like canola oil (see page 98), walnuts are also a good source of an omega-3 fatty acid, linolenic acid, that may have benefits similar to the omega-3s in fish oil. Another asset for nuts is their high fiber content, ranging from 5 to 15 percent by weight.

More research may be needed to evaluate the effects of nuts on atherosclerosis and to identify the responsible constituents. Until these puzzles are cracked, it's premature to rely on nuts — but it would be nutty to deny that they may find a useful niche in the fight against atherosclerosis.

Garlic and Onions

If nuts are the newest health craze, garlic and onions are among the oldest; garlic, in fact, occupied a prominent role among the herbal preparations prescribed in an Egyptian medical papyrus from 1550 B.C. For centuries, garlic (*Allium sativum*) and onions (*Allium cepa*) have been popular as folk remedies for ailments ranging from toothaches to tumors. Recent attention, however, centers on a possible role for these foods in cardiovascular disease.

During the past 30 years, many studies have evaluated garlic and onions, using both animals and humans as subjects. Most studies have reported effects that could help fight atherosclerosis. In particular, feeding experiments have shown that garlic and onions may lower LDL cholesterol, raise HDL cholesterol, reduce platelet activation, and boost the clot-dissolving activity of blood.

It would be nice to report that modern science and folk wisdom agree on a natural way to fight atherosclerosis, but things are not as neat as they seem. For one thing, many of the studies were poorly controlled, and others had methodological shortcomings, rendering them scientifically suspect. Another problem is that results have varied; in general, the results have been more favorable for garlic than onions, and better for the whole food than for extracts. Finally, the amounts needed to affect cardiovascular risk factors are quite large, ranging from 2 to 28 cloves of garlic or 2 ounces of onions per day.

Shakespeare advised his actors in *A Midsummer Night's Dream* to "eat no onions, nor garlic, for we are to utter sweet breath." Indeed, bad breath is the major side effect of garlic and onions; heartburn is the other. To get around the olfactory hurdle, odorless extracts of garlic and onions are sold in powder, pill, and liquid forms. Are they too good to be true? Probably; most analyses of commercial extracts find only very low concentrations of allicin, the active ingredient. Despite many claims made for garlic and onion extracts, most experts believe they just don't have enough allicin to do any good at all.

That may be changing. In Germany, where garlic extracts are the largest-selling nonprescription drugs, new studies suggest that extracts may work. The best studies have used Kwai, a dried garlic powder containing 1.3 percent allicin. A 4-month study of 261 people with high cholesterol levels found that 800 milligrams of Kwai per day lowered blood cholesterol levels by about 12 percent; two much smaller studies reported similar results, and another found that Kwai could reduce the blood pressures of hypertensive subjects.

The German garlic powder is now available without prescription in the United States. A 1993 American study evaluated 900 milligrams of Kwai per day in 42 men and women with high cholesterol. At the end of 12 weeks, the garlic tablets produced an 11 percent fall in LDL cholesterol without changing HDL cholesterol or blood pressure levels. Like the recent German study, the trial from New Orleans was careful and well controlled.

A lot more data will be needed before garlic or onions can assume a scientifically validated role in the fight against atherosclerosis. But there is more than a whiff of evidence to support folk wisdom about garlic, at least with regard to blood cholesterol levels.

Coffee

Popular beliefs have long supported garlic and onions, but doctors have disagreed; folk wisdom may, it seems, prove correct. Popular sentiment and medical views have long condemned coffee; both, it seems, may be wrong.

Most "heart healthy" diets exclude coffee and other sources of caffeine. New evidence, however, suggests that these prohibitions are unnecessary.

Caffeine has been present in the human diet since the Stone Age, when the seeds, bark, and leaves of caffeine-containing plants were chewed for food. The practice of infusing plants in hot water to extract caffeine is, of course, much more recent. The earliest written record of coffee is found in a tenth-century Arabian document; according to legend, the stimulatory properties of caffeine were discovered by an Arabian herdsman who noticed that his goats became unusually frisky after grazing on the berries of the plant that's now called *Coffee arabica*. When Arabians began brewing coffee, they gave it the same name as an early form of wine; as the beverage spread around the world, its name went along, being transformed to café, koffie, and kaffee in various lands. By any name, coffee became popular the world over; the Dutch had established plantations in Java by the end of the seventeenth century, and during the eighteenth century cultivation spread throughout the Caribbean to South America.

Another caffeine-containing beverage, tea, is every bit as widespread and venerable as coffee; cocoa is not far behind. And in twentieth-century America, the cola drink and chocolate bar are additional sources of caffeine.

The enduring popularity of caffeine reflects the fact that it's a drug.

It raises the heart rate and blood pressure. It's a diuretic, increasing the flow of urine. It opens bronchial tubes and can be used medicinally to treat asthma. Much better drugs are available for asthma, but caffeine is used clinically to augment the action of mild pain killers, and it does work. Caffeine is a stimulant; some people become habituated to it, and caffeine withdrawal causes headaches and mild depression.

Caffeine has been blamed for headaches, breast disease, birth defects, pancreatic cancer, ulcers, and heart disease. But careful medical studies have exonerated caffeine in all these cases.

Heart disease deserves special mention because the caffeine jitters persist despite important new data from the 1990s. Early studies suggested that coffee could increase the heart rate and blood pressure, potentially harming patients with heart disease. But new information proves that people who use caffeine regularly are spared from this effect. More to the point, several careful studies have shown that neither drinking coffee nor taking caffeine pills produces cardiovascular harm — even in patients hospitalized for heart disease. And even though early studies suggested that heavy coffee drinking might increase the risk of developing heart disease, recent studies of 6,214 residents of Framingham, Massachusetts and of 45,589 health care professionals found *no* link.

After analyzing the 11 best studies published between 1966 and 1991, Drs. Martin Meyers and Antoni Basinski concluded in 1992 that there is *no* association between coffee consumption and coronary heart disease. A 1993 study of 10,000 people in Scotland confirmed that regular coffee use does not raise blood pressure. Going even further, the study found that people who didn't drink any coffee had *more* heart disease than those drinking 1 to 5 cups a day — and that people who consumed over 5 cups a day had the least heart disease of all. Similarly, a 1993 Dutch study found that drinking 4 or more cups of tea per day was associated with a reduced risk of cardiac death, even after other risk factors were taken into account. The probable cardioprotective element in tea is not caffeine, but a group of antioxidant chemicals called flavenoids — but the caffeine surely didn't hurt.

Decaffeinated coffee has also been controversial. Praised because of its low-caffeine content, it's also criticized because of its chemical processing. To date, there is no hard evidence that decaf is any better — or any worse — than the real thing.

It all boils down to this: when it comes to caffeine, the choice is yours. If you choose to drink coffee, brew it with a filter; perked coffee contains oils that may increase blood cholesterol levels, but filters remove the oils, keeping cholesterol levels steady. If you have insomnia or problems with stress, try doing without caffeine to see if you'll improve. If you have gastritis or ulcers, you should probably also avoid caffeine until diet and medication have corrected the problem. Women who are pregnant or who anticipate pregnancy within a month or two have grounds for concern — and confusion — since two careful studies published in 1993 reach opposite conclusions, with one reporting no effect of coffee on fetal health, the other reporting an increased rate of miscarriages in pregnant women who drank coffee. Patients with high blood pressure or heart disease should use caffeine in moderation, which is pretty good advice for the rest of us as well.

Until the very last drop of data is in, we can't be positive that coffee is completely safe. But filtering fact from fiction, there is no evidence that coffee affects atherosclerosis one way or the other. Don't use coffee to fight atherosclerosis, but don't fight coffee to protect your heart.

Antacids

Coffee may give you heartburn, but it won't harm your heart; antacids can relieve heartburn — can they literally soothe your heart?

It's not quite as silly as it sounds. Two recent studies suggest that antacids may be able to improve blood cholesterol levels.

A 1991 Israeli study of 56 men and women tested chewable antacid tablets containing aluminum and magnesium hydroxide plus simethicone. The administration of 2 tablets 4 times a day lowered LDL cholesterol levels by 10 percent after 2 months and 19 percent after 4 months. But before you dash out to buy antacids, consider the results further: HDL cholesterol levels were also lower after 4 months. Because the fall in HDL was smaller, however, the overall cholesterol ratio improved by 13 percent — hopeful results, but ones that call for confirmation.

A 1992 American study of 56 patients with high blood cholesterol levels evaluated the effects of calcium carbonate tablets. All patients were put on low-fat diets; half were randomly assigned to also receive two 200 milligram antacid tablets 3 times a day with meals, while the other half received placebo tablets. At the end of 6 weeks, calcium carbonate produced only a modest 4 percent fall in LDL cholesterol — but it also increased HDL levels by 4 percent. More intriguing results, more need for additional studies. But since dietary calcium lowers the risk of osteoporosis and may help reduce blood pressure (Chapter 6), you may decide to chew on a few calcium carbonate tablets while you're chewing over this preliminary data.

Lecithin

Antacids are not promoted to improve blood cholesterol levels, but they may eventually prove useful for this purpose. Lecithin is heavily promoted as a nonprescription treatment for high blood cholesterol levels, but it is useless for this purpose.

Lecithin is the common name applied to chemicals called phosphatidylcholines; by either name, they are normal constituents of all cell membranes.

Lecithin is synthesized by humans and is not an essential nutrient. Lecithin supplements, generally derived from soybeans, are widely sold over the counter as a remedy for high cholesterol levels. There is no biological reason to think that lecthin could improve cholesterol levels — and there is absolutely no scientific evidence that it works.

Save your money; lecithin won't save your heart.

Nonprescription Remedies: A Cautionary Note

After you've read this far, I'm sure you'll agree that I'm a firm supporter of nonprescription ways to conquer heart disease. More than most doctors, I'm generally receptive to innovative, nontraditional approaches to cardiovascular disease. But I've also learned that it's easier to promise cures than to deliver results.

Prescription drugs are closely regulated, but nonprescription nutritional supplements are not. Surgical procedures are carefully monitored, but nonmedical manipulations are not. Doctors and druggists are called on to back up their claims, but herbalists and hypnotists are not. I encourage you to learn about new approaches to heart disease — but you should learn a lot before you commit your money, your time, and your body to untried remedies.

Why not spend a few dollars, the argument goes, on nonprescription remedies or nonmedical alternative therapies? Since they don't require prescriptions, they must be safe, particularly if they're "all natural." Doctors don't know everything; why not give some other practitioners a try?

Doctors *don't* know everything. But we do know that medicine is a science and that new therapies can be evaluated objectively to learn if they're helpful — or, for that matter, harmful. We also know that "all natural" products can indeed be harmful; the recent examples of eosinophilia-myalgia syndrome from tryptophan supplements and severe kidney disease from Chinese herbal powders are grim reminders.

Beware of snake oil. Don't let the promise of a quick fix distract you from the things that really work. Keep up with new developments in heart disease; the Appendix will give you a start. Turn to your doctor for information and help; Part III will give you some guidance. Above all, take care of your own heart; the 15 ways to fight atherosclerosis discussed in Part II of this book will give you plenty to do. Use these scientifically proven ways to care for your heart, so you won't be sick enough, frightened enough, or frustrated enough to try unproven remedies that are, in fact, too good to be true.

Panacea Surfing: America's Search for a Quick Fix

Heart disease is common, serious, and frightening. It can be prevented, treated, and, in fact, conquered. But the fight against heart disease may seem as complex and difficult as the disease itself. Once you understand atherosclerosis and how to conquer it, you'll come to understand that the heart-healthy lifestyle advocated throughout these pages is actually both simple and enjoyable. But before you get to this point, you may be tempted to try a shortcut, to put your faith in an instant miracle remedy. Don't kid yourself.

There is no quick fix. Too often, Americans look for the easy way out, popping vitamins with the delusion it will protect them from smoking, taking beta-carotene instead of eating carrots, eating an oat bran muffin with their bacon and eggs, or taking a fish oil capsule instead of a long walk. It won't work.

There is no substitute for the basics: a smoke-free environment, a diet low in saturated fat, cholesterol, and salt, but high in fiber, fish, fruit, and vegetables, and lots of physical exercise without excessive mental stress. People who live this way don't need much more to conquer heart disease. But many of us are starting late, and need extra protection — which is why this book offers 15 ways to fight atherosclerosis.

The basics are for everyone, but the supplements are exactly that — supplements that can help some people but are not suited for everyone. Think them over carefully, and try not to get frustrated by sound bites that tell you oat bran is in, then out, then in, or that antioxidants will save you or harm you. Medical science learns in increments, not break-throughs. Early results are often confusing, even contradictory. But eventually a mosaic of facts emerges, giving us a clear picture of what's right.

Instead of surfing through a bewildering array of miracles and men-aces, consider all the facts, then decide what's best for you. Be alert for changes in your body and in our body of medical knowledge so you can adjust to developments that are really meaningful. Never neglect the basics, but fine-tune your program to incorporate new results when their meaning is clear instead of when they first hit the airwaves to the trumpets of salvation or the sirens of alarm.

Ask your doctor for advice, but make the final decision yourself. Even without a medical degree, you can understand your body and our medical database well enough to make an informed decision. It's the reason why this book's program to conquer heart disease is presented in 15 chapters instead of 15 commandments.

PART III

Conventional Cardiology Can Help

Chapter 18

Understanding Medical Tests and Treatments

W E LIVE IN a rapidly changing world. To keep pace, our language must change as well. Patients are now called health care consumers. They no longer go to doctors, nurses, and clinics, but to health care providers. By whatever name, Americans do go, and they do consume. In 1994, Americans will consume more than $1 billion worth of health care, a record amount; it comes to about 15 percent of the nation's gross domestic product, another record.

America spends far more on health care than any other nation on earth. Are we getting our money's worth? Not entirely; we rank first in spending, but a disappointing sixteenth in life expectancy and a shameful twenty-fourth in infant mortality. We also rank distressingly close to the top in the epidemic of atherosclerosis that's swept through the industrialized world.

The explanations for the gap between what we spend and what we get are numerous and complex, but our updated language reveals part of the problem. Americans are willing to spend huge amounts on their health care because they think they're buying health. It's an expectation that will never be met. No matter what you call them and how much you invest in them, the best doctors, most renowned hospitals, most sophisticated tests, and most advanced treatments can never provide health. Only you can do that, by taking care of yourself — that's what the 15-point program is all about.

Can a doctor really be telling you that doctors and hospitals are a waste of time and money? Not at all. In fact, both are absolutely essential — not as *health* care providers but as providers of *medical* care.

We all need doctors when we're sick. The 15-point program will greatly reduce your risk of atherosclerosis and many other illnesses, but even if you've provided yourself with perfect health, you'll still need a doctor for certain screening tests and preventive services.

Your health is too important to be left to doctors, but you need a doctor as your partner in health, and especially in case of sickness. To help you become an active, informed partner instead of a passive "consumer," you should understand medical tests for healthy hearts as well as the tests and treatments that can do so much for people who are sick at heart.

Choosing a Doctor

It's getting harder all the time. In our new world, your first task will be to select a medical plan or insurance policy. Having done that, you can get back to the basic problem of finding a doctor.

What kind of doctor should you see? For people who are healthy, the answer is clear: a primary care physician. Although some women depend on their gynecologist for primary care, most adults obtain primary care from a family practitioner or internist. Either can do the job, but if sophisticated cardiovascular issues are a concern, an internist might be preferable.

Where does the cardiologist fit in? Cardiologists are all trained as internists, but most are more comfortable concentrating on the heart rather than providing primary care. Since internists are all trained in cardiovascular disease, it's usually best to start with an internist, using a cardiologist if necessary for consultations and advanced care, particularly if invasive tests and treatments seem necessary.

The type of practitioner is less important than the doctor's qualifications, interests, practice style, and personality. Unfortunately, these more important characteristics are more difficult to evaluate. Look for a doctor who was educated at a good American medical school and trained at a well-established medical center. Internists and cardiologists should be certified by their specialty boards, the American Board of Internal Medicine and the American Board of Cardiology; many are elected to membership in the American College of Physicians or the American College of Cardiology.

Don't be afraid to ask doctors about their education and certification; if you prefer, contact your county medical society for information or call the American Board of Medical Specialties (800-776-2378). Ask also about other important matters: hospital affiliations, medical coverage when your personal physician is unavailable, office staffing and hours, telephone access, and availability for unscheduled or urgent care. As a rule of thumb, try to find a physician who is affiliated with a university hospital or large medical center that is convenient and accessible.

Personal chemistry is every bit as important as diplomas and affiliations. You can get the names of well-qualified physicians from a medical society or from the physicians' referral service at medical centers, but you'll have to ask friends or relatives for your chemistry lesson. Better yet, see for yourself. Do all the research you can, then make an appointment for the initial visit and see if the chemistry is there. Look for intelligence and dedication, for professional bearing and human warmth, for someone who can listen as well as talk, for someone who'll take you seriously but has a sense of humor, too. Look for doctors who understand that their patients are more important than they are and that their job is not to tell you what to do, but to help you understand what you should do for yourself.

Medical Tests

Everyone needs a doctor, and everyone needs tests — but if you're taking good care of yourself, you'll need just one doc and remarkably few tests. It's a sad fact that testing has assumed a dominant role in medical practice. Patients go to offices expecting blood and urine tests, EKGs, x-rays, and scans of all sorts. More often than not, they get them. Many of these tests are directed to the heart and circulation. Some are essential, but many are extraneous and some even harmful.

The advantages of tests are obvious. *Screening tests* are designed to detect diseases very early, ideally before they've progressed enough to produce symptoms. The routine blood pressure check is an example of a wonderful screening test; mammograms are high-tech screening tests that are also very effective if used properly. *Diagnostic* tests are used after symptoms have appeared, usually to distinguish among several possible causes of a problem. An EKG, for example, can be very useful to determine the cause of a patient's chest pain, but much more elaborate tests such as scans or even angiograms may be needed in difficult cases.

Tests can do a lot of good, which is why patients want them and doctors order them. But tests have assumed an almost mythical status, which is unrealistic and even dangerous. Like all technologies, medical tests will do more good than harm only if they're used appropriately.

Why not have tests?

Tests are not always the best way to establish a diagnosis. Clinical problem solving should always start with a careful medical history; patients should listen to their bodies, and doctors should listen to their patients. The next step should be a simple physical exam; often, the solution to a puzzle is quite literally close at hand. In this era of echocardiograms and heart scans, unfortunately, the stethoscope is becoming an endangered species.

Tests can be misleading. Even the best test will sometimes miss a diagnosis (a false-negative result) or overdiagnose a condition (a false-positive result). The stress test is a good example: in a 50-year-old man with no symptoms, a positive test is 4 times more likely to be a false positive than to indicate real heart disease. Doctors should use only tests of proven sensitivity and specificity.

Tests are often inconvenient and time consuming — not a big deal for tests that are helpful, but another good reason to avoid superfluous tests. Health is humanity's most precious commodity, but time is not far behind.

Tests may be frightening, uncomfortable, or even painful. They can also have side effects; most are mild, but some side effects are far worse than the original disease. That's why doctors should always start with the simplest, safest tests, moving to invasive procedures only when they're absolutely necessary.

Tests are expensive. Most patients are covered by health plans, which pay the direct costs, so they think tests are "free." Far from it; the tyranny of testing plays a major role in America's runaway medical costs.

Tests can provide a false sense of security to patient and physician alike. Doctors who rely excessively on tests may overlook the basics, such as getting to know their patients. Patients who have exalted confidence in tests may use them as excuses for the bodily abuse and disuse that cause atherosclerosis and so many other diseases in the first place.

Do you still want tests? You should — but only if they're the right tests, done at the right time, for the right reasons. In an ideal world, your doctor would always make the right recommendation for testing. In the real world, that's not always the case, so you should learn as much as you can about tests. One thing to learn, though, is that not all the answers are in; doctors are still learning which tests are best, and there are often legitimate grounds for debate and disagreement. The recommendations offered here are based on the guidelines of the U.S. Preventive Services Task Force, the Canadian Task Force, the American Heart Association, and the American College of Cardiology; since they don't always agree, I've also taken personal clinical experience into account. Remember that these recommendations are only general guidelines, and that specific decisions should always be made collaboratively by patient and physician.

Screening Tests for Healthy Adults

It's your job to take care of your heart. Even if you feel perfectly well, though, you should get a little help from screening tests which may identify potential problems that need extra attention.

Cardiovascular tests are at the heart of the matter. Here are some that can help:

- The complete checkup. It's surprising, perhaps, to think of a doctor's exam as a screening test, but screening is an important function of routine checkups. You'll review your family history and recount any symptoms you may have experienced. Your health habits should be discussed; from the cardiovascular viewpoint, smoking, diet, exercise, and stress are particularly important. Your doctor will measure your height, weight, and blood pressure. A complete physical means a head-to-toe exam, including, of course, your heart and circulation. It may seen old-fashioned, but it's still the best way to screen for unsuspected disease and to detect the poor health habits that can cause problems in the future.

How often should you have a physical? Opinions vary. Healthy people who are able to take good care of themselves can use their age as a guide. It's reasonable to have a physical every 5 years between ages 20 and 30, every 3 years between 30 and 40, every 2 years between 40 and 50, and every year thereafter.

- Blood pressure. Because hypertension is common, silent, dangerous, and treatable, blood pressure checks are among the most useful screening tests. Because blood pressure tends to rise with age (in salt-eating industrialized societies, at least), blood pressure should be checked more often as people age. For individuals with good diet and exercise habits and desirable pressures (see Table 2–4), a reading with every physical should suffice. As discussed in Chapter 2, the presence of risk factors makes more frequent checks desirable.

- Cholesterol. Another valuable screening test. The official recommendation is to have cholesterol levels checked every 5 years. Many physicians who are interested in preventive cardiology suggest more frequent measurements; a cholesterol test with each complete physical seems about right. As with blood pressure, though, patients with abnormal results should have them rechecked more frequently, as should people with major cardiac risk factors and people who experience important changes in their diet and exercise patterns, body weights, or medications.

- Blood sugar. Most major health organizations recommend routine blood sugar determinations only during pregnancy. The American Diabetes Association recommends a test every 3 years in the presence of diabetes risk factors (family history, obesity, etc.). Most physicians order a blood sugar test at the time of each complete physical, arguing that it's an easy and inexpensive test that may motivate patients to eat and exercise properly.

- EKG. The electrocardiogram (EKG) is a time-honored component of the "annual checkup." It's a risk-free test that takes less than 5 minutes: the patient rests quietly on a reclining chair or bed, electrodes are placed on the arms and chest, and a stylus records the electrical activity of the heart on a strip of paper. EKGs are vital for evaluating cardiac symptoms such as chest pain, palpitations, and shortness of breath. Less clear, however, is their role in screening healthy people who have no symptoms. The Canadian Task Force says that routine EKGs are unnecessary; the U.S. Preventive Services Task Force recommends them only for people with major cardiac risk factors; the American Heart Association suggests an EKG at ages 20, 40, and 60; the American College of Cardiology advocates them every 5 years and at the physician's discretion. Faced with such disparities, what's a person to do? Listen to your doctor; many perform EKGs with every complete checkup beyond age 50.

- Stress tests. In simplest terms, the stress test is a procedure in which the EKG is monitored continuously while the patient exercises on a treadmill or bike. In traditional terms, the stress test was part of the standard "executive physical." In modern terms, it has fallen appropriately out of favor as a screening test. As discussed in Chapter 5, routine stress tests are not recommended in the absence of symptoms or other abnormalities indicative of heart disease.
- Chest x-rays. At last, an easy one. All the authorities agree that routine chest x-rays have no role in medical screening evaluations.

General Medical Tests. Healthy hearts need healthy bodies. As you'll learn in the Epilogue, the 15-point program to conquer heart disease will ward off many other leading killers as well. But even if you're taking care of your heart and having the cardiovascular screening tests that are recommended, you should have additional tests to be sure the rest of your body is behaving as it should.

- Complete blood count and urinalysis. Although not considered necessary by most major health organizations, these simple tests are almost always performed at the time of complete physical exams.
- Pap smears are strongly recommended for women every 1 to 3 years, at least until age 65.
- Breast examinations by a physician or nurse specialist are recommended every year beyond age 40; younger women may benefit from a clinical exam every three years. All women should also perform self-examinations at least once a month.
- Mammograms. Although their value is controversial in women younger than 50, annual mammograms are strongly recommended for women older than 50.
- Rectal exams. Generally performed on women at the time Pap smears are obtained, annual rectal exams are also recommended by the American Cancer Society for men older than 40.
- Testing for occult blood in the stool. Although they are simple and inexpensive, these tests are controversial. The American Cancer Society recommends them annually beyond age 50, but the U.S. Preventive Services Task Force does not recommend them at all. More data will be necessary to see which group is right.
- Sigmoidoscopy. Like stool blood testing, this procedure is designed to

screen for colon cancer; it's substantially more accurate than stool blood testing, but it's uncomfortable and expensive. Sigmoidoscopies are recommended every 3 to 5 years beyond age 50 by the American Cancer Society, but they are not recommended as routine screening tests by the U.S. Task Force. New data seems to be favoring the Cancer Society's view, but more studies will be needed to settle the issue.

- Prostate Specific Antigen (PSA). Most urologists recommend this "prostate blood test" annually for men above 50, but most internists don't recommend it for screening purposes. Stay tuned for the final word.

- Dental and eye exams. There is surprisingly little data to support or refute the usual practice of routine dental checks every 6 to 12 months and routine eye exams every 1 to 2 years beyond age 40. In the absence of firm data, these traditional practices seem reasonable.

- Immunizations. Although immunizations are treatments rather than tests, they are valuable preventive medical services. Healthy adults should have a tetanus-diphtheria booster every 10 years, a vaccination for pneumococcal pneumonia at age 65, and an influenza vaccination every year beginning at age 65. Patients with heart disease, lung disease, diabetes, and certain other problems should begin their flu and pneumonia shots earlier. Travelers, of course, often need additional protection.

As you can see, the list of routine screening tests is short, and most of the tests are simple, safe, and inexpensive. These tests, though, are just the tip of the iceberg; patients with medical programs often require tests that healthy people never need. You should know what symptoms raise the need for additional cardiovascular testing, and what tests your doctor is likely to recommend.

The Symptoms of Heart Disease

Chest pain is the most notorious symptom of coronary artery disease; the notoriety is well deserved, but it's important to remember that the pain of angina and heart attacks can be atypical, subtle, or even absent. To make matters even more difficult, many noncardiac conditions ranging from inflamed ribs to gastritis and gallstones can mimic the pain of angina.

In classic cases, though, angina is easy to recognize: when the heart muscle is deprived of the oxygen it needs, its distress signal is a heavy, dull pressure that begins in the mid-chest and often radiates to the neck, jaw, or arms, especially the left arm. Typical angina begins during physical exertion, emotional stress, or exposure to the cold, and it's relieved by rest. When the pain occurs at rest, or when it persists, is very severe, or is accompanied by profuse sweating, nausea, or weakness, it may signal an actual heart attack.

In variant angina, pain occurs at rest, sometimes even interrupting sleep. Some patients don't experience any pain, complaining instead of breathlessness, palpitations, or weakness when their heart muscles are oxygen-deprived. Trickiest of all are patients who have no warning symptoms at all (see silent ischemia, Chapter 1).

Chest pain is the most common symptom of heart disease; the second most common, however, is not one of the atypical forms of angina, but an all-too-typical reaction of the human mind: denial. An astoundingly large number of patients with angina dismiss their pain as "heartburn," "indigestion," or "nothing." It is true that disturbances of the stomach, esophagus, and gallbladder can cause chest pain, but it's a great mistake to deny symptoms because you don't want to find out you have heart disease. Instead, listen to your body and discuss its messages with your doctor. Don't deny symptoms of heart disease; instead, face up to them, have them evaluated medically, and renew your commitment to conquer atherosclerosis.

Another key symptom of heart disease is shortness of breath, which generally reflects impaired pumping by the heart's main chamber, the left ventricle. In mild cases, breathlessness occurs with exertion and is relieved by rest. In more advanced cases, technically called congestive heart failure, shortness of breath occurs when patients lie flat but improves when they use extra pillows or sit up in bed. Ankle swelling is another typical symptom of congestive heart failure; initially, it occurs only in the evening, but in more severe cases, it's day-long and may extend up the body, even producing abdominal swelling.

Palpitations may also signal heart disease. They are sometimes experienced as an unduly rapid pulse, sometimes as an erratic rhythm, sometimes as a skipped beat or prolonged pause between beats. An abnormal heart rhythm may also produce lightheadedness or fainting even without the sensation of an erratic pulse. Arrhythmias can also trigger chest pain or breathlessness.

It's a long list of symptoms, but only a partial list at that. Remember, too, that many noncardiac diseases can produce very similar symptoms; that's why medical school takes four years. Don't try to be your own doctor. Instead, listen to your body and report its distress signals to your doctor, who will work with you to determine if your symptoms are major or minor, cardiac or noncardiac.

A careful history and physical exam are the first steps in evaluating symptoms. But medical tests are often necessary; here are some tests used to evaluate the heart.

Tests for Heart Disease

Many tests can be used to evaluate the heart and circulation, and new procedures are being devised every year. Some tests are complementary, providing information about different aspects of cardiac function. Others are redundant, merely duplicating the information available from previous tests. Some tests are simple and risk-free, but others are invasive, producing discomfort and carrying some risk.

How does your doctor decide which tests to order? The general rule is to start with the easiest, least-invasive test that is likely to provide a diagnosis, moving to more difficult, expensive, or invasive tests only if the first results are inconclusive. It's a good rule, and you should apply it as you negotiate with your doctor. But there is an important exception: in very sick patients, it may be necessary to move directly to invasive tests, since there may not be time to try out less definitive procedures.

Noninvasive Tests

Electrocardiogram (EKG). It's an old standby that has been in use for nearly 100 years, but it's still a very useful test. An EKG can be performed in less than 5 minutes, and it's painless and risk-free. EKGs produce tracings that reflect the heart's electrical activity. As such, they are excellent tools for evaluating cardiac rhythms. Since heart muscles that are deprived of adequate blood supply produce a "current of injury," EKGs are also very useful for detecting angina and heart attacks, particularly if they're performed during an episode of chest pain. EKGs may also reveal scars from prior heart attacks; because large muscles produce large currents, they may also reflect enlargement of the heart's pumping chambers.

Chest x-ray. Another old test, but one that's lost some of its stature in the modern era. Chest x-rays should never be performed as screening tests on apparently healthy people. Still, a simple chest x-ray can help diagnose cardiac enlargement and congestive heart failure as well as many lung disorders. Although a chest x-ray produces only minuscule radiation exposure and is risk-free, excessive x-rays should be avoided.

Stress Test (exercise tolerance test, or ETT). Think of it as an EKG with sneakers. The stress test is conceptually simple: get the heart working hard, and monitor it during exercise to detect abnormalities that are not apparent at rest. The stress test is also technically simple. You'll be asked to avoid food and drink for 4 hours prior to the test, and to report to the lab with sneakers and comfortable clothing. You'll be hooked up to an EKG and asked to walk on a treadmill or pedal a stationary bicycle while your EKG is recorded continuously and your blood pressure is measured periodically. You'll work progressively harder as the treadmill speeds up, stopping only if you develop symptoms or EKG abnormalities or when you tire out. The whole process takes about an hour.

Despite their simplicity, stress tests have drawbacks. They are time consuming and moderately expensive; in rare instances, they can pre-cipitate heart attacks in people with coronary artery disease. In addi-tion, stress tests generate too many false-positive and false-negative results to make them useful screening tests to detect occult heart disease in apparently healthy people. Despite those limitations, stress tests are very helpful when used properly, to diagnose coronary artery blockages in patients who have symptoms suggesting heart disease, and to monitor the progress of patients with known coronary heart disease. Stress tests can also be helpful to diagnose exercise-induced arrhythmias, to evalu-ate exercise capacity, and to provide the information needed for a de-tailed exercise prescription.

Thallium stress test. Think of it as a stress test with pictures. A tiny dose of radioactive thallium is injected intravenously during a stress test, ideally about 1 minute before the exercise is completed. The thallium is taken up by normal heart muscle cells, but not by cells that are not getting enough blood. A scan is performed immediately after exercise, and a second set of images is obtained 4 hours later. Blockages of coronary arteries produce "cold" or pale areas in the early pictures, indicating that the heart muscle is not getting enough blood; if the later images are back to normal, they indicate partial blockages (angina), but pale areas that persist indicate scars in the heart muscle (previous heart attack). Thallium scanning improves the accuracy of stress testing; it does not add to the small risks of stress testing, but it is more expensive and time consuming.

Ambulatory EKG monitoring (Holter monitoring). Think of it as a long EKG — a very long one, at that. A standard EKG can detect only arrhythmias that occur while the machine is recording, a period of perhaps 30 seconds. Stress tests can detect abnormal rhythms that are triggered by exertion. But arrhythmias can occur any time, day or night. To detect them, patients are hooked up to EKG leads attached to a small portable monitor that they carry with them for 24 hours. Since about 10,000 heartbeats are recorded in the course of a day, a computer is used to analyze the results. Holter monitoring is an excellent, risk-free way to detect abnormal heart rhythms. Newer computer programs can also detect insufficient blood flow, or ischemia; it's an important way to detect silent ischemia or "painless angina" during daily life.

Echocardiography (cardiac sonogram). Think of it as a stethoscope with eyes, but it's actually a bit more complex. Instead of listening for sounds from the heart, cardiac echo tests beam sound waves at the heart and record the waves as they're reflected back. The patient lies quietly on a table as a probe is passed across the chest; a special camera is used to record the sound waves, providing images of the heart in action. Cardiac echo tests are painless and risk-free — and they're silent, to boot.

Echocardiography is an extremely powerful diagnostic technique, allowing accurate measurements of the heart's size and thickness, its pumping capacity, and the size and integrity of its valves. Newer echos using Doppler technology provide measurements of the blood flowing through the heart's chambers. Other advances include exercise echocardiography, which combines an echo with a stress test, and transesophageal echocardiography (TEE), which uses a small sound probe that is swallowed to obtain clear images from the rear of the heart.

Echocardiograms are excellent tests, and they're getting even better — which is why more than 4 million are performed in the United States each year. But at about $800 each, they're quite costly, and they're sometimes performed on patients who don't really need them, producing needless worry as well as expense. In general, echos are most valuable for evaluating congestive heart failure and disorders of the heart valves, but they're much less helpful for patients with coronary artery disease.

Many additional noninvasive tests are available, and others are being developed. Each has a role, but in most cases they add little (except expense) to the information that can be gained from the EKG, stress test, thallium scan, Holter monitor, and echocardiogram. Still, your doctor may recommend one of these supplementary studies:

Radionuclide angioradiography (gated blood pool heart scan, MUGA). A radioisotope is used to visualize the blood in the heart's chambers, allowing measurements of the heart's size and its ability to pump blood.

Positron emission tomography (PET scan). A test that measures the metabolism of heart muscle cells and the supply of blood to these cells. PET scans can help distinguish living cells with impaired blood supply (angina) from scarred cells (heart attack).

Magnetic resonance imaging (MRI). High-speed scanners timed precisely to the heart's contractions can provide detailed images of the heart's structure. In the future, perhaps, MRIs will provide a noninvasive way to pinpoint the location and severity of coronary artery blockages.

The noninvasive heart tests are complicated, even for doctors. Perhaps that's why their initials are used as substitutes for their long names. It's a handy shorthand, but it sometimes sounds more like alphabet soup than modern cardiology. By any name, you'll stay out of the soup if you take good care of your heart.

As good as they are, the noninvasive tests have still not eliminated the need for invasive studies.

Invasive Tests

Cardiac catheterization. First used in 1959, cardiac catheterization has been a boon to patients with advanced heart disease; even in the era of scans and echos, it remains the gold standard for evaluating coronary artery blockages, disorders of the heart valves, and congestive heart failure. But because it's an invasive test, it should be reserved for situations in which definitive information is mandatory. Most often, catheterizations are performed on patients who are probable candidates for heart surgery or other invasive treatments.

Cardiac catheterizations are performed in special "cath labs." Patients are awake, but they are often sedated. Under local anesthesia, a thin tube, or catheter, is inserted into an artery, usually in the patient's groin. Doctors advance the catheter through the patient's arteries right into the heart. The catheter can be used to measure the pressure in the heart's pumping chambers, providing the most accurate index of the heart's ability to power blood through the circulation. In most cases, dye is injected through the catheter, after which x-rays are taken to provide pictures of the heart. To evaluate coronary atherosclerosis, dye is injected directly into the coronary arteries in a procedure called *coronary angiography*. Much less often, the catheter can be used to obtain a small piece of heart muscle for analysis in a procedure called a *myocardial biopsy*. In addition to its role in diagnostic testing, cardiac catheterization can be used therapeutically (see angioplasty, page 395, and pacemakers, page 394).

Although cardiac catheterization is the most accurate way to evaluate heart disease, it can create problems of its own. It is expensive and it usually requires an overnight hospitalization. Complications include bleeding at the arterial puncture site and kidney damage from the dye that's injected. The catheter can also dislodge cholesterol plaques from diseased arteries, resulting in heart attacks, strokes, or kidney damage. Despite these concerns, serious complications and deaths are rare, occurring about once in every 1,000 cardiac catheterizations.

More than 1 million cardiac catheterizations are performed in the United States each year at an average cost of more than $4,000. Are all of them really necessary? It's hard to be sure; a 1992 study from Harvard Medical School suggested that only 50 percent of catheterizations are absolutely necessary, but a 1993 study from New York State found that 91 percent of studies were appropriate. The percentages vary, but the moral is clear: before you submit to a cardiac catheterization, be sure it's 100 percent necessary; a second opinion may be helpful.

Electrophysiological studies (EPS). Requiring cardiac catheterization and sophisticated electrical measurements and monitoring, EPS studies allow detailed evaluations of serious cardiac arrhythmias. They are performed only in major cardiology centers on selected patients who may require advanced or experimental treatment of abnormal heart rhythm that have not responded to conventional therapy.

Treatment of Cardiovascular Disease

The best treatment for heart disease is prevention. It sounds utopian, but it works; the 15-point program outlined in *Conquering Heart Disease* will prevent atherosclerosis and its ravages. Even if you already have heart disease, it's not too late to start; in fact, patients with atherosclerosis have the very greatest need for the nonprescription approaches that fight the disease itself. But many patients with heart disease also require prescription drugs or even surgery to manage the complications of atherosclerosis.

Lifestyle interventions and medical therapies are not contradictory, but complementary; if you succeed with the former, you won't need the latter. Still, millions of Americans already have atherosclerosis, so it's important to review some basic medical treatments. Remember, though, that this is just a general review. All medical therapies require individualized consultations and ongoing supervision; your doctor should be providing the details about the benefits and side effects of your medical regimen, as well as information about alternative approaches that may be available.

Drug Therapies

Drugs to lower cholesterol. Nearly every prescription for a cholesterol-lowering drug represents a failure; with the rare exception of inherited abnormalities of cholesterol metabolism, elevated cholesterol levels should respond favorably to reductions in dietary fat and cholesterol (Chapter 4), increases in dietary fiber (Chapter 8), certain nutritional supplements (Chapters 9, 12, and 13), weight control (Chapter 15), and exercise (Chapter 5). Unfortunately, doctors and patients often take the easy way out, turning to drugs that lower blood cholesterol levels. It's no surprise then, that many medications are available.

The "statins." They are new and expensive, but they are probably the most potent and easy-to-use cholesterol-lowering drugs. Four members of this group are currently available, lovastatin (Mevacor), pravastatin (Pravachol), simvastatin (Zocor), and fluvastatin (Lescol). The "statins" act by inhibiting HMG-CoA, a human liver enzyme responsible for producing cholesterol. The four drugs are quite similar in cost and effectiveness. They are also similar in their side effects, which include mild intestinal upset, skin rashes, headaches, and sleep disturbances; less often, the drugs can cause liver inflammation or muscle damage.

Bile acid binding resins. They are the oldest cholesterol-lowering drugs, with a good record for efficacy and safety. Despite their seniority, bile acid binders are expensive. Representative drugs include cholestyramine (Questran, Questran Light, Cholybar) and colestipol (Colestid). They act by sequestering bile acids in the intestines, preventing them from entering the blood and traveling to the liver, where they would ordinarily be converted into cholesterol. Because the medications themselves are not absorbed into the body, serious side effects are rare. But many patients find them unpalatable; others experience constipation, heartburn, belching, or bloating.

Gemfibrozil (Lopid). Another medication that lowers cholesterol by reducing its synthesis in the body, gemfibrozil is particularly useful in patients with high blood triglyceride levels. An older drug belonging to the same chemical group (clofibrate, Atromid-S) has been abandoned because of adverse reactions, but gemfibrozil appears safe; intestinal discomfort is the major side effect, but gallstones may develop in some long-term users. Gemfibrozil is expensive.

Probucol (Lorelco). The good news about probucol is that it lowers LDL cholesterol; the bad news is that it also lowers HDL, or "good," cholesterol levels. Probucol is rarely used to treat elevated cholesterol levels, but it is now attracting research interest because it has antioxidant properties.

Estrogens. Although they are not ordinarily considered cholesterol-improving medications, estrogens are able to lower LDL and raise HDL levels. Only postmenopausal women are candidates for estrogens; Chapter 16 discusses the pros and cons of estrogen replacement therapy.

Drugs Used Principally for Angina

Nitrates. Although they're the oldest anti-anginal medications, the nitrates remain among the most important drugs in modern cardiology — so important, in fact, that new preparations are being developed even today. Nitrates relax blood vessels. Because they widen the coronary arteries, nitrates are very helpful in treating patients with angina; because they relax many other blood vessels, they can also help improve cardiovascular function in certain patients with congestive heart failure.

Short-acting nitrates are used to treat the pain of angina or to provide a half hour of protection in anticipation of physical or mental stress that might precipitate an attack. Long-acting preparations can provide protection against angina throughout the day. The major side effects of the various nitrate preparations are similar: headaches and falling blood pressures, with dizziness or even fainting.

Short-acting nitrates include the classic nitroglycerine tablets, which are placed under the tongue (Nitrostat, other brands), and a new nitroglycerine spray, which is applied under the tongue (Nitrolingual Spray). Long-acting nitrates may be administered as tablets or placed under the tongue (Isordil, many other brands). Long-acting nitrates can also be applied to the skin as an ointment or on a patch (many brands). Nitroglycerine is also available as intravenous medication for the treatment of heart attacks or severe angina in intensive care units.

Drugs Used Principally for Angina and Hypertension

Beta-blockers. Angina and hypertension are the most important uses for this large family of drugs, but they have other major uses as well, including managing certain arrhythmias, preventing migraine headaches, reducing tremors, and even controlling stage fright. We don't know how the beta-blockers can do so many different things, but we do know how they act on the cardiovascular system. Although the details vary from drug to drug, all beta-blockers share the ability to block the effects of adrenaline on the heart and circulation. As a result, the heart rate slows and its contractions become more efficient, so the heart requires less oxygen to keep it pumping. Blood vessels widen, improving blood flow. The net result is to diminish anginal attacks in patients with coronary artery disease and to lower the blood pressure of patients with hypertension.

If the beta-blockers are so great, why don't we all take them? In fact, most patients who have suffered heart attacks are given beta-blockers to reduce the risk of another attack. But beta-blockers are not for healthy people; like all medications, they can produce damaging side effects. Adrenaline, after all, is not all bad, and blocking this natural hormone can be harmful. The heart rate can become too slow and the blood pressure can go too low; the drugs can precipitate congestive heart failure and fluid accumulation in some patients with heart disease. Because the bronchial tubes depend on adrenaline to stay open, beta-blockers can trigger wheezing in folks with asthma. Other side effects may include fatigue or depression, cold extremities, diarrhea, and male erectile dysfunction. Most beta-blockers also raise blood cholesterol levels.

If the beta-blockers are so bad, why does anyone take them? In fact, they must be administered with care, which is why they're prescription drugs. But when they are used appropriately, they do much more good than harm.

Perhaps because so many Americans have cardiovascular disease, the American pharmaceutical industry offers us a large number of beta-blockers. Here's a list of the major members of the family: atenolol (Tenormin, other brands), betaxolol (Kerlone), metoprolol (Lopressor, Toprol XL), nadolol (Corgard), propranolol (Inderal, other brands), timolol (Blocadren), acebutolol (Sectral), carteolol (Cartrol), penbutolol (Levatol), pindolol (Visken), and labetalol (Normodyne, Trandate).

It's quite a list. Don't try to master it, much less the differences among these many drugs. Leave the details to your doctor — better yet, follow the 15-point program to conquer heart disease so your doctor won't have to prescribe any drugs for you.

Calcium channel blockers. Like the hormone adrenaline, the mineral calcium is essential for human health. In fact, diets rich in calcium appear to reduce the risk of hypertension as well as osteoporosis (see Chapter 6). Still, drugs that block calcium's effects on blood vessels are very useful for angina and hypertension.

Calcium plays a crucial role in muscular contraction. By blocking some of calcium's interaction with muscle cells, calcium channel blockers help relax the muscles in the walls of arteries. As the muscles relax, the arteries widen, and blood pressure drops. The heart muscle, too, beats less forcefully under the influence of these drugs; it's why they are so effective in treating angina and certain arrhythmias, but it's also why congestive heart failure is numbered among the side effects of calcium channel blockers. Other side effects may include fluid retention, skin rashes, fatigue, constipation, headaches, and erectile dysfunction.

Despite the potential side effects, most patients who need calcium channel blockers reap important benefits from these drugs with few ill consequences. I hope you'll never need any of them, but if you do, your doctor can choose among diltiazem (Cardizem, Dilacor XR), verapamil (Calan, Verelan), nifedipine (Procardia), nicardipine (Cardene), isradipine (DynaCirc), felodipine (Plendil), and amiodipine (Norvasc).

Drugs Used Principally for Hypertension and Congestive Heart Failure

ACE inhibitors. Like beta-blockers and calcium channel blockers, the ACE inhibitors relax blood vessels, but they have a unique way of going about it. Instead of acting directly on arteries, they block a blood protein (*A*ngiotensin *C*onverting *E*nzyme) that is responsible for producing hormones that narrow blood vessels and promote salt retention. The chemistry is complex, but the clinical results are clear: ACE inhibitors are excellent drugs for treating most types of hypertension as well as the major type of congestive heart failure. Although they have fewer side effects than most other antihypertensives, the ACE inhibitors can cause problems that may include excessive lowering of the blood pressure, abnormalities of kidney function, cough, intestinal symptoms, and skin rashes. Representative ACE inhibitors include captopril (Capoten), enalapril (Vasotec), lisinopril (Prinivil, Zestril), benazepril (Lotensin), fosinopril (Monopril), quinapril (Accupril), and ramipril (Altace).

Diuretics. Better known as "fluid pills," diuretics rid the body of salt and water by stimulating urine flow though the kidneys. By reducing the volume of fluid in the circulation, diuretics lower blood pressure and ameliorate congestive heart failure. Diuretics are the oldest antihypertensive drugs; long a mainstay of drug therapy, they are losing favor because of the greater efficacy and improved safety of new (but much more expensive) antihypertensives.

Diuretics come in three varieties. Thiazide diuretics and the more potent loop diuretics act on different parts of the kidneys to promote salt and water excretion; they also produce potassium excretion, a major side effect of all these drugs. Other side effects include dehydration, fatigue, erectile dysfunction, allergic reactions, gout, and elevated blood sugar and cholesterol levels. The third diuretic category is the potassium-sparing diuretics; their side effects may include high blood potassium levels, breast enlargement or pain in men or women, intestinal disturbances, allergies, and rashes.

With all these side effects, it's obvious that you'd be well advised to reduce your body's sodium burden the old-fashioned way, by eating less salt. Unfortunately, many doctors and patients still opt for diuretics. Your doctor has a wide choice of diuretics. At least 13 thiazides are available, including chlorothiazide (Diuril), hydrochlorothiazide (Hydrodiuril, Esidrix, other brands), and metolazone (Zaroxolyn). The three loop diuretics are furosemide (Lasix), ethacrynic acid (Edecrin), and bumetanide (Bumex); the three potassium-sparing drugs are spironolactone (Aldactone, other brands), triamterene (Dyrenium), and amiloride (Midamor, other brands). And, just in case you're not confused enough, you may also be given combination pills containing both a thiazide and a potassium-sparing drug.

Other antihypertensive medications. The industrialized world is in the midst of an epidemic of hypertension. The pharmaceutical industry seems to be in the midst of an avalanche of antihypertensives. As a way of controlling hypertension, medications are a poor second to the lifestyle modifications embodied in your plan to conquer heart disease. Still, some patients do require medications, and drug therapy is certainly far better than allowing hypertension to go unchecked.

Most doctors now rely on beta-blockers, calcium channel blockers, ACE inhibitors, and diuretics to treat hypertension; when necessary, these medications can even be prescribed simultaneously. But many other antihypertensives are available; each has its pros and cons. Here are just a few of the medications your doctor may prescribe: *drugs that act directly on blood vessels:* hydralazine (Apresoline, other brands), and minoxidil (Loniten, other brands); *alpha blockers:* prazosin (Minipress, other brands), terazosin (Hytrin), and doxazosin (Cardura); *drugs that reduce sympathetic nervous system activity:* clonidine (Catapres, other brands) and guanabenz (Wytensin).

It's quite a list; just reading it may be enough to raise your blood pressure. The list may help you understand your doctor's prescriptions, but another reading assignment will do you much more good: the first 17 chapters of *Conquering Heart Disease.*

Drugs Used Principally for Congestive Heart Failure and Arrhythmias

Digitalis. For hundreds of years, the common folk of England used the foxglove plant, *Digitalis purpurea,* to treat dropsy, a form of congestive heart failure. Observing its efficacy, Dr. William Withering began to investigate digitalis in 1775; after a decade of study he concluded that "it has a power over the motion of the heart to a degree yet unobserved in any other medicine. . . . " Since digitalis is the only FDA-approved oral medication that strengthens the heart's pumping action, Withering's observations remain valid even today.

Digitalis has two major uses. Because it bolsters the contractions of the heart's muscles, it can help treat certain patients with congestive heart failure. Because it influences the electrical activity of the heart, it can slow down the racing pulse in patients with certain rapid or erratic heart rhythms, such as atrial fibrillation.

Although other medications can be used to treat congestive heart failure and arrhythmias, digitalis remains a valuable drug more than 200 years after its first scientific use. In fact, more than 12 million prescriptions for digoxin (Lanoxin, other brands) are issued by American physicians each year. Venerable and valuable as a palliative, digitalis is far from a panacea. In the past, up to 25 percent of all patients taking the drug experienced side effects, including abnormal heart rhythms, nausea, visual disturbances, and even psychiatric symptoms. But modern technology has made digitalis much safer; because doctors are now able to monitor blood digoxin levels, only 2 percent of all patients taking digoxin experience side effects. And modern biotechnology has also produced an effective therapy for massive digitalis overdoses. Still, the safest way to use digitalis is to have a healthy heart so it's not needed at all.

Drugs Used Principally for Arrhythmias

No area of cardiology is more complex than arrhythmias, and none is more controversial. Arrhythmias are common; most are harmless (premature beats, for example) but some can produce discomfort or complications (such as the atrial fibrillation that led to President Bush's hospitalization in 1991), while others can be life-threatening (ventricular tachycardia) or lethal (ventricular fibrillation). Many drugs are available to treat arrhythmias, but some can do more harm than good, even causing new arrhythmias.

Confronted with this complexity, cardiologists often refer patients with complex arrhythmias to other cardiologists who specialize in the area. I won't attempt to explain all the treatment options that may be considered, but I will list some of the oral medications that may be prescribed. Beta-blockers, calcium channel blockers, and digoxin are on the list. Other drugs with anti-arrhythmic properties include quinidine (many brands), procainamide (Pronestyl and other brands), disopyramide (Norpace and other brands), phenytoin (Dilantin and other brands), mexiletine (Mexitil), tocainide (Tonocard), flecainide (Tambocor), propafenone (Rythmol), moricizine (Ethmozine), and amiodarone (Cordarone).

An arrhythmia is not a disease, but the symptom of an underlying heart disease. The best way to treat arrhythmias is, of course, to prevent or correct the heart diseases that cause abnormal pumping rhythms. Your doctor can help — but you can help even more with your 15-point program to conquer heart disease.

Drugs Used to Prevent or Dissolve Clots in Coronary Arteries

Atherosclerosis is a slow and stealthy process that places cholesterol-laden plaques just where you'd want them least, in your coronary arteries. To conquer heart disease, you'll have to win the war against atherosclerosis. But atherosclerotic plaques are not the only things that block coronary arteries; in fact, the final event that leads to most heart attacks is the formation of a blood clot on the surface of the plaque. It's the clot that turns a partial blockage into a complete occlusion.

Two oral medications can be used to inhibit clotting. The first is a nonprescription drug you can get on your own: aspirin; Chapter 7 will help you determine if aspirin is right for you. Although not every healthy person should take aspirin, virtually every patient with coronary heart disease should take low-dose aspirin, providing of course, that there are no other medical problems that might make aspirin dangerous. In some heart patients, though, aspirin may not do the trick. In these cases, doctors can prescribe the other clot-fighting pill, Coumadin. Using Coumadin requires more than just a doctor's prescription; it requires frequent blood tests and dosage adjustments as well as careful attention to diet and to other medications that may interact with Coumadin. Taking aspirin is easier, cheaper, safer, and — in most cases — at least as good as Coumadin. But Coumadin is preferred for all patients with plastic artificial heart valves, most patients with atrial fibrillation, and occasional patients with coronary artery disease.

Doctors can also administer injections of clot-fighting drugs to treat severe angina or new heart attacks in hospitalized patients. One drug (heparin) prevents clot formation, while others (streptokinase, urokinase, tissue plasminogen activator, and anisoylated plasminogen streptokinase-activator complex) are the "clot busters" that can actually dissolve clots and reopen coronary arteries if they are injected within the first 6 hours of a heart attack.

Aspirin costs about a penny; tissue plasminogen activator costs $2,400 for the drug alone, to say nothing of the monetary costs of hospitalization in an acute intensive care unit and the physical and psychological costs of a heart attack. You can pay your money and take your choice. I hope you'll choose prevention. Remember, too, that there's an even cheaper way to stimulate your blood's natural clot-fighting activity: exercise (Chapter 5).

Cardiac Surgery and Invasive Medical Treatments for Heart Disease

It sounds simple: if it's not working right and drugs can't fix it, call a surgeon to repair it or replace it. In practice, of course, it's far from simple. Still, in this era of the bionic man, medical miracles seem almost routine. When it comes to your own heart, though, don't take miracles for granted. As a last resort, heart surgery can do wonders, but it always involves pain, time, expense, and risk.

Procedures for arrhythmias. Many abnormal pumping rhythms resolve without treatment, and many others respond to drug therapy. But refractory arrhythmias can be treated with a variety of electrical devices.

Cardiac pacemakers have excellent records; they are especially useful for speeding up hearts that are beating too slowly. In basic terms, pacemakers consist of a battery, a timer, and a pacing wire. In most cases the power pack can be implanted under the skin using local anesthesia, and the wire can be threaded through the veins into the heart without surgery.

Although pacemakers can sometimes control runaway hearts that are beating too rapidly, other procedures may be necessary. If an abnormal electrical circuit in the heart is responsible for the arrhythmia, it can sometimes be treated at special centers using a new process called radiofrequency catheter ablation. In other cases, cardioversion is necessary. Most often, cardioversion is performed by jolting the heart with an electric current that is passed through paddles placed on the patient's chest; it sounds worse than it is, since mild sedation keeps patients comfortable during the treatment. External cardioversion requires a trip to the hospital, but some arrhythmias are so serious that there's no time to get help. In some such cases, an automatic implantable cardioverter-defibrillator can be used to do the job on its own; these devices have helped over 30,000 patients since they were approved in 1985, but they're available only at special centers and they require chest surgery and careful follow-up care.

Procedures for diseased heart valves. Rheumatic fever, congenital abnormalities, infections, and other processes can damage any of the heart's four delicate valves. The heart muscle can compensate for mild valve damage, and medications can help patients with moderately advanced valve disease. But if valves are severely damaged, they must be repaired or replaced.

The era of open heart surgery began with valve replacement. Because rheumatic fever has declined so dramatically, there has been less and less need for valve jobs, but they are still among the most important and successful heart operations. Damaged valves can sometimes be repaired, but in most cases they have to be replaced. Plastic valves or pig valves can be used; each has its advantages, but neither is as good as the real thing.

Procedures for blocked coronary arteries. It's American medicine at its best: blocked arteries can be reopened, relieving the pain of angina for many patients and prolonging life for some. It's American medicine at its worse, using expensive, high-tech, risky interventions to temporarily correct a problem that should never have occurred in the first place.

Most patients with coronary artery disease respond well to medical treatments, but some patients with angina or heart attacks get better results from procedures that actually restore the flow of blood. The indications for invasive treatment are complex and even controversial; decisions must always be individualized. In general, these procedures should be reserved for patients who fail to improve with drug treatment, for those with severe narrowing of the left main coronary artery, or for those with advanced blockages of multiple coronary arteries.

There are two ways to restore blood flow through blocked coronary arteries: special cardiac catheters can be used to widen the blocked artery, or open heart surgery can be used to bypass the blockage.

First introduced in Switzerland in 1977, catheter treatments have become a mainstay of American cardiology, with about 300,000 procedures performed each year. In the standard approach, called an angioplasty, a balloon-tipped catheter is threaded into the blocked artery; next, the balloon is gently inflated, "squashing" the fatty plaque to widen the artery and restore blood flow. Angioplasties are performed by specially trained cardiologists and radiologists; only local anesthesia is required. The initial results are excellent, with good blood flow in about 90 percent of patients. The complication rate is about 4 percent, but two 1993 studies suggest that complications are somewhat more frequent in women.

Atherotomy is a newer catheter procedure that uses a tiny blade to actually cut away the fatty plaque. Atherotomies were approved for clinical use in 1990, but despite initial enthusiasm, they don't seem any better or safer than angioplasties, and they are more expensive. Still on the horizon are catheter treatments using lasers and balloon angioplasties that are accompanied by the insertion of stents, tiny metal tubes designed to keep arteries open.

Angioplasty is an invasive and expensive treatment for coronary artery disease — but bypass surgery takes the cake in both categories. Most patients who have a choice would prefer an angioplasty, but the 400,000 bypass operations performed in the United States each year testify to the fact that many patients are not candidates for catheter treatment.

Coronary artery bypass surgery can be performed in either of two ways. Most often, a small piece of the saphenous vein is removed from the patient's leg; one end of the vein is sewn into the aorta and the other is sewn into the coronary artery just beyond the blockage. In the other method, the patient's internal mammary artery is moved from its normal location in the chest muscle to bypass the coronary blockage. With either technique, coronary artery bypass surgery is a big deal, but it is successful nearly 90 percent of the time, and significant complications occur in only about 5 percent of patients.

Angioplasties and bypass operations have helped hundreds of thousands of patients. Which is better? Patients have to rely on their own cardiologist to determine which procedure is most likely to succeed. But a 1994 study found that the 1-year outcome of the two treatments was identical in terms of the patient's eventual employment status. And the same study found that drug treatment was just as successful as either invasive treatment.

Why don't procedures that restore blood flow have even better results? The reason is that they are temporary; blood flow is initially restored by 90 percent of the procedures, but as time goes on, the blockages return. After just 6 months, 30 to 50 percent of arteries that have been opened by angioplasties are reoccluded. After 5 years, 40 percent of bypass grafts are at least partially blocked, and after 10 years the failure rate is about 75 percent.

It's good that we have drugs, angioplasties, and bypass operations to treat coronary artery blockages — but it's too bad that we need them. Each of these treatments can help heart patients, but none of them will treat the disease that's really to blame. Atherosclerosis is not a disease of the coronary arteries, but of the entire body. It can't be treated with pills or plumbing, but it can be overcome with a comprehensive lifestyle program. That's what the 15-point plan is all about; it's important for every American, but it is especially critical for patients who have let themselves slide into heart disease.

Cardiologists and cardiac surgeons can treat coronary artery disease, but you are the only one who can conquer atherosclerosis.

Conquering Heart Disease: Ancient Wisdom for the Modern World

Even in the era of thallium scans, beta-blockers, and bypass surgery, there is much we can learn from the ancients — not, perhaps, from their methods of diagnosis and treatment, but from their sense of proportion and balance. The Greeks attributed health to Aesculapius, the god of healing. But he divided his powers between his two daughters; Panacea was in charge of medications, while Hygeia was responsible for wise living and healthful behavior. Our modern world, alas, has devoted much more energy to the search for pharmacological panaceas than to the healthful lifestyle that would make many of them superfluous.

There are no medical panaceas. Find good doctors and work with them to obtain the tests and treatments you really need. But don't stop there. Instead, follow the 15-point program to fight atherosclerosis; if you let Hygeia guide you, you'll conquer heart disease with precious little need for Panacea's remedies.

Epilogue

Healthy Hearts, Healthy Bodies

YOU'VE COME a long way in learning how to conquer heart disease.

In Part I of this book, you learned what causes atherosclerosis and how to assess your personal risks and needs.

In Part II you learned 15 ways to fight atherosclerosis. You should know how each technique works and why it's needed. You should be able to set your goals, and you should know how to achieve those goals while enjoying a vigorous, natural lifestyle.

In Part III you learned how your doctor can help with tests, treatments, and — if you really need them — prescription medications.

Taken together, this program should keep your heart and blood vessels healthy. Atherosclerosis is, after all, a man-made disease; by avoiding the bodily abuse and disuse that characterize the industrialized lifestyle, you'll be able to enjoy the healthy heart that's part of human nature. And even if you're starting late, after cardiovascular disease has set in, you should be able to stop heart disease in its tracks, turning back the relentless course of atherosclerosis.

Needless to say, a healthy heart is a worthy goal in and of itself. Add an enjoyable, even stimulating, lifestyle, and you'll see that incorporating the entire 15-part program into your daily life is really worthwhile.

But is it enough? Will you be like the proverbial chap who gave up

Table 1
HOW TO CONTROL THE 10 LEADING
CAUSES OF DEATH IN AMERICA

Disease	Controllable Risk Factors	Elements of the 15-Point Program That Will Help
1. Heart disease	Tobacco abuse	Chapter 3
	High blood pressure	Chapters 5, 6, 14, 15
	Abnormal cholesterol	Chapters 4, 5, 8, 9, 10, 12, 13, 14, 15, 16
	Lack of exercise	Chapter 5
	Diabetes	Chapters 4, 5, 8, 15
	Obesity	Chapters 4, 5, 8, 14, 15
	Excessive stress	Chapters 5, 14
2. Cancer	Tobacco abuse	Chapter 3
	Radiation and environmental exposure	
	Improper diet	Chapters 4, 8, 11, 15
	Alcohol abuse	Chapters 9, 14
3. Stroke	Tobacco abuse	Chapter 3
	High blood pressure	Chapters 4, 5, 6, 14, 15
	Abnormal cholesterol	Chapters 4, 5, 8, 9, 10, 12, 13, 14, 15, 16
4. Chronic lung disease	Tobacco abuse	Chapter 3
	Environmental exposures	
5. Accidents	Alcohol and drug abuse	Chapters 9, 14
	Tobacco abuse	Chapter 3
	Not using seatbelts	
	Fatigue, stress, and recklessness	Chapter 14
6. Pneumonia and influenza	Tobacco abuse	Chapter 3
	Environmental exposures	
	Alcohol abuse	Chapters 9, 14
	Lack of immunization	
7. Diabetes	Obesity	Chapters 4, 5, 8, 14, 15
	Lack of exercise	Chapter 5
	Improper diet	Chapters 4, 8, 15
8. Suicide	Excessive stress	Chapter 14
	Alcohol and drugs	Chapters 9, 14
9. AIDS	Unsafe sexual practices	
	Drug abuse	Chapter 14
10. Liver disease	Alcohol abuse	Chapters 9, 14
	Exposure to toxins	
	Lack of immunization	

steak and eggs, jogged every day, and had a perfect heart — until he died from cancer at age 45?

Not to worry — this bad dream won't become your reality. In fact, the 15-point program will give you more than a healthy heart; it will give you a healthy body, too.

Table 1 lists the 10 leading causes of death in America today. For all our progress in medical care, the list remained unchanged for many years until 1993, when the continued spread of AIDS brought this tragic disease into ninth place. Don't let all these terrible diseases frighten you; instead let's consider the controllable factors that contribute to each disease — and the ways that the 15-point program can help with each.

As you can see, your 15-point program to conquer heart disease can help protect you against nearly all the controllable risk factors that contribute to America's leading killers. What's left out? Just a few simple guidelines:

First, to reduce your risk of cancer, lung disease, and liver disease, minimize your exposure to radiation, ultraviolet rays, chemical pollutants, and toxins.

Second, to reduce your risk of accidental death, use air bags and seatbelts, drive prudently, and never drink before you drive.

Third, to reduce your risk of AIDS, protect yourself from sexually transmitted diseases.

Fourth, to reduce your risk of pneumonia, viral hepatitis, and other infections, obtain immunizations along with the good medical care and screening tests that can help with all 10 diseases.

It's impressive; by adding 4 simple practices to your 15-point program, you can protect yourself from *all 10* leading causes of death.

How can such a simple plan do so much for your health? It works because it *is* simple; it amounts to getting back to basics, to the lifestyle that suits human genetics. For all its wonderful benefits, the modern world has taken us dangerously far from the way nature intended us to live. You can take advantage of modern technology and still take care of your heart; by adopting this program you'll get back to basics — and you'll enjoy life more than ever.

Take care of your health, so I won't have to.

Appendix

Sources
for Further Information

Harvard Heart Letter
164 Longwood Avenue
Boston, MA 02115
(800) 829-9171

American Heart Association
7272 Greenville Avenue
Dallas TX 75231
(214) 373-6300

National Heart, Lung, and Blood Institute
Information Center
P. O. Box 30105
Bethesda, MD 20824
(301) 251-1222

President's Council on Physical Fitness and Sports
701 Pennsylvania Ave., NW, Suite 250
Washington, D.C. 20004
(202) 272-3430

Office on Smoking and Health
National Centers for Disease Control and Prevention
4770 Buford Highway, NE
Mailstop 50
Atlanta, GA 30341
(800) CDC-1311

Consumer Information Center
Pueblo, CO 81009
Distributes consumer publications on topics such as
education, food and nutrition, health, exercise and
weight control. The Consumer Information Catalog
is available free from the center at the above address.

Index

ACE inhibitors, 389, 390
acetaminophen, 201, 202
acupuncture, 82
Addison, Dr. W. T. L., 183
adrenaline, 55, 59, 291, 294, 295, 296, 309, 319, 388
aerobic dance, 161–162
aerobic sports, 162, 305
Aesculapius, 397
age
    and antioxidants, 266
    as risk factor, 34, 37, 142, 171
AIDS, 399–400
alcohol, 28, 117, 176, 183
    abuse of, 13, 41, 190, 221, 232–234, 235, 256, 302
    addiction to, 231
    in America, 222
    and atherosclerosis, 86–87, 131, 223–229, 235, 297
    calories in, 232
    and cancer, 86–87, 131, 221, 229–230, 234–235
    and cardiovascular disease, 232
    as cause of death, 221, 400
    high-dose, 232–234
    low-dose, 221, 223, 224–225, 226–232, 234, 235, 284, 349
    and medication, 232, 282
Alzheimer's disease, 346
American Cancer Society, 82, 377, 378
    Great American Smoke Out of, 81
American College of Cardiology, 170, 375, 376
American College of Sports Medicine, 165

American Heart Association, 75, 82, 86, 375, 376
    Step Two diet of, 100, 101, 103, 106
American Heart Journal, 303
American Journal of Cardiology, 275, 299
American Journal of Clinical Nutrition, 357
amino acids, 62, 139, 272, 338, 355–356
    and smoking, 72, 76
anemia, 285, 286, 287
    pernicious, 357
aneurysm, 72
anger, 59, 295, 296, 297, 298, 303, 306, 314
angina, 15–16, 17, 29, 99, 141, 198, 293
    and alcohol, 223
    and aspirin, 195, 197
    medication for, 257, 387–389
    and mental stress, 295, 299
    Prinzmetal's, 16
    procedures for, 393
    and smoking, 71, 76, 261
    symptoms of, 151, 378–379
    tests for, 380, 381, 382
    and vitamin E, 262
angiograms, 100, 101, 283, 298, 374, 384
angioplasty, 197, 395–396
Annals of Internal Medicine, 283, 351
antacids, 364–365
antibiotics, 11–12, 119
anticoagulants, 194–195, 198, 199
    See also aspirin
antioxidants, 98, 99, 116, 189, 228, 253–270, 288
    and health, 264–266, 367
    See also olive oil; vitamins: antioxidant

anxiety, 292, 293, 305, 310
aorta, 11, 14, 23, 72, 396
Aquinas, St. Thomas, 305
Armstrong, Mary Anne, 228
arrhythmias, 12–13, 381, 382, 385
  causes of, 13, 19, 20, 58, 71, 76, 232, 294, 299
  procedures for, 394
  treatment of, 388, 389, 391–392
arterial walls, 23–25
  and atherosclerosis, 21, 27, 72, 98, 99, 137, 173, 193, 240
  and cholesterol, 22, 91, 226, 248, 251, 252, 255
  and estrogen replacement, 347
  and stress, 296
arteries, 11, 14, 16, 23, 44, 72, 289, 299
  and atherosclerosis, 23, 173, 198
  blockages in, 15, 17, 18, 19, 252, 382, 395–396
  causes of disease in, 20, 22, 34
  coronary, 11, 236, 395–396
  and smoking, 71
  under stress, 290–291
  See also aspirin; atherosclerosis; blood: pumping of; heart disease: coronary
arteriograms, 29
arthritis, 160, 161, 200, 241, 251
aspirin, 191–204, 226, 240, 279
  adverse effects of, 201–202
  and atherosclerosis, 28, 34, 196–199, 393
  and health, 199–200
  and heart attacks, 32, 191, 192, 193–198, 203, 225
  and illness, 200–201
  prophylactic, and women, 196
asthma, 75, 152, 202, 302, 363, 388
atheroma, 24, 25, 29
  See also plaques
atherosclerosis, 18, 64–65, 236
  and alcohol, 234, 235
  and aspirin, 196–199, 201, 202–204
  beginning of, 42, 228
  causes of, 173, 285, 398
  and cholesterol, 91, 99
  development of, 21–28
  and fiber, 116, 205, 207–210, 213, 214, 215, 220
  incidence of, 295
  and lifestyle, 78, 396–398
  and nutrition, 62, 86, 90, 94, 205, 213
  premature, 35
  prevention of, 20, 25–28, 50, 67, 137–139, 385, 396–398
  progress of, 15, 29, 100
  regression of, 99, 101, 104
  smoking as cause of, 31, 34, 72, 81, 83
  and stress, 61, 295, 296, 303–311
  studies of, 30–31

  three stages of, 21, 193, 225, 251, 296
  See also arterial walls; arteries: coronary; cholesterol; heart disease; risk factors, coronary; stroke
atherotomy, 395
ATH-S (atherosclerosis-susceptible gene), 35

Basinski, Antoni, 363
Bayer Company, 192
beans. See legumes
Beer, Kenneth, 143
Benson, Dr. Herbert, 309
beta-blockers, 237, 283, 284, 387–388, 390
beta-carotene, 127, 253, 254, 256–258, 264, 265, 266, 268, 269, 287
biking, 50, 161
biofeedback, 309–310
biolectric impedance, 56
Blankenhorn, Dr. David, 99, 100
blood, pumping of, 9–11, 15, 16, 18, 44, 138, 142, 173, 232, 290, 294, 384
blood clotting, 24, 25, 27, 99, 135, 252
  and alcohol, 226, 228
  and aspirin, 192, 193, 194, 195, 198, 201, 203
  and dietary fat, 93, 102, 128, 241
  drugs for, 392–393
  and emotions, 59
  and estrogen replacement, 347
  and exercise, 50, 137–138, 146
  and smoking, 72
  and stress, 291, 296
  and strokes, 198
  See also fibrinogen
blood pressure, 43–49, 59, 62, 102, 251, 321
  in America, 172
  control of, 48–49, 116, 145–146, 171, 190, 208
  diastolic, 45, 47, 48
  and drug therapy, 48
  and exercise, 141, 142
  and eyes, 173–174
  home monitoring of, 47
  interpreting, 45
  low, 48, 49, 137
  measuring, 45–48
  and smoking, 72
  and stress, 294, 296, 310–311
  systolic, 44, 47
  understanding, 44–45
  See also hypertension
blood sugar, 275, 278, 283, 291, 320, 337
  and emotions, 59
  evaluating, 53–54
  and exercise, 139, 142, 146
  and glucose tolerance factor (GTF), 282
BMI. See body mass index
body, and mind, 293–297, 315
body mass index (BMI), 103, 148, 183, 317, 322, 327, 334, 335, 336, 341

calculation of, 56–57, 176, 324, 325, 334
  and waist-to-hip ratio, 57, 58, 321, 325, 334
Borg Scale, 155
brain hemorrhages, 41, 42, 72, 193, 195–196, 201, 232, 263
British Aspirin Trial, 196
British Health Education Council, 77
British Medical Journal, 176, 301
Bruhn, Dr. John, 300
Burkitt, Dr. Denis, 213–214

caffeine, 13, 47, 131, 362–364
calcium, 121, 126, 185–188
  and blood pressure, 14, 116, 185–186, 189, 389
  and bones, 139–140, 142, 344–345
calories, 117, 118, 119, 212
  and fat, 86, 87, 93, 98, 102, 103, 104, 105, 107, 122, 336, 338, 339
  and weight loss, 328–329, 334
Canadian National Breast Screening Study, 230
Canadian Task Force, 375, 376
cancer, 58, 223, 251, 400
  and antioxidants, 264–265
  of bladder, 79
  breast, 97, 102, 140, 144, 229–231, 234–235, 348, 349, 350, 351, 352, 354
  of cervix, 79, 140
  and cholesterol, 41, 42
  colon, 84, 97, 140, 144, 188, 199–200, 214, 265, 378
  and diet, 93, 102, 128, 140, 335
  endometrial, 348, 349, 351, 352, 353
  of esophagus, 79
  and grilling meat, 119–120
  lung, 36, 75, 76, 79, 102, 229, 257, 265, 287
  oral, 78, 79
  and pollution, 243
  prostate, 102, 265
  and smoking, 73, 78, 79
  stomach, 265
  and stress, 302
  throat, 79
  uterine, 102, 140, 348, 349, 350, 351, 352, 353
  See also alcohol: and breast cancer
Cannon, Dr. Walter, 291, 309
canola oil, 98, 102, 106, 117, 126
carbohydrates, complex, 116, 123, 126, 206, 334, 336, 337, 338
carbon dioxide, 10, 11
carbon monoxide, 71, 76, 79
cardiac arrests, 20, 150, 151
  See also deaths, sudden
cardiac catheterization, 384–385
cardiomyopathy, 13, 150, 232
CARET trial, 269
cataracts, 251, 266
cells
  endothelial, 23, 25, 251

fat, 55, 317
foam, 23, 24, 25, 252, 255
mitochondria in, 250
muscle, 23, 24, 25
myocardial, 17, 18
red blood, 285, 288, 357
white blood, 23, 251, 252, 255
See also DNA
Centers for Disease Control, 71
cereals, 217, 220
chemicals, 14, 120, 199, 209, 228, 305
  in fish, 240, 243, 244, 245
  in tobacco smoke, 75, 76
chlamydia, 33, 61
chocolate, 126, 130, 131
cholesterol, 21–22, 25, 27, 52, 98, 346
  definition of, 21, 88–91
  and eating habits, 62, 86–87, 106, 107, 117, 119, 121, 123, 208
  and exercise, 50, 137, 142
  good vs. bad, 22, 38, 55, 91
  and heart attacks, 37, 171
  IDL, 22, 39
  levels of, 37–39, 100, 103, 106, 295
  and liver, 22, 23, 39, 91, 93
  low, 40–42, 101
  measurement of, 42–43
  medication for, 49, 273
  and soluble fiber, 206–207, 208, 210
  and stress, 59, 295–296, 299
  studies on, 40–41
  tests for, 36, 42–43
  and U.S. vs. China, 87
  VLDL, 22, 39
  See also fat, dietary; HDL cholesterol; LDL cholesterol
Cholesterol Lowering Atherosclerosis Study (CLAS), 100
chromium, 281–285
  and atherosclerosis, 282–284
  sources of, 282
Cicero, 143, 264
clinical trials, 32, 100, 236, 258, 271, 305
  of antioxidants, 260, 261, 265, 269
coffee. *See* caffeine
collagen, 24, 25
Cooper, Dr. Kenneth, 151
copper, 288
Coronary Drug Project, 274
cortisone, 21, 291, 319
The Costs of Poor Health Habits (Manning et al.), 77, 144
Craven, Dr. Lawrence L., 192–193, 195, 196

dairy products, 117, 121–123
Dalen, Dr. James, 192
death rates. *See* mortality
deaths, sudden, 13, 19–20, 29, 150–152
  causes of, 20, 232, 294, 295, 400

during exercise, 19–20
number of, in United States, 19
time of, 19
See also mortality
depression, 290, 292–293, 297, 298–300, 302, 303
  and exercise, 140, 144, 305, 340
  and heart attacks, 59, 313
desserts, 131, 133–134
diabetes, 16, 36, 39, 40, 52–54, 62, 277
  and atherosclerosis, 199, 251
  and blood sugar, 53–54, 211, 242, 276, 278, 376
  and chromium, 282, 283
  and exercise, 50, 139, 144
  and fiber, 208, 211–212, 214
  genetic basis for, 35
  and obesity, 54, 58, 321
  and smoking, 72
  Type I, 52, 53
  Type II, 52–53, 142
Dickens, Charles, 160
Diet and Reinfarction Trial (DART), 239
diets, 27, 34, 35, 52, 61–64, 236, 332, 333, 344, 359, 365–366
  balanced, 116–117, 220
  changes in, 86
  and cheating, 135
  for children, 42
  in China, 87
  cholesterol-lowering, 37, 43, 91
  and exercise, 139
  liquid, 332, 333
  low-fat, 99, 140
  low-salt, 18
  Mediterranean, 87, 97, 227
  portions in, 107
  vegetarian, 101, 106, 120, 133, 216, 267, 285, 286, 357
  See also fat, dietary; fiber, dietary; weight loss
digitalis, 391–392
dioxins, 243
disease, digestive, 41, 42, 58
disease, periodontal, 78
disease, peripheral vascular, 40
DNA, 251, 264
doctors, 169–170, 372–373
drug abuse, 302
drug therapy. *See* medication

echocardiography (cardiac sonogram), 382–383
edema, 13, 18, 294
eggs, 121, 123, 125
electrocardiograms (EKGs), 16, 18, 29, 150, 153, 374, 376–377
  ambulatory, 382
electrophysiological studies (EPS), 385
emotions, and health, 293–303

emphysema, 36, 76–77
endocarditis, 12
endorphins, 305
Environmental Protection Agency (EPA), 73, 75, 76, 243
enzymes, 18, 55, 138, 194, 206, 217, 250, 253, 337
EPA. *See* Environmental Protection Agency
estrogen, 35, 55, 58, 140, 229, 230, 341–354, 387
estrogen replacement therapy, 35, 230, 272, 341, 344, 345–354, 387
  drawbacks of, 348–350
  medication, 353
exercise, 35, 49–52, 62, 97, 117, 136–170
  aerobic, 50, 137, 138, 145, 146, 147, 148, 154–164, 194, 229, 304–305, 307, 339–340
  and aging, 34, 142–144
  amount of, 147–148
  autoregulation, 307–311
  behavioral, 306–307
  best type of, 145–147
  and blood pressure, 14, 47, 190
  for children, 42, 144
  and cholesterol, 43, 282, 284, 386
  complications of, 152
  death during, 19–20, 149–152
  and doctors, 169–170
  flexibility, 146, 147, 164–165, 166
  and health, 9, 139–140, 236, 339–340, 366
  intensity of, 155–159
  lack of, 49, 52, 53, 54, 137, 143–145, 149, 170, 171, 297, 319
  medical complications of, 149–152
  mental, 305
  and mind, 304–305
  and osteoporosis, 344
  preventing injuries in, 166–167
  research on, 32, 101
  resistance, 305
  setting goals for, 51–52, 148–149
  and speed training, 147
  for strength, 165
  and treatment of atherosclerosis, 140–142, 194, 197
exercise machines, 162–164, 165
eye damage, 14, 199, 251

family history, as risk factor, 35–36
fat, body, 55–57, 161, 317, 322, 335, 338
  of Americans vs. Chinese, 87
  and exercise, 52, 142, 146
  and hypertension, 14
  See also obesity
fat, dietary, 14, 27, 42, 43, 62, 237, 321
  around the world, 86–87
  chemical structure of, 87–88
  and cholesterol, 84–135
  goals for, 103–116, 149

and health, 102–103, 229, 281, 334
in human history, 85–86
reduction of, 100–102, 197, 212, 334–335, 337, 386
saturated, 22, 84, 87–88, 90, 91, 93, 94, 96, 97, 98, 100, 101, 106, 107, 118, 119, 121, 128, 190
in United States, 84–85
unsaturated, 87, 88, 93, 94, 97, 98, 106, 128, 239, 360
See also calories
FDA. *See* Food and Drug Administration
fiber, dietary, 87, 107, 115, 117, 136, 205–220, 321
and cholesterol, 43
definition of, 206
and health, 213–214, 265, 334, 336, 339
in human history, 85, 86
and hypertension, 14
increase in, 116, 126, 190, 337, 386
setting goals for, 214–215
sources of, 123, 124, 125
types of, 206–207
See also under specific diseases
fibrillation
atrial, 198, 390, 391, 392, 393
ventricular, 20, 392
See also arrhythmias
fibrinogen, 62, 137–138, 194, 226, 347
fish, 98, 123, 124, 129, 133, 190, 236–247
and aquaculture, 244
and atherosclerosis, 27, 86, 116, 187, 237, 239–241, 268
and cholesterol, 246
consumption of, 238, 239–241, 245–247
cooking, 247
raw, 244
safety of, 242–245, 246
smoked, 247
vs. fish oil, 241–242
fish oils, 88, 93, 98–99, 99, 239, 240, 241–242, 268, 360
fitness programs, 167–169
Fixx, Jim, 150
Fleck, John, 143
folic acid, 355, 357
food
Chinese, 87, 134
and discipline, 339
fresh, 217
Italian, 134
junk, 338–339
Mexican, 134
natural, 184
restaurant, 132–135
Food and Drug Administration (FDA), 179, 243, 266–267, 272
food labeling, 104, 106, 107, 131–132, 220

Framingham Heart Study, 30, 36, 55, 223, 224, 296, 298, 310, 321, 358
free radicals, 249–253, 255, 260, 262, 264, 286, 288
Freud, Sigmund, 317
Friedman, Dr. Meyer, 59, 297–298, 303
fruits, 116, 123, 126, 128–129, 205, 207
and fiber, 205
and vitamins, 258, 264, 265, 266, 267, 268, 269

Galbraith, John Kenneth, 321
gallstones, 102–103, 333, 376
gangrene, 16, 72, 199
garlic, 360–362
Gathers, Hank, 150
Gay, John, 144
gender, as risk factor, 34–35
genetic factors, 86, 97, 227, 318
Goldman, Dr. Lee, 36
Gordon, Albert, 143
gout, 61, 277, 278
grains, whole, 116, 123–126, 205, 207, 213, 216, 222, 267, 268, 272
granola, 107, 123
Greece, 86, 87, 97, 98, 143, 397
Greenland, 238

Harvard Cardiovascular Health Center, 140
Harvard Medical School, 229–230, 385
Harvard School of Public Health, 50, 148, 324
HDL cholesterol, 22–23, 38, 248, 251
and age, 142
and alcohol, 225–226, 227, 228, 234
and estrogen replacement therapy, 347, 349, 350, 351
and exercise, 52, 137, 145, 148, 235
levels of, 40, 43, 54
lowering, 72, 93, 94, 95, 97, 102, 364
and medication, 271, 273–274, 278, 282, 283, 284, 285
and obesity, 320
raising, 35, 137, 141, 212, 235, 240, 361, 365, 387
Health Professionals Follow-up Study, 224
heart
healthy, 9–11
pumping chambers of, 9–11, 13–14
heart attacks, 16–18, 27, 29, 87
and blood pressure, 45, 48
causes of, 31, 44, 75, 252, 295, 298–299
and cholesterol, 22
consequences of, 18
and diabetes, 53
and dietary fat, 102, 135
and exercise, 50, 141
heart attacks, *continued*
expense of, 18
increase in, 78

and obesity, 55, 57, 84, 102, 321
procedures for, 393–396
rates of, 97
and risk profiles, 64–68, 103
and smoking, 71, 79, 80
and stress, 293, 297
symptoms of, 151, 378
in women, 342, 344, 351, 354
See also alcohol; aspirin; smoking: and cardiovas-
    cular disease
heart disease
    and age, 27–28, 35
    and alcohol, 221
    and antioxidant vitamins, 264
    and behavior, 14, 20, 27, 28
    and blood pressure, 171, 172–173
    case control studies of, 30, 32
    causes of, 9–27, 72
    cohort analysis in, 30, 32
    congenital, 12, 13
    coronary, 13, 14, 15–20, 22, 27, 28, 29, 33, 37,
        39, 40, 99
    family history of, 35–36, 40
    and fiber, 207–208
    as leading cause of death, 102, 140, 229
    and nutrition, 86
    prevention of, 26–27, 385, 393
    rheumatic, 11–12, 394
    symptoms of, 376–378
    treatment of, 385–397
    types of, 11–20
heart failure, congestive, 293, 299, 379, 383, 384,
        387
    causes of, 11, 13, 14, 18, 19, 173, 232
    drugs for, 389–392
    symptoms of, 379
heart muscle (myocardium), 9, 11, 13, 15
Heberden, Dr. William, 223
hepatitis, 275, 276, 278
Hippocrates, 136, 143, 191, 213, 303
Hoffman, Felix, 192
Hollman, Dr. Arthur, 191
Homer, 222
homocysteine, 355–358
Honolulu Heart Study, 223
hormones, 14, 19, 21, 35, 55, 119, 139, 185, 319,
        336, 350, 351, 352
    female, 343
    male, 346
    and stress, 55, 291
    See also adrenaline; estrogen
Huang Ti (Emperor of China), 176, 183
hydrogenation, of vegetable oils, 93–97, 106, 117,
        122, 124, 125, 205
hypertension, 13–14, 23, 31, 40, 52, 146, 172,
        294
    and alcohol, 232
    control of, 14, 44, 171, 186

and diabetes, 53
drugs for, 387–391
and exercise, 144
and fiber, 212, 214
and fish oil capsules, 241
genetic basis for, 35, 36
and heart disease, 172
labile, 47
measurement of, 45–48
and obesity, 54, 58
research on, 14, 283
risk of, 43–44
white coat, 47, 296
See also blood pressure
hyperthyroidism, 302
hypnosis, 81, 82, 364

immunizations, 376, 400
Institute of Aerobics Research, 151
insulin, 52, 53, 62, 139, 212, 262, 291, 336, 337
INTERSALT Study, 176, 183
Iowa Women's Health Study, 230, 269, 359, 360
Iribarren, Dr. Carlos, 41
iron, 285–288, 337
ischemia, silent, 16, 17, 18, 19, 20, 76, 197, 198,
        379, 382
isolation, social, 59, 298, 299–301, 303, 314

Jacobs, Dr. Daniel, 40
Japan, 238, 247
    coronary artery disease in, 28
jogging, 50, 150, 151, 160
Johannesen, Herman, 143
Johns Hopkins University, 143
Joint National Committee on Detection, Evalua-
        tion, and Treatment of High Blood Pressure,
        178
Journal of the American Medical Association, 275

Kaiser Permanente Study, 224
Kessler, David, 73
kidney disease, 14, 40, 48, 52, 116, 139, 174, 184,
        199, 202, 366
kidney stones, 116, 188, 260
Klatsky, Dr. Arthur, 228
Kromhout, Dr. Daan, 238

Lancet, 303
LDL cholesterol, 22, 38, 142, 240
    and atherosclerosis, 22, 193, 228, 251
    and dietary fat, 93, 94, 95, 97, 102, 104, 106
    and dietary fiber, 209, 210, 215
    and estrogen replacement therapy, 347, 350,
        351
    and exercise, 137, 141
    lowering, 35, 39, 43, 361, 364, 387
    and medication, 271, 273, 278, 283
    and obesity, 54, 321

oxidation of, 23, 91, 98, 173, 226, 248, 252, 253, 255, 256, 262, 286, 288, 347
lecithin, 365
legumes, 123, 126, 127, 205, 209, 216–217
Leiden Intervention Trial, 101
Lewis, Reggie, 150
lifestyle, 35, 49, 65, 68, 190
 changes in, 28, 55, 67, 171, 172, 287, 312, 348–349, 385, 398
Lifestyle Heart Trial, 101
Lind, Dr. James, 258, 260, 261
lipoproteins, 22, 39–40, 55, 225–226, 262
 high density (HDL), 22, 23, 25
 intermediate density (IDL), 22
 low density (LDL), 22, 23, 25
 very low density (VLDL), 22, 39
 See also cholesterol
liver disease, 58, 221, 223, 228, 232, 277, 400
Loma Linda University, 359
lungs, 10
 diseases of, 16, 400
 fluid in, 18, 19
 See also cancer: lung

Maclagan, Dr. Thomas, 192
magnesium, 188–189
magnetic resonance imaging (MRI), 56, 383
Male Health Professionals Study, U.S., 257, 260–261, 263, 264
mammograms, 229, 235, 347, 373, 377
Manning, Dr. Willard, 77, 144–145
Maravich, Pete, 150
margarine, 94, 95, 96, 122, 123, 125
meat, 117, 119–120, 123, 182, 267, 285
medication, 18, 20, 32, 43, 99, 101, 189, 247, 385–393, 396
 for diabetes, 52
 for high blood pressure, 44, 47, 48, 49, 172, 387–391
 hormone, 353
 as last resort, 277
 to lower cholesterol, 385–387
 over-the-counter, 276, 365–366
 self, 313
 and stress control, 315
 vs. diet, 102
 and weight loss, 333
 See also aspirin
meditation, 309–310
menopause, 35, 139–140, 343–346, 352
mental health, 302–303
meta-analysis, 41–42, 141, 176, 183, 197, 209
Metropolitan Life Insurance Company, 324
Meyers, Dr. Martin, 363
microwave ovens, 115, 120, 127, 247
Miller, Dr. George, 135
minerals, dietary, 171, 215, 281
 See also specific minerals

Morris, J. N., 169, 207
mortality, 40–41, 48, 57–58, 145, 295, 322
 infant, 371
mortality rates, 18, 83, 223, 237, 301, 351
MRI. See magnetic resonance imaging
Multiple Risk Factor Intervention Trial (MR. FIT), 224, 238, 298
Murray, Dr. Paul, 151
muscular activity, two categories of, 146–147
myocardial infarction. See heart attack
myocarditis, 13, 150

National Academy of Sciences, 178, 184, 186
 Food and Nutrition Board of, 282
National Cholesterol Education Program, 170
 guidelines of, 38–39, 42, 103, 106
National Health Examination Follow-up Study, 299
National High Blood Pressure Education Program, 45
National Institute of Mental Health, 302
New England Journal of Medicine, 94, 188, 200, 238, 263
niacin, 271–280
 and atherosclerosis, 274–275
 and cholesterol, 273–274, 282, 284
 as a medication, 273–280
 toxicities of, 275–276, 280
 using, 279–280
 as a vitamin, 272
nicotine
 and addiction, 73, 77, 78, 80, 82
 and blood pressure, 47, 79
 See also smoking
nicotine patches, 49, 82
Niebuhr, Reinhold, 304
nitrates, 387
nitroglycerin, 16, 387
Nurses' Health Study, U.S., 32, 95, 186, 196, 224, 257, 260, 263, 264, 266
nutrition, 9, 96, 116, 117, 247, 268, 281, 386
 and atherosclerosis, 62, 86, 90, 94, 205, 213
 and eating out, 132–135
 See also atherosclerosis: and nutrition; diets
nuts, 358–360

oat bran, 208–209, 220, 367
obesity, 39, 54–58, 317–324, 328
 in America, 322
 causes of, 317–321, 339
obesity, continued
 definition of, 317, 324
 and diabetes, 52, 53
 and diet, 62, 84, 86, 102
 and exercise, 50, 139, 144
 and fiber, 208, 212–213, 214
 genetic basis of, 35
 and health, 322–323, 332

O'Connor, Dr. Gerald, 141
Oldridge, Neil, 141
olive oil, 96, 97–98, 121, 125, 127, 227, 254
  and atherosclerosis, 93, 98
  and dietary fat, 87, 102, 106, 117, 118
omega-3 fatty acids, 98–99, 100, 102, 106, 129
  and fish, 129, 194, 240–241, 242, 243, 245,
    247, 360
Ornish, Dr. Dean, 101
Osler, Sir William, 295
osteoporosis, 116, 144, 161, 345
  and calcium, 139–140, 185, 187, 188, 345,
    365, 389
  and estrogen therapy, 348, 352, 354
  and menopause, 344
  and thin women, 58, 327
oxidation, 91, 98, 173, 193, 226, 228, 248, 250
  See also cholesterol
oxygen, 10, 11, 13, 79, 248, 250, 388
  and exercise, 138
  lack of, 15, 16, 17, 18, 71, 76, 142, 143,
    194, 199
  in red blood cells, 285
  and stress response, 290, 291
  See also blood: pumping of; free radicals

pacemakers, 13, 19, 394
Paffenbarger, Dr. Ralph, 50, 145, 148
Pap smears, 348, 377
PCBs (polychlorinated biphenyls), 243, 244
pellagra, 272
Peto, Dr. Richard, 197
PET scan (positron emission tomography),
  383
Physicians' Health Study, U.S., 32, 195–196,
  199, 200, 201, 257, 269, 286, 356
plaques, 16, 17, 24–25, 236, 252, 392, 393
  and blood clots, 194, 195, 198, 393
  and cholesterol, 91, 137, 173, 226, 255, 392
  and chromium, 283
  treatment of, 20, 99, 100, 101, 199, 392,
    395–397
platelets, 25, 194, 201, 228, 240, 241, 252,
  255, 296, 361
  and smoking, 72, 76
  See also blood: clotting of
Plato, 303, 304
pollution, environmental, 85, 137, 243, 400
Pope, Alexander, 304
potassium, 13, 14, 116, 176, 182–184, 189,
  212, 338
poultry, 117–119, 123
pregnancy, 54, 186, 200, 267, 358, 363, 364
  and alcohol, 231, 235
  and smoking, 75, 79
Preventive Services Task Force, U.S., 375,
  376, 377, 378
progesterone, 343, 349–350, 352, 353
prostaglandins, 199, 201, 240

proteins, 61–62, 116, 119, 121, 124, 126, 139,
  185, 194, 241, 250, 251, 253, 337–338
  in diet, 116, 119, 121, 124, 126, 337–338
  See also fibrinogen
psyllium, 210, 215
Public Health Service, U.S., 37
pulse, 59, 158, 290, 294, 307, 310, 379, 391

quinine, 191–192

radiation, 400
radionuclide angioradiography, 383
Red Cross, CPR program of, 20
research, 208–209, 236, 298
  in China, 265
  in Denmark, 224, 237, 298
  in England, 135, 169
  on Eskimos, 237–238, 240
  in Finland, 86, 257, 263–264, 265, 286,
    287, 289
  in Germany, 101, 361, 362
  in Hawaii, 41, 223, 224
  in Holland, 94, 208, 238, 343, 363
  in Iceland, 287
  in India, 212, 213, 360
  in Italy, 294
  in Norway, 238
  in Sweden, 135, 238, 301, 303
  in Texas, 95
  at University of Toronto, 130, 143
Reye's syndrome, 202
risk factors, coronary, 29–33, 65, 224, 298
  and age, 203
  and alcohol, 230, 235
  and exercise, 49, 51, 52, 138
  and family history, 35–36
  and fat, 57, 86, 95, 321
  for hypertension, 296
  and iron, 285, 286, 287
  psychological, 58–61, 314
  and rumor, 61–62
  See also cholesterol; obesity; smoking
risk scores, cardiac, 234, 277, 284, 304, 334,
  335
Roeback, Dr. John, 283
Rosenman, Dr. Ray, 59, 297–298
running, 160–161

St. Thomas Atherosclerosis Study (START),
  100–101
salicylic acid. See aspirin
salt, 115, 118, 120, 124, 126, 174–182, 247
  in American diet, 27, 86, 177–178
  and blood pressure, 14, 116, 174, 175–177,
    183, 212, 390
  and body fluids, 174–175
  and dairy products, 121, 123
  and food labeling, 107
  in primitive societies, 177–178

Sartre, Jean-Paul, 311
sauces, 124, 133, 134, 182
sedentary living. *See* exercise: lack of
selenium, 288
Selye, Dr. Hans, 291
Seven Countries Study, 86
Seventh Day Adventists, 358, 359
Shakespeare, William, 160, 332, 361
shopping, 131–132
    See also food labeling
shortness of breath, 13, 16, 18, 173, 379
Siscovick, Dr. David, 151
skiing, cross-country, 50
sleep, 313–314
smoking, 34, 41, 43, 58, 71–83
    and cardiovascular disease, 23, 27, 71–76,
        80, 86, 171, 251
    as cause of death, 221, 229, 257
    cessation of, 79–82, 190, 197, 282, 284,
        341
    costs of, 76
    in developing countries, 73, 83
    and exercise, 138
    and health, 72–73
    passive, 35, 36, 73, 75, 76, 83, 221
    and quitting techniques, 81–82
    as risk factor, 30, 31, 35, 36, 37, 49, 52,
        297, 299
    and society, 83
    and vitamins, 263, 265
snacks, 129–130
snuff, 78
social networks, 59, 300–301, 303, 314
sodium. *See* salt
Spertner, Jim, 150
Springsteen, Bruce, 339
Stanford University, 50
Stanley, Edward (Earl of Derby), 170
Stone, Reverend Edward, 191
strep throats, 11, 12
stress, 14, 15, 16, 27, 35, 59, 85, 296
    control of, 50, 61, 190
    and exercise, 140, 164, 304–311, 339,
        367
    and fight or flight reaction, 291–292
    and loss, 292–293
    reduction of, 49, 101, 303–315
    sources of, 311
    and technology, 137
stroke
    and alcohol, 232
    and antioxidants, 264
    and aspirin, 193, 196, 198, 203
    and blood pressure, 14, 16, 44, 45, 48, 171,
        173, 174
    as cause of death, 102, 144, 173, 174, 223,
        347–348
    and eating fish, 238
    and fat, 57, 84, 102

and smoking, 72, 79
    in women, 344, 351, 354
sugar, 15, 116, 125, 126, 211, 321, 334,
    336–337, 338
Surgeon General's report (1964), 81, 83
surgery, 18, 20, 384, 385, 393–396
    open heart, 393–395
SU.VI.Max study (France), 269
Swift, Jonathan, 143
swimming, 50, 159, 161, 340

tests, 371–385, 398
    blood, 18, 39–40, 42, 53–54, 76, 88, 174,
        278, 373, 376
    blood pressure, 376
    blood sugar, 376
    cardiovascular, 375
    cholesterol, 36, 42–43, 376
    diagnostic, 373
    fitness, 51
    for heart disease, 380–385
    invasive, 384–385
    screening, 373, 375–377
    stress, 153, 381–382
    for triglycerides, 39–40
Thompson, Dr. Paul, 151
thyroid disease, 13
TIAs. *See* transient ischemic attacks
tobacco, 13, 78–79, 138
tobacco industry, 73, 75, 77, 83
tobacco taxes, 77, 83
trans-fatty acids, 94, 95, 96, 97, 100, 102, 122,
    125. *See also* hydrogenation
transient ischemic attacks (TIAs), 198
trauma, 41, 42, 221, 230, 317
triglycerides, 39–40
    See also lipoproteins
Trowell, Dr. H. C., 213–214
Tufts University, 95, 130, 143
Type A personality, 59, 297–298, 303, 305,
    306

U. S. Department of Agriculture, 118
ulcers, peptic, 276, 277
U.S. Pharmacopoeia, 188

vegetables, 116, 123, 126–128, 207
    and calcium, 187
    and fat, 239
    lack of, in diet, 27, 86, 205
    and stroke, 264
vegetables, *continued*
    and vitamins, 258, 265, 266, 267, 268,
        269
ventricular tachycardia, 20
    See also arrhythmias
vitamin A, 102, 116, 253, 254, 256–258, 265,
    317
vitamin B, 123, 126, 355, 357, 358

vitamin C, 116, 127, 253, 254, 258, 260–261, 263, 264, 265, 266, 269
vitamin D, 102, 121, 185, 188, 317
vitamin E, 32, 98, 102, 250, 254, 260, 261–264, 265, 268, 269, 317
vitamin K, 102, 317
vitamins, 86, 115, 229, 317, 338, 355–358
  antioxidant, 190, 253–270
  and fiber, 215
  and food labels, 107
  See also antioxidants; niacin
vitamin supplements, 62, 257, 263, 264, 266–268, 366

walking, 50, 151, 154, 160
weight control, 49, 52, 55, 103, 190, 229, 284, 316–341, 386

weight loss, 57–58, 105, 282, 324–326
  and behavior modification, 329–330
  and crash diets, 331
  and fibrinogen, 62, 194
  and medication, 331
  and surgery, 333
  traditional options for, 328–329
wine, 97, 118, 207, 222, 226, 235
  red, 227–228, 235, 254
Withering, Dr. William, 391
Wolf, Dr. Stewart, 299
World War II, 238

x-rays, chest, 376, 381

yoga, 309